Hematopathology

Editor

MINA L. XU

SURGICAL PATHOLOGY CLINICS

www.surgpath.theclinics.com

Consulting Editor

JASON L. HORNICK

September 2019 • Volume 12 • Number 3

ELSEVIER

1600 John F. Kennedy Boulevard • Suite 1800 • Philadelphia, Pennsylvania, 19103-2899

http://www.theclinics.com

SURGICAL PATHOLOGY CLINICS Volume 12, Number 3
September 2019 ISSN 1875-9181, ISBN-13: 978-0-323-68227-5

Editor: Stacy Eastman
Developmental Editor: Donald Mumford

Surgical Pathology Clinics (ISSN 1875-9181) is published quarterly by Elsevier Inc., 360 Park Avenue South, New York, NY 10010. Months of issue are March, June, September, and December. Business and Editorial Office: Elsevier Inc., 1600 John F. Kennedy Blvd., Ste. 1800, Philadelphia, PA 19103-2899. Accounting and Circulation Offices: Elsevier Inc., 3251 Riverport Lane, Maryland Heights, MO 63043. Periodicals postage paid at New York, NY and at additional mailing offices. Subscription prices are $213.00 per year (US individuals), $279.00 per year (US institutions), $100.00 per year (US students/residents), $272.00 per year (Canadian individuals), $318.00 per year (Canadian Institutions), $263.00 per year (foreign individuals), $318.00 per year (foreign institutions), and $120.00 per year (international & Canadian students/residents). Foreign air speed delivery is included in all *Clinics'* subscription prices. All prices are subject to change without notice. **POSTMASTER:** Send address changes to *Surgical Pathology Clinics*, Elsevier, 3251 Riverport Lane, Maryland Heights, MO 63043. **Customer Service: 1-800-654-2452 (US). From outside the United States, call 1-314-447-8871. Fax: 1-314-447-8029. E-mail: JournalsCustomerServiceusa@elsevier.com (for print support) and JournalsOnlineSupport-usa@elsevier.com (for online support)**.

Reprints. For copies of 100 or more, of articles in this publication, please contact the Commercial Reprints Department, Elsevier Inc., 360 Park Avenue South, New York, NY 10010-1710. Tel. 212-633-3874; Fax: 212-633-3820; E-mail: reprints@elsevier.com.

Surgical Pathology Clinics of North America is covered in *MEDLINE/PubMed (Index Medicus)*.

Contributors

CONSULTING EDITOR

JASON L. HORNICK, MD, PhD
Director of Surgical Pathology and
Immunohistochemistry, Brigham and Women's
Hospital, Professor of Pathology, Harvard
Medical School, Boston, Massachusetts

EDITOR

MINA L. XU, MD
Director of Hematopathology, Associate
Professor, Department of Pathology and
Laboratory Medicine, Yale School of Medicine,
New Haven, Connecticut

AUTHORS

ALEX CHAN, MD
Hematopathology Diagnostic Service,
Department of Pathology, Memorial
Sloan Kettering Cancer Center, New York,
New York

MARGARET COCKS, MD, PhD
Dermatopathology Fellow, Department of
Pathology, University of Virginia,
Charlottesville, Virginia

AHMET DOGAN, MD, PhD
Hematopathology Diagnostic Service,
Department of Pathology, Memorial
Sloan Kettering Cancer Center, New York,
New York

YURI FEDORIW, MD
Associate Professor, Department of
Pathology and Laboratory Medicine, Director
of Hematopathology, University of North
Carolina School of Medicine, Chapel Hill,
North Carolina

ALEJANDRO A. GRU, MD
Associate Professor, Department of
Pathology, University of Virginia,
Charlottesville, Virginia

SARMAD H. JASSIM, MD
Hematopathology Fellow, Pathology
Department, University of Michigan,
Ann Arbor, Michigan

JASON H. KURZER, MD, PhD
Clinical Assistant Professor, Department of
Pathology, Stanford University School of
Medicine, Stanford, California

AMY J. LILLY, MD
Department of Pathology and Laboratory
Medicine, University of North Carolina
School of Medicine, Chapel Hill, North Carolina

SANAM LOGHAVI, MD
Department of Hematopathology, The
University of Texas MD Anderson Cancer
Center, Houston, Texas

L. JEFFREY MEDEIROS, MD
Department of Hematopathology, The
University of Texas MD Anderson Cancer
Center, Houston, Texas

ZENGGANG PAN, MD, PhD
Associate Professor, Department of Pathology,
Yale School of Medicine, New Haven,
Connecticut

KYLE PARKER, MD
Department of Pathology, Section of Hematopathology, The University of Chicago Medical Center, Chicago, Illinois

DENIZ PEKER, MD
Associate Professor, Department of Pathology, University of Alabama at Birmingham, Birmingham, Alabama

SUDHIR PERINCHERI, MBBS, PhD
Assistant Professor, Department of Pathology, Yale School of Medicine, New Haven, Connecticut

KSENIYA PETROVA-DRUS, MD, PhD
Department of Pathology, Hematopathology Diagnostic Service and Diagnostic Molecular Pathology, Memorial Sloan Kettering Cancer Center, New York, New York

PIERLUIGI PORCU, MD
Professor, Division of Hematologic Malignancies and Hematopoietic Stem Cell Transplantation, Department of Medical Oncology, Sidney Kimmel Cancer Center, Thomas Jefferson University, Philadelphia, Pennsylvania

SHERIF A. REZK, MD
Chief of Laboratory Medicine, Department of Pathology and Laboratory Medicine, University of California Irvine (UCI) Medical Center, Orange, California

MIKHAIL ROSHAL, MD, PhD
Department of Pathology, Hematopathology Diagnostic Service, Memorial Sloan Kettering Cancer Center, New York, New York

GENE P. SIEGAL, MD, PhD
Mowry Professor, Department of Pathology, University of Alabama at Birmingham, Birmingham, Alabama

LAUREN B. SMITH, MD
Professor, Section Head, Hematopathology Fellowship, University of Michigan, Ann Arbor, Michigan

GIRISH VENKATARAMAN, MD
Associate Professor, Director, Clinical Immunohistochemistry Laboratory, Department of Pathology, Section of Hematopathology, The University of Chicago Medical Center, Chicago, Illinois

SA A. WANG, MD
Department of Hematopathology, The University of Texas MD Anderson Cancer Center, Houston, Texas

WEI WANG, MD, PhD
Department of Hematopathology, The University of Texas MD Anderson Cancer Center, Houston, Texas

SHI WEI, MD, PhD
Professor, Department of Pathology, University of Alabama at Birmingham, Birmingham, Alabama

OLGA K. WEINBERG, MD
Assistant Professor, Department of Pathology, Boston Children's Hospital, Boston, Massachusetts

LAWRENCE M. WEISS, MD
Department of Pathology and Laboratory Medicine, University of California Irvine (UCI) Medical Center, Orange, California; Medical Director and Director of Pathology Services, NeoGenomics Laboratories, Aliso Viejo, California

MARK R. WICK, MD
Professor, Department of Pathology, University of Virginia, Charlottesville, Virginia

WENBIN XIAO, MD, PhD
Department of Pathology, Hematopathology Diagnostic Service, Memorial Sloan Kettering Cancer Center, New York, New York

MINA L. XU, MD
Director of Hematopathology, Associate Professor, Department of Pathology and Laboratory Medicine, Yale School of Medicine, New Haven, Connecticut

Contents

Defining the Boundary Between Myelodysplastic Syndromes and Myeloproliferative Neoplasms   651

Sanam Loghavi and Sa A. Wang

In this article we provide a practical and comprehensive review of myeloid neoplasms with overlapping myelodysplastic (MDS) and myeloproliferative (MPN) features, with emphasis on recent updates in classification, particularly the utility of morphologic, cytogenetic, and molecular findings in better defining and classifying these disease entities. We provide the reader with a summary of the most recent developments and updates that have helped further our understanding of the genomic landscape, clinicopathologic features, and prognostic elements of myeloid neoplasms with MDS/MPN features.

Optimal Measurable Residual Disease Testing for Acute Myeloid Leukemia   671

Wenbin Xiao, Kseniya Petrova-Drus, and Mikhail Roshal

Increasing evidence supports the prognostic significance of measurable residual disease (MRD) in acute myeloid leukemia (AML). Dynamic MRD assessment for patients with AML complements baseline patient risk assessment factors in determining patient prognosis. MRD status may also be helpful in informing therapeutic decisions. The European Leukemia Net MRD working party recently issued consensus recommendations for the use of MRD in AML. The Food and Drug Administration also issued advice for using MRD in trials of hematologic malignancies. This article discusses MRD testing, highlights the challenges in adopting MRD testing in clinical practice, and provides insights into the future of the field.

Acute Leukemias of Ambiguous Lineage: Clarification on Lineage Specificity 687

Jason H. Kurzer and Olga K. Weinberg

Acute leukemias of ambiguous lineage (ALAL) include acute undifferentiated leukemia and mixed-phenotype acute leukemia (MPAL). This article provides an overview of the diagnosis of ALAL and focuses on the data accounting for the current lineage-assignment criteria for blasts harboring more than one lineage-associated marker. In addition, the currently known molecular data are reviewed, which show that MPAL-associated gene mutations, methylation signatures, and expression profiles are a mixture of those seen in both acute myeloid leukemia and acute lymphoblastic leukemia. Finally, the prognosis and current treatments of MPAL are briefly discussed.

Prognostic and Predictive Biomarkers in Diffuse Large B-cell Lymphoma   699

Alex Chan and Ahmet Dogan

Diffuse large B-cell lymphoma is the most common lymphoid malignancy in the world at 25% to 40% of all adult non-Hodgkin lymphomas. The disease is remarkably heterogeneous in terms of pathogenesis, presentations, and outcomes. Approximately 60% of patients are curable with current first-line therapies, but the remaining patients have poor outcomes. Extensive research has been performed to stratify patients on prognosis, identify patients who would be cured, and identify others who would benefit from novel therapies. This article synthesizes this research.

Challenges in the Diagnosis of Gray Zone Lymphomas   709

Kyle Parker and Girish Venkataraman

The diagnosis of B-cell lymphoma unclassifiable with features intermediate between diffuse large B-cell lymphoma and classical Hodgkin lymphoma, also called gray zone lymphoma (GZL), is frequently challenging. Incorrect diagnosis as either classic Hodgkin lymphoma or diffuse large B-cell lymphoma has significant implications for choice of upfront therapy based on recent large multi-institutional series from the United States and Europe. These studies have clarified some diagnostic challenges and provided guidance on the spectrum of morphologic features in this entity. This article clarifies some of the diagnostic conundrum surrounding GZL and provides an evidence-based approach to GZL diagnosis using morphology and immunohistochemistry.

Early Events in Lymphoid Neoplasms and Indolent Follicular Lymphomas   719

Sudhir Perincheri

Technical advances in diagnostic modalities have led to the characterization of indolent lymphoid disorders similar to the in situ lesions described in epithelial malignancies. These early and indolent lymphoid lesions share clinicopathologic characteristics with well-characterized lymphoid malignancies such as chronic lymphocytic leukemia and follicular lymphoma. The in situ lesions have an indolent clinical course with only a minor subset shown to progress to frank malignancies. In addition to the in situ lesions, new indolent lymphoproliferative disorders have been recently characterized. Diagnosis and characterization of these indolent lesions is necessary to prevent overtreatment with aggressive therapeutic regimens.

New/Revised Entities in Gastrointestinal Lymphoproliferative Disorders   733

Sarmad H. Jassim and Lauren B. Smith

The gastrointestinal tract is a common extranodal site of involvement by lymphomas. These may be diagnostically challenging because they can mimic a variety of benign conditions and may be difficult to subclassify when malignant. The classification of gastrointestinal lymphomas is an evolving area with some recent changes. Although some of these entities are rare, they are important to recognize because of the variable clinical presentations, comorbidities, and treatment implications. This article explores new and revised entities in gastrointestinal lymphoproliferative disorders.

EBV–Associated Lymphoproliferative Disorders: Update in Classification   745

Sherif A. Rezk and Lawrence M. Weiss

Although about 90% of the world's population is infected by EBV only a small subset of the related infections result in neoplastic transformation. EBV is a versatile oncogenic agent involved in a multitude of hematopoietic, epithelial, and mesenchymal neoplasms, but the precise role of EBV in the pathogenesis of many of the associated lymphoid/histiocytic proliferations remains hypothetical or not completely understood. Additional studies and use of evolving technologies such as high-throughput next-generation sequencing may help address this knowledge gap and may lead to enhanced diagnostic assessment and the development of potential therapeutic interventions.

Human Immunodeficiency Virus-Associated Lymphoproliferative Disorders

Amy J. Lilly and Yuri Fedoriw

HIV infection is associated with an increased risk for developing B-cell lymphoproliferative disorders. The spectrum of disease differs in HIV-infected versus HIV-uninfected persons, with aggressive B-cell non-Hodgkin lymphomas constituting a higher proportion of all lymphoproliferative disorders in the HIV-positive population. Although antiretroviral therapy (ART) has significantly changed the landscape of lymphomas arising in HIV-infected persons, population growth and aging are reflected in the steady increase in non–AIDS-defining cancers. In the ART era, outcomes for HIV-infected lymphoma patients are similar to those of HIV-negative patients. This article reviews the diagnostic features and summarizes current biologic understanding of HIV-associated lymphomas.

Recent Advances in Cutaneous T-cell Lymphoma: Diagnostic and Prognostic Considerations

Margaret Cocks, Pierluigi Porcu, Mark R. Wick, and Alejandro A. Gru

This review describes the latest advances in the diagnosis of cutaneous T-cell lymphoma focusing on the most clinically useful features introduced since the publication of the World Health Organization revision in 2017. Clinical entities described include mycosis fungoides, Sézary syndrome, lymphomatoid papulosis, primary cutaneous anaplastic large cell lymphoma, primary cutaneous gamma delta T-cell lymphoma, primary cutaneous acral $CD8^+$ T-cell lymphoma, primary cutaneous $CD4^+$ small/medium T-cell lymphoproliferative disorder, and hydroa-vacciniforme-like lymphoproliferative disorder. Distinguishing histologic clues to diagnosis are discussed, and important molecular advances are described. Key prognostic indicators that may assist clinicians with timely and appropriate management options are presented.

Histiocytic and Dendritic Cell Neoplasms

Zenggang Pan and Mina L. Xu

Histiocytic and dendritic cell neoplasms are very rare, belonging to a group that share morphologic, immunophenotypic, and ultrastructural characteristics of mature histiocytic/dendritic neoplasms. Histiocytic and dendritic cell neoplasms may arise de novo or in association with B-cell, T-cell, or myeloid neoplasms. Recent molecular findings, particularly the discoveries of the mutations in the RAS-RAF-MEK-ERK pathway, have greatly advanced the diagnosis and treatment options. Histiocytic and dendritic cell neoplasms may closely resemble each other, non-hematopoietic neoplasms, and even reactive processes. Therefore, it is essential to understand the clinicopathologic characteristics, differential diagnoses, and pitfalls of each entity.

Bone Pathology for Hematopathologists

Deniz Peker, Shi Wei, and Gene P. Siegal

Bone pathology can be challenging because the skeleton is a living tissue prone to developing a diverse array of inflammatory, metabolic, genetic, reactive, circulatory, and neoplastic abnormalities. Several areas of bone pathology are particularly difficult or problematic for hematopathologists given the close resemblance of some hematologic entities to primary/metastatic bone lesions; examples include plasmacytic disorders versus osteoblastic tumors and lymphoma/leukemia versus round cell tumors of bone. This article provides a conceptual and practical overview of selective bone disorders commonly encountered in the differential diagnosis of hematologic diseases.

Wei Wang and L. Jeffrey Medeiros

Castleman disease (CD) is divided clinically into unicentric or multicentric type. Pathologically, CD is divided into hyaline-vascular and plasma cell variants. Unicentric CD is most common, about 75% of these cases are hyaline-vascular variant, and surgical excision is often curative. In contrast, there are a number of types of multicentric CD including HHV8-associated, idiopathic, and a subset of cases that arise in association with POEMS syndrome. Therapy is required for most patients with multicentric CD, but there is no consensus approach currently. As is evidence, the designation Castleman disease encompasses a heterogeneous group of diseases of varied pathogenesis and which require different therapies.

SURGICAL PATHOLOGY CLINICS

SERIES OF RELATED INTEREST

Clinics in Laboratory Medicine

THE CLINICS ARE AVAILABLE ONLINE!
Access your subscription at:
www.theclinics.com

Preface
Hematopathology

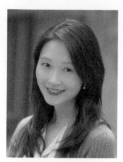

Mina L. Xu, MD
Editor

While hematopathology has long required the melding of morphology, routine laboratory test results, and advanced molecular/genetic data, recent years have brought an explosion of new ideas and information to the field. It has become ever more challenging for those in practice to sort out the emerging data for clinically relevant and actionable knowledge.

In this issue of *Surgical Pathology Clinics*, the authors hope to examine some of the controversial topics in hematopathology and also to provide a useful reference in areas that are not often systematically addressed. With regard to the former, these experts in the field have provided guidance in navigating the murky boundaries between mediastinal gray zone lymphomas and its mimics as well as between MDS, MPN, and MDS/MPN overlap syndromes. In addition, an in-depth assessment of optimal AML MRD testing is included. With regard to the latter, there are pathologic conditions of the bone for hematopathologists, establishment of criteria in Castleman lymphadenopathy as well as

a comprehensive overview of prognostic and predictive biomarkers in diffuse large B-cell lymphomas, some of which could lead to optimal selection of targeted therapeutics. Finally, important recent changes to the classification of specific lymphoid and myeloid neoplasms are presented with numerous illustrations.

I am excited to share this collection of select updates in and around our evolving field of hematopathology.

Mina L. Xu, MD
Director of Hematopathology
Associate Professor
Department of Pathology and Laboratory
Medicine
Yale School of Medicine
310 Cedar Street
New Haven, CT 06510, USA

E-mail address:
mina.xu@yale.edu

Surgical Pathology 12 (2019) xi
https://doi.org/10.1016/j.path.2019.05.001
1875-9181/19/© 2019 Published by Elsevier Inc.

Defining the Boundary Between Myelodysplastic Syndromes and Myeloproliferative Neoplasms

Sanam Loghavi, MD, Sa A. Wang, MD*

KEYWORDS

• MDS • MPN • MDS/MPN • Atypical CML • CMML • Ring sideroblasts • Cytopenia • Cytosis

Key Points

- A subset of myeloid neoplasms shows clinical, laboratory, and pathologic features overlapping between myelodysplastic syndromes (MDS) and myeloproliferative neoplasms (MPN).

- Although a large proportion of these overlapping neoplasms has been assigned to well-known disease entities, some remain to be defined.

- Recent molecular profiling has helped in understanding these disease entities, which has also challenged the current classification scheme.

- A meaningful classification of these overlap neoplasms requires comprehensive laboratory, morphologic, cytogenetic, and molecular workup.

ABSTRACT

In this article we provide a practical and comprehensive review of myeloid neoplasms with overlapping myelodysplastic (MDS) and myeloproliferative (MPN) features, with emphasis on recent updates in classification, particularly the utility of morphologic, cytogenetic, and molecular findings in better defining and classifying these disease entities. We provide the reader with a summary of the most recent developments and updates that have helped further our understanding of the genomic landscape, clinicopathologic features, and prognostic elements of myeloid neoplasms with MDS/MPN features.

OVERVIEW

Myeloid neoplasms with clinical and laboratory features between myelodysplastic syndrome (MDS) and myeloproliferative neoplasm (MPN) have long been recognized. In the 2008 World Health Organization (WHO), myelodysplastic/myeloproliferative neoplasms (MDS/MPN) were first introduced as a new disease category to include several well-defined entities, namely chronic myelomonocytic leukemia (CMML), juvenile myelomonocytic leukemia (JMML), atypical (*BCR/ABL1*-negative) chronic myeloid leukemia (aCML), and a provisional entity refractory anemia with ring sideroblasts and marked thrombocytosis (RARS-T). The discovery of frequent association of RARS-T with spliceosome gene *SF3B1* mutations[1] as well as mutations in *JAK2* V617F[2–7] or less frequently (<10%)[8,9] with *CALR*, or *MPL* genes provides sufficient evidence to support RARS-T as a true hybrid myeloid neoplasm not only clinicopathologically but also at the molecular level. In the 2017 WHO revision, RARS-T becomes a formally recognized entity, and renamed as MDS/MPN with ring sideroblasts and thrombocytosis

The authors have no conflicts of interest to disclose.

Department of Hematopathology, The University of Texas, MD Anderson Cancer Center, Houston, TX, USA

* Corresponding author. Department of Hematopathology, The University of Texas MD Anderson Cancer Center, 1515 Holcombe Drive, Box 0072, Houston, TX 77030.

E-mail address: swang5@mdanderson.org

Surgical Pathology 12 (2019) 651–669
https://doi.org/10.1016/j.path.2019.03.010

(MDS/MPN-RS-T), under the MDS/MPN category. There are still cases that do not meet diagnostic criteria for any of the aforementioned entities; such cases are currently placed under the term "unclassifiable" MDS/MPN (MDS/MPN-U).

The laboratory and morphologic features of MDS/MPN are characterized by ineffective and/or dysplastic hematopoiesis of one or more myeloid lineages with concurrent proliferation (with or without dysplasia) of one or more myeloid lineage(s). Unlike MDS, MDS/MPN by definition must show proliferative features that are defined by the presence of cytoses, which could be monocytosis ($\geq$10%, and $\geq$10 $\times$ 10^9/L monocytes), thrombocytosis ($\geq$450 $\times$ 10^9/L platelets), or leukocytosis ($\geq$13 $\times$ 10^9/L white blood cells [WBCs]). In addition, MDS/MPN must show certain degree of dysplasia that is often associated with cytopenia as a result of ineffective hematopoiesis. Applying these defining criteria, most of the myeloid neoplasms with hybrid MDS and MPN features would fall into several well-recognized disease entities, such as CMML, JMML, aCML, and MDS/MPN-RS-T. Cases of MDS/MPN-U are more heterogeneous, not forming a unique subset of diseases; however, similar to other entities, these cases must present with cytosis as well as cytopenia that is not attributable to a known antecedent history of MDS or MPN. A diagnosis of MDS/MPN requires the exclusion of cases with a recurrent/specific molecular genetic lesion, such as BCR-ABL1, PDGRBA, PDGFRB, FGFR1, and PCM1-JAK2, as well as cases with $\geq$20% blasts that meet the criteria of acute leukemia.

The diagnosis and classification of these chronic myeloid neoplasms with hybrid features can be challenging despite applying the above mentioned criteria. Some MDS cases may initially present with thrombocytosis, whereas some patients with MPN may have significant cytopenia(s). The proliferative features commonly observed in MPNs, including clustering of large atypical megakaryocytes, hepatosplenomegaly, extramedullary hematopoiesis, and thrombotic events, are not currently included in the diagnostic criteria of MDS/MPN, but are liberally used by some clinicians and diagnosticians as MPN-associated features. Furthermore, dysplastic features as well as monocytosis can be secondarily acquired in MPNs, further complicating our ability to distinguish MPNs from MDS/MPNs or even MDS, particularly when the initial diagnostic material is not available for review.

Recent advances in next generation sequencing (NGS) and messenger RNA sequencing have furthered our understanding of these overlapping syndromes, and provided additional insight for disease diagnosis, classification, risk stratification, and management. The molecular genetic data will continue to shed light onto this challenging area. Here we perform a systemic review of well-defined disease entities mainly diagnosed in adult patients with focus on recent updates; and highlight some problematic areas within the scope of myeloid neoplasms with hybrid MDS and MPN features.

CHRONIC MYELOMONOCYTIC LEUKEMIA

CMML is a myeloid neoplasm with features overlapping MDS and MPN features and an inherent risk for transformation to acute myeloid leukemia defined by persistent relative (>10%) and absolute monocytosis ($\geq$1 $\times$ 10^9/L) in the peripheral blood (PB).[10] It has an annual incidence rate of ~0.4 cases per 100,000 persons; men are affected more than women with a male:female ratio of ~2.5:1.0. The reported median age at diagnosis ranges from 65 to 75 years, but the highest incidence of disease is in patients older than 80.[10–13] Patients may present with constitutional symptoms, cytopenias, hematosplenomegaly, cutaneous lesions, infection, bleeding, and/or various inflammatory or autoimmune processes.[14] In most cases, hematopoietic precursors exhibit morphologic dysplasia in at least 1 cell lineage; however, in rare instances, dysplasia maybe absent or subtle. The cytopenias associated with CMML, similar to other MDSs, are a result of ineffective hematopoiesis. The diagnostic criteria according to 2017 WHO classification is shown in Box 1.

If a diagnosis of CMML is suspected in the setting of PB or bone marrow (BM) eosinophilia, it is essential to investigate for rearrangements in PDGFRA, PDGFRB, FGFR1, and the PCM1-JAK2 translocation, as identification of any of these alterations excludes the diagnosis of CMML. Among these, PDGFRB rearrangements are most likely to present with monocytosis.[15] Identification of these alterations has great clinical significance because of available targeted therapeutic options. Imatinib has shown excellent efficacy in cases with PDGFRA and PDGFRB rearrangements.[16] Of note, eosinophilia may evolve during the course of CMML or at progression, which also may be associated with acquisition the same genetic alterations.[17]

A small subset (~3%) of patients with CMML present with moderate to severe reticulin fibrosis at initial diagnosis.[18] These patients tend to present with a higher WBC count with more frequent MP-CMML phenotype, higher absolute monocytosis, higher BM blast percentage, higher serum lactate dehydrogenase (LDH) levels, and more frequently have splenomegaly and a significantly higher frequency of *JAK2* p.V617F mutations (up to 50%). The overall features have significant clinicopathologic overlap with primary myelofibrosis. A recent study has shown that megakaryocytic morphology (dysplastic vs large atypical MPN-like) and *JAK2* V617F allelic burden are useful features in distinguishing the two entities, as PMF tends to have higher *JAK2* V617F allele burden compared with CMML.[19] Unlike cases of MDS with fibrosis in which the frequency of *TP53* mutations is high,[20] the frequency of *TP53* alterations is not increased compared with CMML without fibrosis. CMML-F is independently associated with a shorter overall survival by multivariate analysis; therefore, it is essential to evaluate for and report significant BM fibrosis in patients with CMML.[18]

The 2017 revision of the WHO classification includes 2 updates to the classification of CMML. It subclassifies CMML based on a WBC cutoff of 13×10^9/L into myeloproliferative (MP)-CMML and myelodysplastic (MD)-CMML subtypes and introduces a 3-tiered blast-based subgrouping scheme that includes a novel "CMML-0" category (PB <2% and/or BM <5%). We recently sought to validate these 2 subclassification schemes in a large (n = 629) cohort of patients with CMML diagnosed and treated at our institution. Not surprisingly, patients with MP-CMML had shorter

overall survival (OS) (21 vs 34 months) and leukemia-free survival (LFS) (15.2 vs 22.0 months) and included more CMML-2 cases (5%–19% blasts in PB <2 and/or 10%–19% blasts in BM or blasts with Auer rods)[10] and more frequent *RAS* mutations (37% vs 17%) compared with MD-CMML. These results further validate the need to distinguish MP-CMML from MDS-CMML and its recognition as a distinct clinical and biologic subgroup. In contrast, our findings did not show a clear benefit for using the proposed 3-tiered blast-based system.[21] We were able to demonstrate in our patient cohort that a blast percentage cutoff of 10% correlates with OS, but we noted that the CMML-0 group included a large subset ($\sim$36%) of patients with higher-risk CMML-specific Prognostic Scoring System (CPSS)[22] scores and $\sim$11% of patients with high-risk cytogenetic alterations. Overall, the newly proposed CMML-0 and CMML-1 categories were similar in terms of their CPSS risk profile, cytogenetic risk groups, and mutation profiles. The 3-tiered blast-based subgroups did not improve the prognostic power of CPSS.[21] Given these results and the low concordance rate for blast enumeration in CMML,[23,24] we suggest that adding the CMML-0 subcategory does not have clear prognostic benefits.[25]

Multicolor/multiparameter flow cytometry immunophenotyping (FCI) is a useful tool in distinguishing reactive monocytosis from CMML; however, the changes observed in CMML may be seen in other myeloid stem cell disorders as well. Myeloid blasts in CMML exhibit frequent antigenic aberrancies (median of 6 aberrancies per case) including increased intensity of CD117, CD123, CD13, and CD34 expression and decreased intensify of CD38 expression as well as aberrant expression of lineage infidelity markers including CD2, CD5, CD7, CD19, and CD56, and asynchronous expression of mature myelomonocytic markers, such as CD64 and CD15. Monocytes and granulocytes show frequent immunophenotypic aberrancies (96% and 83%, respectively). Hematogones are absent in more than 90% of cases.[26]

Evaluation of monocytic "partitions" has also proven helpful in the diagnosis of CMML. Normal PB monocytes are immunophenotypically subdivided into 3 functional categories, including classic monocytes (CD14+/CD16−), intermediate monocytes (CD14+/CD16+), and nonclassic monocytes (defined as CD14−/CD16+). Approximately 90% of monocytes in healthy individuals are composed of the classic subtype. This classic monocyte population is expanded in CMML; rendering monocytes partitioning a quite specific tool for distinguishing CMML from reactive monocytosis.[27] Expansion of classic monocyte subsets (≥94%) has also been shown to be able to discriminate CMML from other MDS subtypes with a sensitivity of 72% and specificity of 86%. Using a classic monocyte fraction cutoff of 92% FCI is reportedly able to distinguish CMML from other MPNs with monocytosis with a sensitivity of 93% and specificity of 100%.[28]

Chromosomal alterations are seen in up to 30% of CMML cases and are a powerful indicator of outcome and prognosis. The most frequent chromosomal abnormalities include + 8 (23%), − Y (20%), −7/del 7q (14%), +21(8%), del20q (8%), and der(3q) (8%).[29,30] In 2011, Such and colleagues[29] introduced a cytogenetic risk stratification system in which 3 cytogenetic risk categories were recognized as independent prognostic predictors: a diploid karyotype or −Y were considered to be low risk; trisomy 8, alterations of chromosome 7, and complex karyotype were considered high-risk, and all other karyotypes were considered intermediate risk. More recently, our group[31] was able to demonstrate in a large patient cohort (n = 417) that patients with trisomy 8 as a sole abnormality had a median OS similar to that of the patients with the intermediate-risk category proposed by Such and colleagues[29] and significantly longer than patients with other high-risk karyotypes. We also showed that a complex karyotype with ≥3 chromosomal alterations predicted for a significantly shorter OS compared with cases harboring 3 chromosomal abnormalities. Based on these findings, we proposed a modification to the cytogenetic risk stratification system by Such and colleagues[29] with an enhanced prognostic power with respect to OS and LFS prediction in which patients with isolated trisomy 8 are classified as intermediate risk.

Recurrent somatic mutations have been identified in CMML. These mutations involve genes across several functional categories including epigenetic and transcriptional regulators, such as TET2 (60%), and ASXL1 (40%), EZH2 (<5%), DNMT3A (~5%), IDH1 (<2%), and IDH2 (~5%),[32–35] and the spliceosome machinery including SRSF2 (50%), U2AF1 (7%), SF3B1 (5%–10%), ZRSR2 (3%), and PRPF8[35] frequently combined with mutations in genes involved in cell signaling (overall frequency ~30%) including NRAS (10%–20%), KRAS (5%–10%), CBL (13%), BRAF (7%),[36] JAK2 (5%), PTPN11 (<5%), FLT3 (<5%), and NPM1 (<3%).[35,37] Cell signaling and EZH2 mutations are more common in MP-CMML. Co-occurrence of SRSF2 and TET2 mutations has been shown to be highly specific (~98%)

to myeloid neoplasms with a CMML-like phenotype.[38]

Gene mutations have specific prognostic implications in CMML. Truncating ASXL1 mutations (frameshift and nonsense) have been shown to independently predict a poor outcome and shorter OS.[33,34,37,39] Loss-of-function EZH2 mutations frequently co-occur with ASXL1 mutations in CMML. Although EZH2 mutations alone do not appear to independently influence outcome, patients with ASXL1/EZH2 co-mutated CMML have a shorter median OS in comparison with CMML cases with ASXL1 mutation alone,[35] but LFS seems to be unaffected.[35] Clonal TET2 mutations in ASXL1 wild-type CMML are associated with favorable outcome.[34] DNMT3A mutations have also been shown be associated with a shorter OS in CMML.[35]

RUNX1 mutations are seen in up to 37% of CMML cases and are associated with more profound cytopenia. It appears that OS is unaffected by RUNX1 mutations; however, some studies have suggested that C-terminal RUNX1 mutations may be associated with more frequent and rapid progression to acute leukemia.[40]

TP53 mutations (clonal and subclonal) are present in ~4% of CMML cases and are more common in MP-CMML. As opposed to MDS in which TP53 mutations tare highly associated with complex karyotype, TP53 mutated CMML usually has a noncomplex karyotype. The prognostic significance of TP53 mutations in CMML remains unclear, but some studies have shown an adverse impact on OS.[35,41]

Several CMML-specific risk stratification systems are currently available, all using various combinations of hematologic indices, and cytogenetic and molecular alterations.[22,42–45] A summary of the features used in the commonly used risk stratification models is provided in **Box 2**.

Allogeneic hematopoietic stem cell transplantation (AHSCT) remains the only curative treatment option for patients with CMML. A wait and watch approach is acceptable in patients with low-risk and clinically stable disease. Other therapeutic measures are commonly used to alleviate the symptoms related to cytopenias and cytoses (erythropoiesis-stimulating agents, cytoreductive chemotherapy, and hypomethylating agents).[46] AHSCT remains the treatment of choice in younger patients with CMML (<65 years). It is recommended to begin cytoreductive chemotherapy or HMAs before AHSCT, particularly in patients with increased BM blast count (>10%) and patients with high-risk disease. Ruxolitinib may be used in patients with MP-CMML to abrogate the effects of aberrant RAS signaling.[47]

Box 2
Variables used in the current prognostication models for CMML

MDAPS[43]

Hemoglobin less than 12 gm/dL

Circulating immature myeloid cells

Absolute lymphocyte count greater than 2.5×10^9/L

$\geq$10% BM blasts

Global MDAPS[45]

Older age

Poor performance status

Thrombocytopenia

Anemia

Increased BM blasts

Leukocytosis (>20 $\times$ 10^9/L)

−7/del7q, complex karyotype

Prior transfusion

CPSS[29]

WHO subgroups (CMML-1 and CMML-2)

Myelodysplastic (MD)-CMML versus myeloproliferative (MP)-CMML

RBC transfusion dependency or hemoglobin level

Karyotype

Diploid karyotype or −Y: low risk

+8 and −7/del7q and complex karyotype: high risk

All other karyotypes: intermediate risk

CPSS-Mol[112]

WBC count

Transfusion dependency

BM blast count

CPSS cytogenetic risk groups

ASXL1, NRAS, SETP1, and RUNX1 status

Groupe Francophone des Myelodysplasies[37]

ASXL1 mutation

Age older than 65 years,

WBC greater than 15 $\times$ 10^9/L

Thrombocytopenia less than 100 $\times$ 10^9/L

Hemoglobin less than 10 g/dL in women and less than 11 g/dL in men.

(Continued)

Mayo Prognostic Model[44]

Hemoglobin less than 10 g/dL

Thrombocytopenia less than 100 $\times$ 10^9/L,

Absolute monocyte count greater than 10 $\times$ 10^9/L

Circulating immature myeloid cells

Mayo Molecular Model[33]

ASXL1 mutation

Circulating immature myeloid cells

Thrombocytopenia less than 100 $\times$ 10^9/L

Hemoglobin less than 10 g/dL

Absolute monocyte count greater than 10 $\times$ 10^9/L

Abbreviations: CPSS, CMML-specific prognostic scoring system; CPSS-mol, molecular CPSS; MDAPS, The MD Anderson Prognostic System; RBC, red blood cell; WBC, white blood cell.

ATYPICAL CHRONIC MYELOID LEUKEMIA, BCR-ABL1 NEGATIVE

aCML is an exceedingly rare MDS/MPN with a reported incidence of approximately 0.01 to 0.04 per 100,000 persons. This disease is characterized by the concurrent presence of myelodysplastic and myeloproliferative features including dysplastic neutrophilic leukocytosis with increased left-shifted neutrophilic precursors ($\geq$10%) in circulation. BCR-ABL1 and rearrangements of PDGFRA, PDGFRB, FGFR1, or PCM1-JAK2 are absent by definition.[48] The WHO 2017 diagnostic criteria for aCML are summarized in Box 3.

Patients are generally older and the median reported age at presentation is 72 years.[48–50] Men are affected more than women with a male:female ratio of 2:1. Organomegaly (45%), anemia, thrombocytopenia, and leukocytosis are common; circulating blasts are seen in a subset ($\sim$17%) of patients. aCML is characterized by the presence of dyspoietic leukocytosis as well as circulating neutrophil precursors, which distinguish aCML from MDS/MPN-U.[49,50] Older age (>65 years) and leukocytosis greater than 50 $\times$ 10^9/L have been reported to be associated with shorter OS, and palpable hepatosplenomegaly, monocytosis, BM blasts in excess of 5%, and transfusion dependency have been linked to increased rate of acute myeloid leukemia (AML) transformation.[51]

PB shows neutrophilic leukocytosis with increased granulocytic precursors comprising $\geq$10% of leukocytes. Dysgranulopoiesis is virtually

---

Box 3

WHO 2017 diagnostic criteria for atypical chronic myeloid leukemia (aCML), *BCR-ABL1* negative

Neutrophilic leukocytosis with neutrophilic precursors (promyelocytes, myelocytes, metamyelocytes) representing ≥10% of leukocytes

Dysplastic granulopoiesis including abnormal chromatin clumping

No or minimal absolute basophilia; basophils typically less than 2% of WBCs

No or minimal absolute monocytosis; monocytes less than 10% of WBCs

Hypercellular BM with dysplastic granulocytic hyperplasia ± erythroid and megakaryocytic dysplasia

Less than 20% blasts in the PB and BM

No evidence of *BCR-ABL1*, *PDGFRA*, *PDGFRB*, or *FGFR1* rearrangement, or *PCM1-JAK2*

Not meeting WHO criteria for PMF, PV, or ET and no previous history of these disease

Presence of *SETBP1* and/or *ETNK1* mutations and absence of *CSF3R* mutation[a]

[a] These features are not required but are highly suggestive of aCML.

---

always present and is often prominent (**Fig. 1A**). In addition to typical features of dysgranulopoiesis (hypogranulation, nuclear hypolobation) a characteristic form of dysgranulopoiesis in aCML is the presence of hypersegmented neutrophils with seemingly normal granulation with twisted and abnormally branched nuclear lobes. Chromatin is often dense and clumping. This form of dysgranulopoiesis is observed in approximately 20% to 30% of aCML cases and is quite helpful in establishing the diagnosis. The WHO has recognized this a "variant" dysgranulopoiesis. Eosinophilia, basophilia, and relative monocytosis are uncommon.

The BM is often hypercellular for age with a disproportionate increase in myeloid lineage cells and decreased erythroid precursors (**Fig. 1B**). Severe granulocytic dysplasia is invariably present and is helpful in distinguishing aCML from its mimics, particularly chronic neutrophilic leukemia (CNL). Dyserythropoiesis is present in approximately half of cases. Dysmegakaryopoiesis with or without megakaryocytic hyperplasia is frequently seen. Blasts may be increased (commonly <5%) but should be less than 20% of all nucleated cells by definition. Various degrees of BM reticulin fibrosis may be present at the time of initial diagnosis or appear later in the course of disease.

An abnormal karyotype is identified in 40% to 50% patients; however, specific recurrent cytogenetic abnormalities have not been identified. Trisomy 8 is the most common cytogenetic abnormality (18%).[50] Other alterations, including del(20q) and abnormalities of chromosomes 12, 13, 14, 17, and 19, have also been reported.[48] Complex karyotype, monosomy 7, or del(7q) and i17(q) have been reported in approximately 8% of cases.[50] Rare cases with *BCR-JAK2* have been reported,[50,52–54] and such cases have been proposed to be variants of *PCM-JAK2*, and assigned to the category of "myeloid lymphoid neoplasm with eosinophilia and a specific gene rearrangement" in the 2017 WHO classification. In contrast to other myeloid neoplasms, there is no established prognostic significance for alterations of chromosome 7 or a complex karyotype.[49]

Somatic mutations across various functional gene categories are present in aCML, including those involved in epigenetic regulation (*SETBP1* [up to 33%]; *ASXL1* [25%]; *TET2* [25%]; *EZH2* [up to 15%]) and cell signaling (*NRAS/KRAS* [up to 35%]; *ETNK1* [9%]; *JAK2* [7%]; *CBL* [7%]).[49,55,56] *CSF3R* mutations that are commonly present in CNL are notably uncommon (<10%) in aCML.[57,58] *CALR* and *MPL* mutations are also typically absent.[59] The detailed mechanistic role of *SETBP1* in aCML has not been well characterized; however, some studies have suggested that the stabilization of SET results in inhibition of the tumor suppressor protein phosphatase 2A (PP2A), which in turn leads to uncontrolled cellular proliferation.[56] Patients with *SETBP1*-mutated aCML have an shorter OS (22 vs 77 months, $P = .01$) compared with those with wild-type *SETPB1*.[56]

aCML should be distinguished from reactive or secondary neutrophilia as a result of smoking, infections, inflammation, drugs including growth factors, stress (physical or emotional), hemorrhage, myelophthisis, paraneoplastic syndromes, and asplenism.[60–71] Dysplastic features are not seen in reactive or secondary leukocytosis with neutrophilia and neutrophils often show toxic granules, Döhle bodies, and hypersegmentation. Granulocytic left-shift is typically seen in the form of increased bands, and although a few granulocytic precursors, including promyelocytes, myelocytes, and metamyelocytes, may be present, they rarely surpass more than 10% of leukocytes. The BM may show slight hypercellularity with increased neutrophils and their precursors but significant dyspoiesis should be absent.

Among other neoplastic conditions, the differential diagnostic considerations for aCML include chronic myeloid leukemia (CML) that also presents with marked leukocytosis with increased neutrophil

Fig. 1. (*A*) PB smear of a patient with aCML showing left-shifted granulocytic maturation and characteristic neutrophilic dysplasia with hyperchromatic and twisted nuclei (Wright-Giemsa, original magnification ×1000). (*B*) The BM core biopsy is hypercellular and shows markedly increased myeloid:erythroid ratio with dysplastic megakaryopoiesis (hematoxylin and eosin, original magnification ×40).

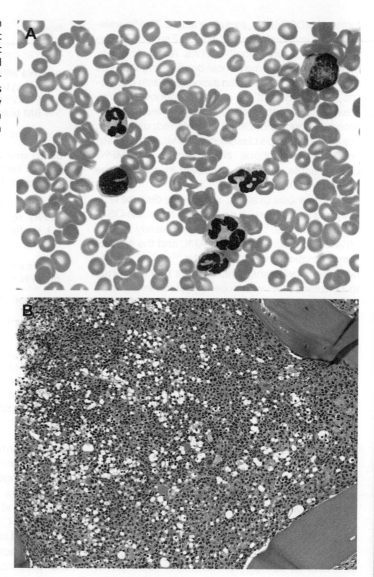

precursors in PB. Dysgranulopoiesis is not a typical feature in CML. Increased neutrophils are typically associated with increased eosinophils and basophils. The megakaryocytes of CML may resemble those seen in aCML (small, hypolobated). The ultimate differentiating feature is the presence of *BCR-ABL1* fusion, which defines CML. CNL is a myeloproliferative neoplasm that is also characterized by neutrophilic leukocytosis; however, in CNL the PB leukocytes are predominantly composed of mature neutrophils and band forms (≥80% of WBCs) and other granulocytic precursors comprise less than 10% of WBCs (often less than 5%). Toxic granulation and Döhle bodies are often seen; however, significant dysgranulopoiesis is not. Similar to aCML the BM of patients with CNL is hypercellular due to granulocytic hyperplasia composed predominantly of metamyelocytes to mature neutrophils. Megakaryocytes are usually normal in number or can be slightly increased, but there is no significant megakaryocytic dysplasia. Megakaryocytes may be large and multilobated. Mutation in *CSF3R* is virtually a disease-defining molecular marker of CNL.[57,59] In contrast to CNL, *CSF3R* mutations are uncommon (<10%) in aCML. In rare instances, a case may carry the hot-spot canonical T618I *CSF3R* mutation and exhibit prominent neutrophilic dysplasia; experts in the field have suggested that these cases may be biologically distinct and should not be pushed into either of these diagnostic categories but should rather be referred to as CNL with dysplasia.[72] CMML is described earlier in this article in detail. In general, the presence of persistent relative and absolute monocytosis takes precedence of a diagnosis of CMML over other forms of MDS/MPNs, including aCML. The "persistent monocytosis" requires at least 2 sets of CBC in a minimum of one month interval. A subset of patients with CMML may show overlapping features with aCML at presentation associated with borderline monocytosis. If the degree of monocytosis increases and becomes a persistent feature over time, a diagnosis of CMML is preferred; otherwise, the case should be classified as aCML. Other diagnostic considerations also include MDS/MPN-unclassifiable which is discussed in detail in the following in this review.

The prognosis of aCML is poor. The disease typically has an aggressive course with a median OS of 14 to 30 months.[48,51,56,73,74] Approximately 15% to 40% of patients progress to AML and the median transformation time is 18 months.[48,51,56,75] Allogeneic stem cell transplantation has been reported to be associated with superior outcomes In these patients compared with conventional therapies.

MYELODYSPLASTIC/MYELOPROLIFERATIVE NEOPLASM WITH RING SIDEROBLASTS AND THROMBOCYTOSIS

MDS/MPN with ring sideroblasts and thrombocytosis (MDS/MPN with RS-T) is a de novo MDS/MPN characterized by the simultaneous presence of dyserythropoiesis, ≥15% ring sideroblasts, and an elevated platelet count of greater than 450 × 10⁹/L. PB blasts should be less than 1% and BM blasts should be less than 5%.[76] This was a provisional entity referred to as "refractory anemia with ring sideroblasts associated with marked thrombocytosis" in the previous iteration of the WHO classification, but is now recognized as a distinct category of MDS/MPN (Box 4). The discovery of recurrent SF3B1 mutations in this disease has contributed, at least in part, to its recognition as a distinct disease subtype. In general, increased ring sideroblasts are present at initial diagnosis. Other well-established MPNs may show increased ring sideroblasts as a result of therapy or disease progression; these cases should not be classified as MDS/MPN RS-T.

The clinical presentation of MDS/MPN RS-T overlaps with other Philadelphia-negative MPNs including essential thrombocythemia (ET). Splenomegaly is common (~40%) and hepatomegaly also may occur.[6] Anemia is invariably present and is often macrocytic, which is helpful in distinguishing MDS/MPN RS-T from ET. The degree of cytopenias is typically milder compared with patients with MDS-RS.

Microscopic examination of the PB shows platelet anisocytosis including increased forms

with abnormal shape and hypogranulation. The leukocyte count and distribution is typically within normal range, although mild leukocytosis may be seen in rare cases. The BM often shows megaloblastoid and dysplastic erythroid hyperplasia and increased (≥15%) ring sideroblasts (Fig. 2). RSs are formed as a result of abnormal perinuclear mitochondrial accumulation of iron. They are defined by the presence of at least 5 siderotic granules covering at least one-third of the nuclear circumference. Multilineage dysplasia may be present but is not required for the diagnosis. Megakaryocytes are typically increased and resemble those observed in other Philadelphia-negative MPNs. Increased reticulin fibrosis may be seen in a subset of patients.

Approximately 10% of cases present with an abnormal karyotype and ~80% have evidence of clonality by mutation analysis.[76] Myeloid neoplasms fulfilling criteria for MDS with isolated del(5q) and those harboring t(3;3) (q21.3;q26.2), inv(3) (q21.3q26.2) are excluded from this category by definition, as are cases with BCR-ABL1 fusion.

SF3B1, a component of the RNA splicing machinery, is the most common somatic mutation encountered in MDS/MPN with RS-T (>80%). SF3B1 K700E is the most common variant (~50%) but codons 622, 625, 666, and 666 are also hot spot regions.[77,78] SF3B1 mutations are

Fig. 2. (*A*) BM trephine biopsy in a patient with MDS/MPN with ring sideroblasts and thrombocytosis showing atypical mega-karyocytic hyperplasia with megakaryocytic clustering and dilated sinusoids; the BM is hypercellular for age (hematoxylin and eosin, original magnification ×200). (*B*) The BM aspirate smear shows megaloblastoid erythroid precursors with dysplastic features including basophilic stippling of cytoplasm; the granulocytes are also dysplastic characterized by abnormal distribution of cytoplastic granules (Wright-Giemsa, original magnification ×1000). (*C*) An iron stain shows increased ring sideroblasts in the BM aspirate (iron, original magnification ×1000).

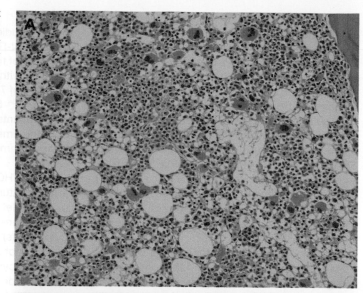

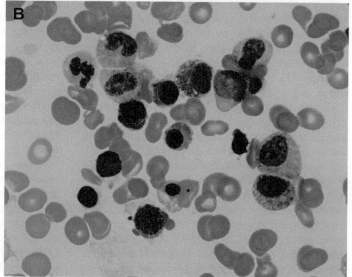

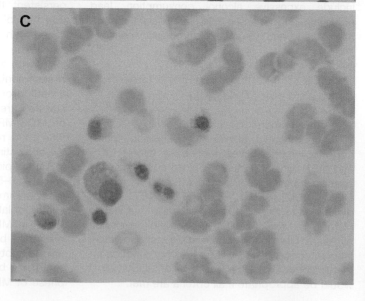

often associated with *JAK2* V617F ($\sim$30%–50%) and less frequently with *MPL* or *CALR* mutations. Concurrent *JAK2* and *MPL* mutations have been reported in rare cases, but they appear to be present in mutually exclusive clones.[79] *JAK2* and *MPL* mutations may be acquired throughout the course of disease and are usually associated with increased platelet counts. Other recurrent mutations include those involved in the spliceosome machinery: *SRSF2* ($\sim$7%), *U2AF1* ($\sim$5%), *ZRSR2* ($\sim$3%); in signaling pathways: *SETBP1* ($\sim$13%), *CBL*($\sim$4%); epigenetic modulators: *ASXL1* ($\sim$15–30%), *TET2* ($\sim$10–25%), *EZH2* ($\sim$7%), *DNMT3A* ($\sim$15%), *IDH2* ($\sim$4%); and transcription regulators: *ETV6* ($\sim$3%), *RUNX1* ($\sim$1).[1,80]

The reported median OS for patients with MDS/MPN RS-T ranges from 76 to 128 months, which is significantly shorter compared with the OS of patients with ET but longer than patients with MDS-RS.[2,81] Most patients fall into the lower risk group when stratified by the revised-International Prognostic Scoring System (R-IPSS).[42] The presence of *SF3B1* mutation is an independent predictor of longer OS in this disease (6.9 years in mutated cases vs 3.3 years in wild-type cases). *JAK2* mutations also predict a more indolent clinical course and favorable outcomes.[81] In contrast, anemia and an abnormal karyotype, *SETBP1* and *ASXL1* mutations are associated with an inferior survival.[80,82]

The major differential diagnosis of MDS/MPN RS-T includes ET. Unlike MDS/MPN-RS-T, patients with ET generally do not present with anemia, BM cellularity is typically normal, and there is no morphologic dysplasia in the erythroid or granulocytic series in ET.[59] MDS/MPN RS-T should be distinguished from other non-neoplastic conditions associated with increased ring sideroblasts. These include excessive alcohol consumption, lead poisoning, copper and pyridoxine deficiency, isoniazid therapy, and congenital sideroblastic anemia.[83]

MYELODYSPLASTIC/MYELOPROLIFERATIVE NEOPLASM-UNCLASSIFIABLE

Like other hematological malignancies, the 2017 WHO classification allows an unclassifiable category to include cases that have hybrid MDS and MPN clinical features, but do not fit into any specific type of well-defined MDS/MPN, namely CMML, aCML, JMML, and MDS/MPN-RS-T. This disease category excludes patients with a known history of MDS or MPN who have developed hybrid features in the course of disease. However, if an antecedent MDS or MPN history is not documented or confirmed, a diagnosis of MDS/MPN-U would be appropriate if all criteria are met.

The studies on MDS/MPN-U, not including MDS/MPN-RS-T, are limited,[50,84–88] likely due to the rarity of these cases and difficulty in diagnosis. Patients with MDS/MPN-U are elderly, with a median age of 71 years and showing a male predominance.[50,84] Splenomegaly is reported in 20% to 30% patients. The survival is poor, 21.8 months[50] from the time of initial diagnosis and 12.4 months from the time being referred to a tertiary cancer centers.[84]

In the WHO definition of MDS/MPN-U, the proliferative features are defined by a WBC $\geq$13 $\times$ 10^9/L or a platelet count $\geq$450 $\times$ 10^9/L, and dysplastic features are by the presence of dyspoiesis and cytopenia(s). Dysplasia can be observed in any lineage(s), not necessarily corresponding to the lineage with cytopenia; conversely, cytosis may not always correlate with the proliferation of the respective lineage in BM. The cases that are classified as MDS/MPN-U are composed of a group of neoplasms with laboratory and BM morphologic features that could be quite heterogeneous. PB may show dysplastic neutrophils, left-shifted neutrophil precursors, nucleated red cells, and circulating blasts (<20%). Mild basophilia or eosinophilia may be seen in some patients. BM often shows a hypercellularity, and moderate to marked fibrosis can be observed in 20% to 30% cases. Myeloid:Erythroid (M:E) ratio may vary from case to case, ranging from markedly increased to markedly decreased/reversed. Although many of the cases show dysplastic megakaryocytes, approximately 20% to 30% of cases show large megakaryocytes with clustering, mimicking MPN megakaryocytes, or a mixture of MDS-like and MPN-like megakaryocytes. Some cases are classified as MDS/MPN-U due to the presence of persistent thrombocytosis and or leukocytosis that would be otherwise classified as MDS. In cases with significant myelofibrosis,[50] dysplasia should be demonstrated in at least one lineage even with limited aspirate material available for assessment. If a case of MDS/MPN coexists with a benign or neoplastic BM infiltrate, and the full features are difficult to characterize, a diagnosis of MDS/MPN-U would be appropriate at the time, and reclassification may be needed after the coexisting condition resolves.

Karyotypic abnormalities are reported in approximately 20–50% of patients.[50,84] Trisomy 8 is the most common, occurring in 15% to 20% of patients. Isolated 17q (i[17]q) is reported in 5% or less[50] in MDS/MPN-U. Isolated i(17)q has been proposed by some investigators to represent a unique subtype of MDS/MPN[89]; however, isolated i(17)q has been reported in CMML, aCML, blast phase of MPN, and AML, not unique. Cases that meet the criteria for MDS with isolated del(5q) are excluded irrespective of the presence of thrombocytosis or leukocytosis. However, it is known that leukocytosis is very uncommon in MDS with isolated del(5q). and it has been suggested to classify accordingly by disease phenotype.

In the recent studies of mutation landscape of MDS/MPN,[86,87] genes found frequently mutated in MDS/MPN-U are ASXL1, TET2, followed by JAK2, SRSF, EZH2, U2AF1, RUNX1, SETBP1, and SF3B1. Similar to earlier studies,[50] JAK2 V617F mutations are detected in approximately 20% to 30% patients with MDS/MPN-U, significantly more frequent in MDS/MPN-U than in aCML and CMML, but less frequent than MDS/MPN-RS-T.[86,87] MPL and CALR are reported in a much lower frequency (5% or less) in MDS/MPN-U. Bose and colleagues[86] showed that SF3B1 mutations were 12% in their cohort of MDS/MPN-U. Meggendorfer and colleagues[87] sequenced 177 patients with various subtypes of MDS/MPN, and the mutation profiles showed that RAS pathway was more frequently affected in aCML and CMML and JAK-STAT pathway was more often affected in MDS/MPN-RS-T. MDS/MPN-U seemed to be a mixture, involving genes in epigenetic regulation, JAK-STAT pathway, and splicing machinery, but marginally involving the RAS pathway. The findings indicate that MDS/MPN-U might be better segregated by a specific mutation profile rather than by the disease phenotype.

How might the molecular characteristics of MDS/MPN-U be translated in this clinical and morphologically defined entity? A high frequency of JAK2 V617F in MDS/MPN-U suggests that some patients might have had an undetected phase of MPN, and developed dysplastic features that were found at the first time of diagnosis. In the phase II trial of ruxolitinib in combination with azacytidine in MDS/MPN, responders were more frequently JAK2-mutated and had splenomegaly compared with nonresponders.[90] It is known that some MDS/MPN-U cases are closely resembling aCML, presenting with leukocytosis, anemia, and/or thrombocytopenia, but lack one of the stringent required criteria of aCML, such as marked dysgranulopoiesis or the presence of 10% or more circulating granulocytic precursors (promyelocytes, myelocytes, and metamyelocytes).[50] The latter feature has been shown to be an independent prognostic risk regardless of the diagnosis either as aCML or MDS/MPN-U. In such cases, if mutations frequently associated with aCML, such as SETBP1 and/or NRAS/KRAS, are detected, this subset of MDS/MPN cases might be more close to aCML biologically. It is noteworthy that in MDS, if an SF3B1 mutation is detected, a diagnosis of MDS-RS only requires RS ≥5%. However, this rule does not apply to MDS/MPN-RS-T, an entity with a high frequency of SF3B1 mutations,[91,92] which requires the presence of 15% or more RS to make such a diagnosis. The question arises that in the presence of SF3B1 mutations, a case with thrombocytosis, macrocytic anemia, and 5% to 14% RS, would it be more appropriately classified as MDS/MPN-RS-T than its current assignment of MDS/MPN-U? It was recently shown that myeloid neoplasms with relative but not absolute monocytosis[93] had a mutation profile similar to CMML with frequent mutations in ASXL1, TET2, and SRSF2, and a significant proportion of the cases evolved to CMML in a short period of time. This suggests that if a case of MDS/MPN-U later demonstrates persistent monocytosis, a reclassification as of CMML might be appropriate.

In summary, the MDS/MPN-U category includes cases that fulfill the criteria of a hybrid MDS and MPN, but are not perfect for a specific subtype of MDS/MPN. Cytogenetic abnormalities are seen in approximately one third to half of the patients, but nothing unique. Molecular profiling of MDS/MPN-U reveals frequent mutations that affect various pathways. The molecular characteristics may be more informative than morphology for further subgrouping, and provide insightful references for therapeutic consideration.[90]

OVERLAP WITH THE OVERLAP NEOPLASMS

Ironically, MDS and MPN may show clinical, pathologic, and molecular genetic features overlapping with the disease entities categorized under MDS/MPN. The boundary between MDS, MPN, and MDS/MPN could be rather blurry. The recent understandings of molecular genetic profiling have challenged the current classification scheme.

Myelodysplastic Syndrome with Relative Monocytosis

CMML was considered as a form of MDS in the French-American-British (FAB) classification system. However, these cases are characterized by a proliferation of monocytes, both in proportions (≥10%) as well as in absolute counts (≥10 × 10⁹/L). These cases have been included as a form of MDS/MPN in the 2001 WHO classification. In the 2017 classification, CMML is further divided into 2 types: a dysplastic type (MD) and a proliferative type (MP) with a dividing WBC count of 13 × 10⁹/L. MP-CMML presents with more frequent constitutional symptoms and organomegaly, and shows a shorter OS, whereas MD-CMML closely resembles MDS. Although NRAS/KRAS mutations are significantly more frequent in MP-CMML,[22,94,95] the presence of both *TET2* and *SRSF2* mutations is a common molecular feature of both MP-CMML and MD-CMML.[96]

Recently, Geyer and colleagues[58] studied 44 patients who had relative monocytosis (16.8%, 10%–48%) but due to a low WBC, the absolute monocytes were less than 10×10^9/L. Of the 44 patients, more than 90% were classified as MDS, with MDS multilineage dysplasia being the most common (39%). The clinicopathological features of these patients were strikingly similar to MD-CMML. The "signature" CMML mutations of *TET2, ASXL1* and *SRSF2* were similarly frequent in these patients. In a median interval of 12 months, 38% of patients progressed to CMML. The investigators proposed to classify such cases as oligomonocytic CMML to allow patients being stratified according to CPSSs and have the benefit of participating in CMML clinical trial therapies.

Del(5q) Syndromes with Thrombocytosis and Leukocytosis

The interstitial deletion of chromosome 5q (del[5q]) is the most common cytogenetic abnormality in MDS. Del(5q) syndrome is used to define MDS with del(5q) either in isolation or with one other cytogenetic abnormality that is not monosomy 7 or del(7q); and with less than 5% blasts in BM and less than 1% blasts in PB. Thrombocytosis greater than 350×10^9/L was reported in nearly one-third of patients with del(5q). Deficiency of miR-145 and miR-146a, mapped within and adjacent to the common deleted region, may underlie the thrombocytosis in some patients with 5q-syndrome.[97] A small subset of patients (6%–7%) with isolated del(5q) may have concomitant *JAK2* V617F mutations.[98,99] Cases with *JAK2* V617F mutations might more frequently present with marked thrombocytosis (>450×10^9/L).[98,99] In one study, *MPL* W515L mutations were detected in 3 (3.8%) of 79 patients; all 3 patients had normal platelets and none had leukocytosis.[99] *JAK2* or *MPL* mutations, if positive, were detected at the time of diagnosis, indicating an early event. In some of these cases, the *JAK2* mutation and del(5q) were found in genetically discordant clones.[100] The presence of *JAK2* V617F and *MPL* W515L does not appear to alter the disease phenotype or prognosis, and these cases are currently retained in the 5q-syndrome in the 2017 WHO classification. A subset of cases of 5q-syndrome (10%–20%), usually cases with ring sideroblasts, have been found to have *SF3B1* mutations.[101,102]

The confusion and challenge arise in dealing with del(5q) abnormalities, either in isolation or associated with another karyotypic abnormality that is not -7 or -7q, when patients present with thrombocytosis ($\geq 450 \times 10^9$/L) and or leukocytosis ($\geq 13 \times 10^9$/L) with or without RS. Should such cases be classified as MDS with isolated del(5q), or MDS/MPN? According to the recent 2017 WHO classification scheme (**Fig. 3**), if blasts are increased, $\geq 5\%$ in BM and $\geq 1\%$ in PB, such cases are no longer isolated del(5q) syndrome, and cases should be classified according to their clinical morphologic features regardless of del(5q). If blasts are not increased (<5% in BM and <1% in PB), and patients have leukocytosis with or without thrombocytosis, should such cases be classified as aCML, CMML, MDS/MPN-RS-T, or MDS/MPN-U according to BM, PB, and clinical features? The 2017 WHO classification scheme has no clear instruction for cases that otherwise met the diagnostic criteria for CMML

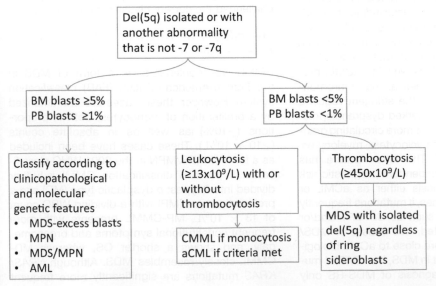

Fig. 3. Diagnostic algorithm for myeloid neoplasms with del(5q) cytogenetic abnormality.

and aCML but does recommend to exclude such cases from MDS/MPN-U or MDS/MPN-RS-T. It is noteworthy that leukocytosis is extremely uncommon in MDS with isolated del(5q); whereas, del(5q) is extremely uncommon in CMML or aCML, 1% to 2% or less.[22,31,103] For cases with thrombocytosis but no leukocytosis, the cases would be retained in MDS del(5q) syndrome regardless of *JAK2* and *MPL* mutation status.

Myeloproliferative Neoplasms Overlapping with Myelodysplastic Syndrome and Myelodysplastic Syndrome/Myeloproliferative Neoplasm

Philadelphia-negative classic MPNs include essential thrombocythemia (ET), P Vera (PV), and primary myelofibrosis (PMF). At the time of diagnosis, cytosis is one of the major criteria in the diagnosis of ET and PV, but it is not required for a diagnosis of PMF. In PMF,[104,105] leukocytosis ($\geq$13 $\times$ 10^9/L) is seen in approximately half of the patients, and thrombocytosis ($\geq$450 $\times$ 10^9/L) in 20%. Anemia with hemoglobin less than 10 g/dL is seen in approximately 50% of patients with PMF and less than 8 g/dL in 20%. Approximately 10% to 15% of patients may have leukopenia or thrombocytopenia, respectively. However, severe cytopenia involving 2 or 3 (pancytopenia) lineages is extremely uncommon at the time of initial diagnosis of PMF, which should raise the possibility of an alternative diagnosis, such as MDS with fibrosis or MDS/MPN. PMF is also characterized by several other typical MPN features, such as thrombotic events, a proliferation of abnormal megakaryocytes, and granulocytes in the BM, associated with gradual/progressive myelofibrosis, high LDH, and extramedullary hematopoiesis. The latter is manifested as leukoerythroblastosis in the blood, hepatomegaly, and splenomegaly. However, these MPN features, if not associated with cytosis in PB, are insufficient to define "proliferative" nature in the diagnosis of MDS/MPN according to the WHO criteria., It is noteworthy that this definition has been challenged with recent understanding of genomic landscape of MPN and MDS/MPN.[106] The vast majority of patients with PMF demonstrate one of the MPN driver mutations[106,107] in *JAK2* (50%–75%), *MPL* (5%–10%), or *CALR* (10%–15%). There are approximately 10% of cases that are negative for all 3, also known as triple-negative PMF.

Theoretically, none of the MPNs should show morphologic dysplasia at initial BM evaluation. However, some "MDS-like" megakaryocytes (small, monolobated, or hypolobated forms) are commonly found in PMF, in a spectrum with other large cloudlike megakaryocytes in PMF. On the other hand, mild dysplasia is common in patients treated with hydroxyurea; and significant dysplasia can be acquired as a sign of disease progression in MPN.[108] The latter is often associated with significant cytopenia(s). PMF with *SF3B1* mutations may present with ring sideroblasts associated with severe anemia.

One of the challenges is to assess dysplasia in cases with significant BM fibrosis, which often produces poor-quality BM aspirates. Approximately 10% to 15% of MDS cases may present with significant myelofibrosis ($\geq$MF-2),[20,109,110] and approximately 5% to 15% of these fibrotic MDSs have *JAK2* V617F mutations. On the other hand, a subset of MPN cases can have mutations in chromatin and spliceosome (*SF3B1*, *SRSF2*, and *U2AF1*) regulators, Loss of heterozygosity (LOH) at chromosome 4q, and aberrations in chromosomes 7 and 7q. These genetic alterations are enriched in patients with MPN with myelofibrosis and dyspoiesis.[106,111] Due to significant overlapping in morphology, hematology laboratory features (cytopenia vs cytosis), as well as mutational profiles, a differential diagnosis among MDS, MPN, and MDS/MPN can be extremely difficult in cases with significant myelofibrosis (**Fig. 4**). One of the common mistakes is to diagnose any case with significant myelofibrosis as PMF, not considering other clinical, morphologic, and molecular genetic features. Some may call a case that otherwise would be MDS with fibrosis (MDS-F) as MDS/MPN due to the presence of increased large megakaryocytes in BM.

Some features may help in the differential diagnosis. Compared with patients with PMF, patients with MDS-F[20,109,110] often have more profound cytopenia(s) and lower circulating CD34+ cell count. Leukoerythroblastic blood features and hepatosplenomegaly are much less common in patients with MDS-F. Patients with MDS-F have higher BM cellularity and, more frequently, multilineage dysplasia. By contrast, patients with PMF more frequently presented megakaryocytic hyperplasia, megakaryocyte clusters, "cloudlike" or "balloon-shaped" megakaryocytic nuclei, dilation of marrow sinuses, and intrasinusoidal hematopoiesis. P53 by immunohistochemistry stain as well as *TP53* mutations are more common in MDS-F.[20] *JAK2* V617F mutation in MDS-F shows a lower variant allele frequency (VAF) than patients with PMF.[109]

In summary, of the cases crossing the boundary of MDS and MPN, there include well-defined entities with characteristic clinical, laboratory, and morphologic features. NGS data have demonstrated recurrent molecular genetic alterations in these clinically and morphologically defined

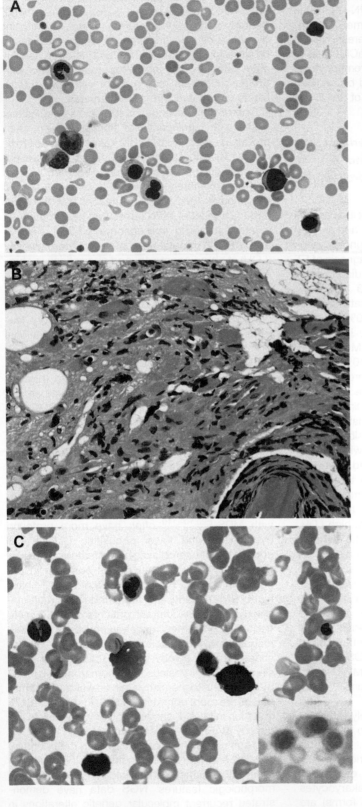

Fig. 4. A case in the twilight zone of PMF, MDS with fibrosis, and MDS/MPN) A 74-year-old patient, without an antecedent history of MDS or MPN, presented with WBC 11.8 × 10⁹/L, hemoglobulin 8.6 g/dL, MCV 103 fL, platelets 130 × 10⁹/L, and requiring red cell transfusion. The patient was also found to have massive hepatosplenomegaly and high LDH, positive *JAK2* V617F (VAF 19%), and *SF3B1* mutation (VAF 33%). PB (*A*) shows leukoerythroblastosis, dysgranulopoiesis, rare blasts, and many tear drops (wright Giemsa, original magnification ×1000). BM biopsy (*B*) shows a proliferation of megakaryocytes, and MF3 fibrosis (hematoxylin and eosin, original magnification ×500). Aspirate smears (*C*) show dysgranulopoiesis and dyserythropoiesis (wright Giemsa, original magnification ×1000). with ring sideroblasts (*inset*) (Perl iron stain, original magnification ×1000). This case shows hybrid clinical, morphologic, and molecular features of MDS and MPN and highlights the difficulty in classification.

entities, further supporting the categorization. For MDS/MPN-U, identification of unique subset of diseases would help for diagnosis and patient management. There cases remain difficult to classify based on our current approach to disease classification. Recent advances in genomic studies have revealed hybrid molecular genetic features in a subset of neoplasms that are currently classified either under MPN or MDS, questioning if these diseases are biologically akin to MDS/MPN. This leads to further debates if other features of MPN, such as organomegaly, high LDH, thrombosis, a proliferation of large megakaryocytes and granulocytes, and the presence of MPN driver mutations should be considered as "proliferative" features in addition to cytosis in the assessment of a potential case of MDS/MPN. This is a field that is fast evolving with our increased understanding of the genomic landscape of diseases and emerging innovative therapies.

REFERENCES

1. Jeromin S, Haferlach T, Weissmann S, et al. Refractory anemia with ring sideroblasts and marked thrombocytosis cases harbor mutations in SF3B1 or other spliceosome genes accompanied by JAK2V617F and ASXL1 mutations. Haematologica 2015;100(4):e125–7.

2. Wang SA, Hasserjian RP, Loew JM, et al. Refractory anemia with ringed sideroblasts associated with marked thrombocytosis harbors JAK2 mutation and shows overlapping myeloproliferative and myelodysplastic features. Leukemia 2006;20(9):1641–4.

3. Schmitt-Graeff AH, Teo SS, Olschewski M, et al. JAK2V617F mutation status identifies subtypes of refractory anemia with ringed sideroblasts associated with marked thrombocytosis. Haematologica 2008;93(1):34–40.

4. Boissinot M, Garand R, Hamidou M, et al. The JAK2-V617F mutation and essential thrombocythemia features in a subset of patients with refractory anemia with ring sideroblasts (RARS). Blood 2006;108(5):1781–2.

5. Remacha AF, Nomdedeu JF, Puget G, et al. Occurrence of the JAK2 V617F mutation in the WHO provisional entity: myelodysplastic/myeloproliferative disease, unclassifiable-refractory anemia with ringed sideroblasts associated with marked thrombocytosis. Haematologica 2006; 91(5):719–20.

6. Szpurka H, Tiu R, Murugesan G, et al. Refractory anemia with ringed sideroblasts associated with marked thrombocytosis (RARS-T), another myeloproliferative condition characterized by JAK2 V617F mutation. Blood 2006;108(7): 2173–81.

7. Ceesay MM, Lea NC, Ingram W, et al. The JAK2 V617F mutation is rare in RARS but common in RARS-T. Leukemia 2006;20(11):2060–1.

8. Broseus J, Lippert E, Harutyunyan AS, et al. Low rate of calreticulin mutations in refractory anaemia with ring sideroblasts and marked thrombocytosis. Leukemia 2014;28(6):1374–6.

9. Visconte V, Tabarroki A, Hasrouni E, et al. Molecular and phenotypic heterogeneity of refractory anemia with ring sideroblasts associated with marked thrombocytosis. Leuk Lymphoma 2016;57(1):212–5.

10. Orazi A, Bennett JM, Germing U, et al. Chronic myelomonocytic leukemia. In: Swerdlow SH, Campo E, Harris NL, et al, editors. WHO classification of tumours of haematopoietic and lymphoid tissues. Lyon (France): International Agency for Research on Cancer; 2017. p. 82–6.

11. Dinmohamed AG, van Norden Y, Visser O, et al. The use of medical claims to assess incidence, diagnostic procedures and initial treatment of myelodysplastic syndromes and chronic myelomonocytic leukemia in the Netherlands. Leuk Res 2015; 39(2):177–82.

12. Germing U, Gattermann N, Minning H, et al. Problems in the classification of CMML—dysplastic versus proliferative type. Leuk Res 1998;22(10): 871–8.

13. Solal-Celigny P, Desaint B, Herrera A, et al. Chronic myelomonocytic leukemia according to FAB classification: analysis of 35 cases. Blood 1984;63(3): 634–8.

14. McCullough KB, Patnaik MM. Chronic myelomonocytic leukemia: a genetic and clinical update. Curr Hematol Malig Rep 2015;10(3):292–302.

15. Patnaik MM, Lasho TL, Finke CM, et al. Targeted next generation sequencing of PDGFRB rearranged myeloid neoplasms with monocytosis. Am J Hematol 2016;91(3):E12–4.

16. Helbig G, Stella-Holowiecka B, Grosicki S, et al. The results of imatinib therapy for patients with primary eosinophilic disorders. Eur J Haematol 2006; 76(6):535–6.

17. Shah S, Loghavi S, Garcia-Manero G, et al. Discovery of imatinib-responsive FIP1L1-PDGFRA mutation during refractory acute myeloid leukemia transformation of chronic myelomonocytic leukemia. J Hematol Oncol 2014;7:26.

18. Gur HD, Loghavi S, Garcia-Manero G, et al. Chronic myelomonocytic leukemia with fibrosis is a distinct disease subset with myeloproliferative features and frequent JAK2 p.V617F mutations. Am J Surg Pathol 2018;42(6):799–806.

19. Hu Z, Ramos CB, Medeiros LJ, et al. Utility of JAK2 V617F allelic burden in distinguishing chronic myelomonocytic leukemia from primary myelofibrosis with monocytosis. Hum Pathol 2018;85:290–8.

20. Loghavi S, Al-Ibraheemi A, Zuo Z, et al. TP53 overexpression is an independent adverse prognostic factor in de novo myelodysplastic syndromes with fibrosis. Br J Haematol 2015;171(1):91–9.

21. Loghavi S, Sui D, Wei P, et al. Validation of the 2017 revision of the WHO chronic myelomonocytic leukemia categories. Blood Adv 2018;2(15):1807–16.

22. Such E, Germing U, Malcovati L, et al. Development and validation of a prognostic scoring system for patients with chronic myelomonocytic leukemia. Blood 2013;121(15):3005–15.

23. Goasguen JE, Bennett JM, Bain BJ, et al. Morphological evaluation of monocytes and their precursors. Haematologica 2009;94(7):994–7.

24. Droin N, Jacquel A, Hendra JB, et al. Alpha-defensins secreted by dysplastic granulocytes inhibit the differentiation of monocytes in chronic myelomonocytic leukemia. Blood 2010;115(1):78–88.

25. Loghavi S, Curry JL, Garcia-Manero G, et al. Chronic myelomonocytic leukemia masquerading as cutaneous indeterminate dendritic cell tumor: expanding the spectrum of skin lesions in chronic myelomonocytic leukemia. J Cutan Pathol 2017;44(12):1075–9.

26. Shen Q, Ouyang J, Tang G, et al. Flow cytometry immunophenotypic findings in chronic myelomonocytic leukemia and its utility in monitoring treatment response. Eur J Haematol 2015;95(2):168–76.

27. Selimoglu-Buet D, Wagner-Ballon O, Saada V, et al. Characteristic repartition of monocyte subsets as a diagnostic signature of chronic myelomonocytic leukemia. Blood 2015;125(23):3618–26.

28. Patnaik MM, Timm MM, Vallapureddy R, et al. Flow cytometry based monocyte subset analysis accurately distinguishes chronic myelomonocytic leukemia from myeloproliferative neoplasms with associated monocytosis. Blood Cancer J 2017;7(7):e584.

29. Such E, Cervera J, Costa D, et al. Cytogenetic risk stratification in chronic myelomonocytic leukemia. Haematologica 2011;96(3):375–83.

30. Wassie EA, Itzykson R, Lasho TL, et al. Molecular and prognostic correlates of cytogenetic abnormalities in chronic myelomonocytic leukemia: a Mayo Clinic-French Consortium Study. Am J Hematol 2014;89(12):1111–5.

31. Tang G, Zhang L, Fu B, et al. Cytogenetic risk stratification of 417 patients with chronic myelomonocytic leukemia from a single institution. Am J Hematol 2014;89(8):813–8.

32. Merlevede J, Droin N, Qin T, et al. Mutation allele burden remains unchanged in chronic myelomonocytic leukaemia responding to hypomethylating agents. Nat Commun 2016;7:10767.

33. Patnaik MM, Itzykson R, Lasho TL, et al. ASXL1 and SETBP1 mutations and their prognostic contribution in chronic myelomonocytic leukemia: a two-center study of 466 patients. Leukemia 2014;28(11):2206–12.

34. Patnaik MM, Lasho TL, Vijayvargiya P, et al. Prognostic interaction between ASXL1 and TET2 mutations in chronic myelomonocytic leukemia. Blood Cancer J 2016;6:e385.

35. Patnaik MM, Vallapureddy R, Lasho TL, et al. EZH2 mutations in chronic myelomonocytic leukemia cluster with ASXL1 mutations and their co-occurrence is prognostically detrimental. Blood Cancer J 2018;8(1):12.

36. Zhang L, Singh RR, Patel KP, et al. BRAF kinase domain mutations are present in a subset of chronic myelomonocytic leukemia with wild-type RAS. Am J Hematol 2014;89(5):499–504.

37. Itzykson R, Kosmider O, Renneville A, et al. Prognostic score including gene mutations in chronic myelomonocytic leukemia. J Clin Oncol 2013;31(19):2428–36.

38. Malcovati L, Papaemmanuil E, Ambaglio I, et al. Driver somatic mutations identify distinct disease entities within myeloid neoplasms with myelodysplasia. Blood 2014;124(9):1513–21.

39. Abdel-Wahab O, Adli M, LaFave LM, et al. ASXL1 mutations promote myeloid transformation through loss of PRC2-mediated gene repression. Cancer Cell 2012;22(2):180–93.

40. Kuo MC, Liang DC, Huang CF, et al. RUNX1 mutations are frequent in chronic myelomonocytic leukemia and mutations at the C-terminal region might predict acute myeloid leukemia transformation. Leukemia 2009;23(8):1426–31.

41. Wang W, Routbort MJ, Loghavi S, et al. Characterization of chronic myelomonocytic leukemia with TP53 mutations. Leuk Res 2018;70:97–9.

42. Greenberg PL, Tuechler H, Schanz J, et al. Revised international prognostic scoring system for myelodysplastic syndromes. Blood 2012;120(12):2454–65.

43. Onida F, Kantarjian HM, Smith TL, et al. Prognostic factors and scoring systems in chronic myelomonocytic leukemia: a retrospective analysis of 213 patients. Blood 2002;99(3):840–9.

44. Patnaik MM, Padron E, Laborde RR, et al. Mayo prognostic model for WHO-defined chronic myelomonocytic leukemia: ASXL1 and spliceosome component mutations and outcomes. Leukemia 2013;27(7):1504–10.

45. Kantarjian H, O'Brien S, Ravandi F, et al. Proposal for a new risk model in myelodysplastic syndrome that accounts for events not considered in the original International Prognostic Scoring System. Cancer 2008;113(6):1351–61.

46. Solary E, Itzykson R. How I treat chronic myelomonocytic leukemia. Blood 2017;130(2):126–36.

47. Solary E. Unplugging JAK/STAT in chronic myelomonocytic leukemia. Clin Cancer Res 2016;22(15):3707–9.

48. Vardiman JW, Bennett JM, Bain B, et al. Atypical chronic myeloid leukaemia, BCR-ABL1 negative. In: Swerdlow SH, Campo E, Harris NL, et al, editors. WHO classification of tumours of haematopoietic and lymphoid tissues. Lyon (France): IARC; 2008. p. 80–1.

49. Talati C, Padron E. An exercise in extrapolation: clinical management of atypical CML, MDS/MPN-unclassifiable, and MDS/MPN-RS-T. Curr Hematol Malig Rep 2016;11(6):425–33.

50. Wang SA, Hasserjian RP, Fox PS, et al. Atypical chronic myeloid leukemia is clinically distinct from unclassifiable myelodysplastic/myeloproliferative neoplasms. Blood 2014;123(17):2645–51.

51. Breccia M, Biondo F, Latagliata R, et al. Identification of risk factors in atypical chronic myeloid leukemia. Haematologica 2006;91(11):1566–8.

52. Xu Y, Yin J, Pan J, et al. A BCR-JAK2 fusion gene from ins(22;9)(q11;p13p24) in a patient with atypical chronic myeloid leukemia. Leuk Lymphoma 2013;54(10):2322–4.

53. Bellesso M, Santucci R, Dias DF, et al. Atypical chronic myeloid leukemia with t(9;22)(p24,11.2), a BCR-JAK2 fusion gene. Rev Bras Hematol Hemoter 2013;35(3):218–9.

54. Muta T, Osaki K, Yamano Y. Translocation t(9;22) (p23;q11) in atypical chronic myeloid leukemia (aCML) presenting osteolytic lesions. Int J Hematol 2002;76(4):344–8.

55. Gambacorti-Passerini CB, Donadoni C, Parmiani A, et al. Recurrent ETNK1 mutations in atypical chronic myeloid leukemia. Blood 2015;125(3):499–503.

56. Piazza R, Valletta S, Winkelmann N, et al. Recurrent SETBP1 mutations in atypical chronic myeloid leukemia. Nat Genet 2013;45(1):18–24.

57. Maxson JE, Gotlib J, Pollyea DA, et al. Oncogenic CSF3R mutations in chronic neutrophilic leukemia and atypical CML. N Engl J Med 2013;368(19): 1781–90.

58. Geyer JT, Orazi A. Myeloproliferative neoplasms (BCR-ABL1 negative) and myelodysplastic/myeloproliferative neoplasms: current diagnostic principles and upcoming updates. Int J Lab Hematol 2016;38(Suppl 1):12–9.

59. Arber DA, Orazi A, Hasserjian R, et al. The 2016 revision to the World Health Organization classification of myeloid neoplasms and acute leukemia. Blood 2016;127(20):2391–405.

60. Park HJ, Ha YJ, Pyo JY, et al. Delta neutrophil index as an early marker for differential diagnosis of adult-onset Still's disease and sepsis. Yonsei Med J 2014;55(3):753–9.

61. Lawrence YR, Raveh D, Rudensky B, et al. Extreme leukocytosis in the emergency department. QJM 2007;100(4):217–23.

62. Juturi JV, Hopkins T, Farhangi M. Severe leukocytosis with neutrophilia (leukemoid reaction) in alcoholic steatohepatitis. Am J Gastroenterol 1998;93(6):1013.

63. Kawada T. Smoking-induced leukocytosis can persist after cessation of smoking. Arch Med Res 2004;35(3):246–50.

64. Biezeveld MH, van Mierlo G, Lutter R, et al. Sustained activation of neutrophils in the course of Kawasaki disease: an association with matrix metalloproteinases. Clin Exp Immunol 2005;141(1):183–8.

65. Meyerson HJ, Farhi DC, Rosenthal NS. Transient increase in blasts mimicking acute leukemia and progressing myelodysplasia in patients receiving growth factor. Am J Clin Pathol 1998;109(6): 675–81.

66. Dale DC, Fauci AS, Guerry DI, et al. Comparison of agents producing a neutrophilic leukocytosis in man. Hydrocortisone, prednisone, endotoxin, and etiocholanolone. J Clin Invest 1975;56(4): 808–13.

67. Christensen RD, Hill HR. Exercise-induced changes in the blood concentration of leukocyte populations in teenage athletes. Am J Pediatr Hematol Oncol 1987;9(2):140–2.

68. Marinella MA. Extreme leukemoid reaction associated with retroperitoneal hemorrhage. Arch Intern Med 1998;158(3):300–1.

69. Ascensao JL, Oken MM, Ewing SL, et al. Leukocytosis and large cell lung cancer. A frequent association. Cancer 1987;60(4):903–5.

70. Kayashima T, Yamaguchi K, Akiyoshi T, et al. Leukemoid reaction associated with diabetic ketoacidosis—with measurement of plasma levels of granulocyte colony-stimulating factor. Intern Med 1993;32(11):869–71.

71. Kohmura K, Miyakawa Y, Kameyama K, et al. Granulocyte colony stimulating factor-producing multiple myeloma associated with neutrophilia. Leuk Lymphoma 2004;45(7):1475–9.

72. Dao KT, Tyner JW, Gotlib J. Recent progress in chronic neutrophilic leukemia and atypical chronic myeloid leukemia. Curr Hematol Malig Rep 2017; 12(5):432–41.

73. Hernandez JM, del Canizo MC, Cuneo A, et al. Clinical, hematological and cytogenetic characteristics of atypical chronic myeloid leukemia. Ann Oncol 2000;11(4):441–4.

74. Kurzrock R, Bueso-Ramos CE, Kantarjian H, et al. BCR rearrangement-negative chronic myelogenous leukemia revisited. J Clin Oncol 2001; 19(11):2915–26.

75. Koldehoff M, Beelen DW, Trenschel R, et al. Outcome of hematopoietic stem cell transplantation in patients with atypical chronic myeloid leukemia. Bone Marrow Transplant 2004;34(12): 1047–50.

76. Orazi A, Hasserjian R, Cazzola M, et al. Myelodysplastic/myeloproliferative neoplasm with ring

sideroblasts and thrombocytosis. In: Swerdlow SH, Campo E, Harris NL, et al, editors. WHO classification of tumours of haematopietic and lymphoid tissues. Lyon (France): IARC; 2017. p. 93–4.

77. Patnaik MM, Lasho TL, Hodnefield JM, et al. SF3B1 mutations are prevalent in myelodysplastic syndromes with ring sideroblasts but do not hold independent prognostic value. Blood 2012;119(2): 569–72.

78. Papaemmanuil E, Cazzola M, Boultwood J, et al. Somatic SF3B1 mutation in myelodysplasia with ring sideroblasts. N Engl J Med 2011;365(15): 1384–95.

79. Malcovati L, Della Porta MG, Pietra D, et al. Molecular and clinical features of refractory anemia with ringed sideroblasts associated with marked thrombocytosis. Blood 2009;114(17): 3538–45.

80. Patnaik MM, Lasho TL, Finke CM, et al. Predictors of survival in refractory anemia with ring sideroblasts and thrombocytosis (RARS-T) and the role of next-generation sequencing. Am J Hematol 2016;91(5):492–8.

81. Broseus J, Florensa L, Zipperer E, et al. Clinical features and course of refractory anemia with ring sideroblasts associated with marked thrombocytosis. Haematologica 2012;97(7):1036–41.

82. Patnaik MM, Tefferi A. Refractory anemia with ring sideroblasts (RARS) and RARS with thrombocytosis (RARS-T): 2017 update on diagnosis, risk-stratification, and management. Am J Hematol 2017;92(3):297–310.

83. Camaschella C. Hereditary sideroblastic anemias: pathophysiology, diagnosis, and treatment. Semin Hematol 2009;46(4):371–7.

84. DiNardo CD, Daver N, Jain N, et al. Myelodysplastic/myeloproliferative neoplasms, unclassifiable (MDS/MPN, U): natural history and clinical outcome by treatment strategy. Leukemia 2014;28(4): 958–61.

85. Sochacki AL, Fischer MA, Savona MR. Therapeutic approaches in myelofibrosis and myelodysplastic/myeloproliferative overlap syndromes. Onco Targets Ther 2016;9:2273–86.

86. Bose P, Nazha A, Komrokji RS, et al. Mutational landscape of myelodysplastic/myeloproliferative neoplasm-unclassifiable. Blood 2018;132(19): 2100–3.

87. Meggendorfer M, Jeromin S, Haferlach C, et al. The mutational landscape of 18 investigated genes clearly separates four subtypes of myelodysplastic/myeloproliferative neoplasms. Haematologica 2018;103(5):e192–5.

88. Mughal TI, Cross NC, Padron E, et al. An International MDS/MPN Working Group's perspective and recommendations on molecular pathogenesis, diagnosis and clinical characterization of myelodysplastic/myeloproliferative neoplasms. Haematologica 2015;100(9):1117–30.

89. Kanagal-Shamanna R, Bueso-Ramos CE, Barkoh B, et al. Myeloid neoplasms with isolated isochromosome 17q represent a clinicopathologic entity associated with myelodysplastic/myeloproliferative features, a high risk of leukemic transformation, and wild-type TP53. Cancer 2012;118(11): 2879–88.

90. Assi R, Kantarjian HM, Garcia-Manero G, et al. A phase II trial of ruxolitinib in combination with azacytidine in myelodysplastic syndrome/myeloproliferative neoplasms. Am J Hematol 2018; 93(2):277–85.

91. Broseus J, Alpermann T, Wulfert M, et al. Age, JAK2(V617F) and SF3B1 mutations are the main predicting factors for survival in refractory anaemia with ring sideroblasts and marked thrombocytosis. Leukemia 2013;27(9):1826–31.

92. Visconte V, Rogers HJ, Singh J, et al. SF3B1 haploinsufficiency leads to formation of ring sideroblasts in myelodysplastic syndromes. Blood 2012; 120(16):3173–86.

93. Geyer JT, Tam W, Liu YC, et al. Oligomonocytic chronic myelomonocytic leukemia (chronic myelomonocytic leukemia without absolute monocytosis) displays a similar clinicopathologic and mutational profile to classical chronic myelomonocytic leukemia. Mod Pathol 2017;30(9): 1213–22.

94. Schuler E, Schroeder M, Neukirchen J, et al. Refined medullary blast and white blood cell count based classification of chronic myelomonocytic leukemias. Leuk Res 2014;38(12): 1413–9.

95. Cervera N, Itzykson R, Coppin E, et al. Gene mutations differently impact the prognosis of the myelodysplastic and myeloproliferative classes of chronic myelomonocytic leukemia. Am J Hematol 2014;89(6):604–9.

96. Bacher U, Haferlach T, Schnittger S, et al. Recent advances in diagnosis, molecular pathology and therapy of chronic myelomonocytic leukaemia. Br J Haematol 2011;153(2):149–67.

97. Kumar MS, Narla A, Nonami A, et al. Coordinate loss of a microRNA and protein-coding gene cooperate in the pathogenesis of 5q- syndrome. Blood 2011;118(17):4666–73.

98. Ingram W, Lea NC, Cervera J, et al. The JAK2 V617F mutation identifies a subgroup of MDS patients with isolated deletion 5q and a proliferative bone marrow. Leukemia 2006; 20(7):1319–21.

99. Patnaik MM, Lasho TL, Finke CM, et al. WHO-defined 'myelodysplastic syndrome with isolated del(5q)' in 88 consecutive patients: survival data, leukemic transformation rates and prevalence of

JAK2, MPL and IDH mutations. Leukemia 2010; 24(7):1283–9.

100. Sokol L, Caceres G, Rocha K, et al. JAK2(V617F) mutation in myelodysplastic syndrome (MDS) with del(5q) arises in genetically discordant clones. Leuk Res 2010;34(6):821–3.

101. Malcovati L, Karimi M, Papaemmanuil E, et al. SF3B1 mutation identifies a distinct subset of myelodysplastic syndrome with ring sideroblasts. Blood 2015;126(2):233–41.

102. Malcovati L, Papaemmanuil E, Bowen DT, et al. Clinical significance of SF3B1 mutations in myelodysplastic syndromes and myelodysplastic/myeloproliferative neoplasms. Blood 2011;118(24): 6239–46.

103. Patnaik MM, Vallapureddy R, Yalniz FF, et al. Therapy-related chronic myelomonocytic leukemia (CMML): molecular, cytogenetic, and clinical distinctions from de novo CMML. Am J Hematol 2018;93(1):65–73.

104. Dupriez B, Morel P, Demory JL, et al. Prognostic factors in agnogenic myeloid metaplasia: a report on 195 cases with a new scoring system. Blood 1996;88(3):1013–8.

105. Visani G, Finelli C, Castelli U, et al. Myelofibrosis with myeloid metaplasia: clinical and haematological parameters predicting survival in a series of 133 patients. Br J Haematol 1990; 75(1):4–9.

106. Grinfeld J, Nangalia J, Baxter EJ, et al. Classification and personalized prognosis in myeloproliferative neoplasms. N Engl J Med 2018;379(15):1416–30.

107. Klampfl T, Gisslinger H, Harutyunyan AS, et al. Somatic mutations of calreticulin in myeloproliferative neoplasms. N Engl J Med 2013;369(25): 2379–90.

108. Hidalgo Lopez JE, Carballo-Zarate A, Verstovsek S, et al. Bone marrow findings in blast phase of polycythemia vera. Ann Hematol 2018;97(3):425–34.

109. Fu B, Jaso JM, Sargent RL, et al. Bone marrow fibrosis in patients with primary myelodysplastic syndromes has prognostic value using current therapies and new risk stratification systems. Mod Pathol 2014;27(5):681–9.

110. Della Porta MG, Malcovati L, Boveri E, et al. Clinical relevance of bone marrow fibrosis and CD34-positive cell clusters in primary myelodysplastic syndromes. J Clin Oncol 2009;27(5):754–62.

111. Delic S, Rose D, Kern W, et al. Application of an NGS-based 28-gene panel in myeloproliferative neoplasms reveals distinct mutation patterns in essential thrombocythaemia, primary myelofibrosis and polycythaemia vera. Br J Haematol 2016; 175(3):419–26.

112. Elena C, Galli A, Such E, et al. Integrating clinical features and genetic lesions in the risk assessment of patients with chronic myelomonocytic leukemia. Blood 2016;128(10):1408–17.

Optimal Measurable Residual Disease Testing for Acute Myeloid Leukemia

Wenbin Xiao, MD, PhD*, Kseniya Petrova-Drus, MD, PhD, Mikhail Roshal, MD, PhD

KEYWORDS

- Acute myeloid leukemia • Minimal/measurable residual disease • Flow cytometry
- Molecular assays • RT-qPCR • Next-generation sequencing • Droplet digital PCR

Key Points

- Measurable residual disease (MRD) monitoring should be routinely integrated into clinical practice of acute myeloid leukemia

- An integrated approach combining immunophenotyping and molecular detection techniques improves sensitivity and specificity of MRD

- Many obstacles exist in implementing MRD detection in clinical practice

ABSTRACT

Increasing evidence supports the prognostic significance of measurable residual disease (MRD) in acute myeloid leukemia (AML). Dynamic MRD assessment for patients with AML complements baseline patient risk assessment factors in determining patient prognosis. MRD status may also be helpful in informing therapeutic decisions. The European Leukemia Net MRD working party recently issued consensus recommendations for the use of MRD in AML. The Food and Drug Administration also issued advice for using MRD in trials of hematologic malignancies. This article discusses MRD testing, highlights the challenges in adopting MRD testing in clinical practice, and provides insights into the future of the field.

OVERVIEW

Morphologic complete remission (CR) (<5% blasts by differential count in the bone marrow) after induction therapy is a historically established measure of treatment response in acute myeloid leukemia (AML). It is often incorporated with genetic and pretreatment clinical parameters to guide further therapy in patients with AML.[1–4] However, at least half of the patients who achieve morphologic CR ultimately relapse. It is clear that the measure is imperfect at best, with poor sensitivity and specificity. Residual treatment-resistant leukemia cells, less than the cytomorphologic detection limit, are considered responsible for the relapse.[5] Moreover, some patients with recovering blast counts in excess of 5% show no evidence of disease by more specific methods.[6] Increasing evidence indicates that identifying minimal/measurable residual disease (MRD) less than the cytomorphology-based 5% blast threshold and excluding patients with transient nonleukemic regenerating blast increase can redefine risk stratification.[6,7] Depending on the methodology, MRD analysis can detect leukemia cells down to levels of 10^{-3} to 10^{-6} of white blood cells (WBCs), approximately 2 to 5 log higher sensitivity, compared with 1:20 in cytomorphology-based assessments.[8,9]

Disclosures: This study was supported in part through the National Institutes of Health, National Cancer Institute (Cancer Center Support Grant P30 CA008748).
Department of Pathology, Hematopathology Diagnostic Service, Memorial Sloan Kettering Cancer Center, 1275 York Avenue, New York, NY 10065, USA
* Corresponding author.
E-mail address: xiaow@mskcc.org

Surgical Pathology 12 (2019) 671–686
https://doi.org/10.1016/j.path.2019.03.009

Most studies, regardless of specific technique used to evaluate MRD, report a robust association of MRD with inferior outcomes in patients with AML with an average hazard ratio (HR) of 2 to 4.[9–12] These differences are noted as early as 2 weeks after beginning induction chemotherapy[13,14] and are associated with increasing risk thereafter with failure to clear MRD at later time points conferring the highest risk.[7] As early as day 28 postinduction, MRD independently predicts overall survival (OS) and relapse-free survival (RFS).[15–20] MRD after consolidation is generally associated with even higher risk of relapse and shorter OS and RFS.[16,21–27] The difference persists despite allogeneic hematopoietic stem cell transplant (HSCT) and holds up across age groups and risk categories.[23,28,29] Patients with AML who undergo HSCT with any level of MRD by flow cytometry before HSCT are at significantly increased risk of relapse and death.[7,30–32] Data in older patients (>65 years old)[15] and children[6,14,17,20,33] with AML undergoing standard induction have also shown the prognostic relevance of MRD. Multivariable regression modeling consistently indicates that MRD is an independent, and frequently the only, posttreatment prognostic variable for relapse and survival.[15–17,23,30,33,34]

Given the prognostic significance of MRD across the AML treatment continuum, the 2017 European Leukemia Net (ELN) recommends comprehensive MRD monitoring following induction and consolidation courses to assess kinetics of disease response, and then monitoring sequentially after consolidation to detect impending relapse.[35] Dynamic MRD assessment for patients with AML complements baseline patient risk assessment factors such as age, karyotype, and molecular alterations in determining patient prognosis. More importantly, MRD status may be helpful in informing therapeutic decisions.[16,29] A recent survey in the United States confirmed that MRD is frequently used in making treatment decisions and in estimating prognosis. However, there is lack of uniformity in these practices.[36] Standardization of assays, adoption of requisite technology, and dissemination of data about the value of MRD use would likely increase usage of MRD in the care of patients with AML. To guide the development of a standardized or harmonized approach to MRD testing, the ELN MRD working party recently issued consensus recommendations for the measurement and application of MRD in AML.[9] The US Food and Drug Administration (FDA) also issued a road map for drug companies looking to use MRD in trials of patients with hematologic malignancies.[37] This article discusses the current methods of MRD detection, highlights the challenges in adopting MRD testing in routine clinical practice, and provides some insights into the future of the field.

MINIMAL/MEASURABLE RESIDUAL DISEASE DETECTION METHODS

A perfect MRD test should accurately identify the smallest populations of leukemia cells in patients with AML in morphologic CR, which, if left untreated, cause relapse while being indifferent toward residual leukemia/preleukemic cells that do not cause relapse.[8] Current MRD testing methods have not achieved this ideal state, except perhaps for real-time quantitative polymerase chain reaction (RT-qPCR) testing in chronic myeloid leukemia. The most commonly used methods of MRD assessment are multicolor flow cytometry (MFC) and RT-qPCR of specific mutations or gene fusions detected at diagnosis. Recently, next-generation sequencing (NGS) has emerged as a promising technology to expand on these methodologies (**Table 1**).

MULTICOLOR FLOW CYTOMETRY

MFC techniques are based on the expression of antigens that characterize diverse lineages of hematopoietic cells. In MRD detection, MFC can be used to evaluate cell populations that deviate from an antigen-expression pattern typical of normal or regenerating cells of similar lineage and maturation stage. Such deviations include cross-lineage expression, overexpression, reduced or absent expression, and asynchronous expression of multiple antigens. AML blasts may then be defined by expression of distinct leukemia-associated immunophenotypes (LAIPs; **Fig. 1**),[26,38,39] or by manifesting an immunophenotypic maturation profile detected using a fixed antibody panel that is different from normal (DfN; **Fig. 2**).[10] In an LAIP approach, a comprehensive panel is run to identify several phenotypes that are infrequent in normal bone marrow. These phenotypes are then used to follow the patient longitudinally. In a DfN-type approach, the same panel is used to both evaluate and follow patients with AML. The approach relies both on identifications of populations that are infrequent in normal marrows and understanding maturational patterns that can deviate from normal. With expansion of use of 8-color to 10-color flow cytometry, these 2 approaches are increasingly closely related because fixed comprehensive multicolor panels used in state-of-the-art DfN approaches are usually sufficient to detect common LAIPs and also allow for substantial posttreatment antigenic changes (immunophenotypic shifts). In a strict LAIP approach, assessment of the diagnostic

Table 1
Comparison of methods for measurable residual disease detection

Method	Sensitivity (%)	Pros	Cons
Cytomorphology	5–10	Short turnaround time Relatively easy to perform	Difficult to differentiate between marrow recovery Low sensitivity
Cytogenetics, conventional	3–10	Routinely used Provide global genetic information	Low sensitivity
Cytogenetics, FISH	0.2–10	Routinely used	Dependent on presence of a previously identified cytogenetic abnormality
MFC	∼0.1–0.001	Short turnaround time Applicable to 90% of patients with a large antibody panel Can evaluate cellular composition of entire sample High specificity when using DfN/LAIP approach and many combinations of antibodies	High level of expertise needed Sensitivity varies dependent on immunophenotype Detection may be challenging when shifts in leukemia immunophenotype are present Unclear whether preleukemia immunophenotype can be differentiated
General molecular techniques		Amenable to standardization Serial measurements may be used to assess kinetics of MRD	Longer turnaround time
RT-qPCR	0.01–0.001	High sensitivity High specificity for leukemic cells	Need a dedicated assay for each fusion/mutation (specific primer sets) May not detect atypical fusion products (eg, p230 of BCR-ABL1) Applicable to ∼50% of younger and ∼35% of older patients
Locked nucleic acid RT-qPCR	0.001–0.0001	Very high sensitivity High specificity for leukemic cells Amenable to standardization	Same as RT-qPCR
Droplet digital PCR (ddPCR)	∼0.01–0.0001	Absolute quantitation, no need for standard curves for each mutation/primer set High sensitivity	Same as RT-qPCR
NGS, conventional	2–2.5	Evaluate large number of mutated genes at once Evaluation of clonal heterogeneity at diagnosis and clonal evolution during disease course	Requires batching, long turnaround time Mutation detection depends on depth of sequencing at specific loci Clone responsible for relapse may be a minor component during disease diagnosis Difficult to distinguish leukemic vs preleukemic mutations
NGS, error corrected	0.01	Same as conventional NGS with higher sensitivity	Same as conventional NGS

Abbreviations: DfN, different from normal; FISH, fluorescence in situ hybridization.

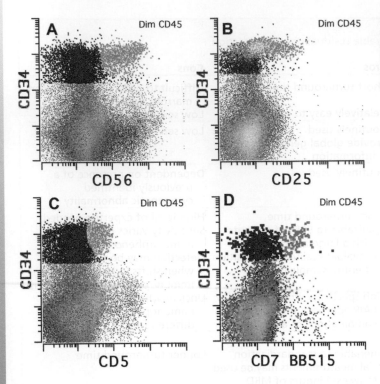

Fig. 1. MFC MRD detection by LAIP approach. A subset of blasts aberrantly expresses cross-lineage markers such as CD56 (*A*), CD25 (*B*), CD5 (*C*), and CD7 (*D*). Green, granulocytes; red, blasts; yellow, LAIP-identified blasts.

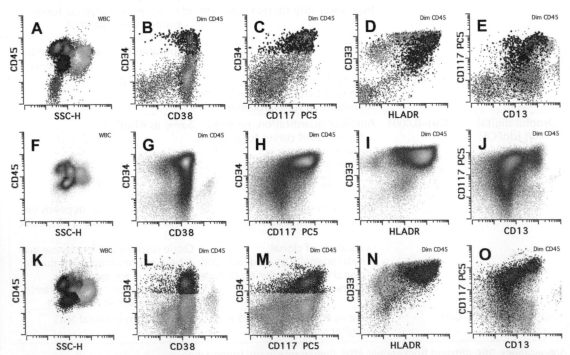

Fig. 2. MFC MRD detection by DfN approach. (*A–E*) An example of the immunophenotype of normal blasts in the marrow. The blasts (red) show normal maturation pattern by expressing CD45 (dim), CD38, CD117, CD33, and CD13. (*F–J*) AML blasts. The blasts show aberrant expression of CD117 (bright), CD33 (bright), and CD13 (dim). (*K–O*) MRD detection after induction therapy for the same patient. The blasts (1.0% of WBC) show similar aberrant expression of CD117 (bright), CD33 (bright), and CD13 (dim).

sample is required for defining leukemic populations to follow. In contrast, DfN does not restrict MRD determination to specific LAIPs present at diagnosis and takes immunophenotypic shifts over time into account, but is also informed by LAIPs present at diagnosis when available. Therefore, if sufficiently broad antibody panels are used for detection, the differences between LAIPs and DfN may be minimized and LAIPs become part of DfN. Therefore, an integrated LAIP-based DfN approach has recently been recommended by the ELN MRD working party.[9]

The major advantages of MFC are its wide applicability, assay availability, relative affordability, and rapid turnaround time, which facilitates prompt decision making for therapeutic intervention.[10] MFC also allows simultaneous evaluation of expression levels of multiple antigens on the leukemic blasts, which are relevant for potential targeted immunotherapy.[40]

There are several limitations inherent to MFC MRD testing. Not all leukemia cells have a readily identifiable abnormal phenotype within the context of commonly used panels, and phenotypes may change over time with gains/losses of specific abnormalities or patterns of abnormalities because of disease evolution, subclone selection, and/or progression through the cell cycle.[41] Therefore, sensitivity for detection of MRD by MFC varies from case to case and from time point to time point, although

in general it is not less than 0.1% for greater than 95% of cases.[16] The MFC approach requires a very high level of expertise for data interpretation, which is not widely available.[10] In addition, the MFC method has considerable variability in the equipment, reagents, data analysis methods, and reporting used in MRD evaluation, confounding reproducibility and applicability outside of a limited number of expert centers with high level of analytical expertise.[42–44] Appropriate instrumental compensation and fluorochrome selection/combinations are also key for success.[45] Some, but not all, of these problems can be reduced with standardized laboratory procedures, including sample processing and instrument settings, single-tube approaches with a preconfigured and stable assay, automated interpretation software, central review, and continuous quality assessment.[8,9] Researchers continue to work on improving MFC methodology and technology. Zeijlemaker and colleagues[46] have developed a simple 1-tube assay with a marker cocktail (CLL-1/TIM-3/CD7/CD11b/CD22/CD56) in 1 fluorescence channel that seems to accurately detect CD34+CD38− leukemic stem cells (LSCs). Our own recent study suggests that simply measuring plasmacytoid dendritic cells (PDC) predicts the outcome with a power of the same magnitude to MRD detection at the time points such as postinduction as well as pretransplant (**Fig. 3**).[47] However, despite variations in

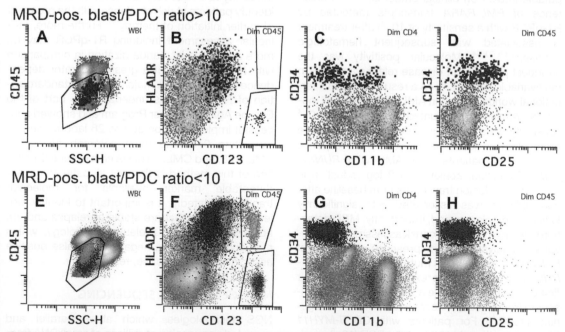

Fig. 3. MFC blast/PDC ratio. (*A–D*) MRD-positive case with blast/PDC ratio greater than 10. The blasts show aberrant expression of CD11b and CD25. Note the marked reduction in PDC gate. (*E–H*) MRD-positive case with blast/PDC ratio less than 10. Only a small subset of blasts shows aberrant expression of CD25. In this case, the PDC number is within normal range. PDC, plasmacytoid dendritic cells.

technology, specific antibody composition, and other factors, several studies have shown a very high degree of concordance across the time spectrum for risk assessment of AML.[6,7,16,30,48]

REAL-TIME QUANTITATIVE POLYMERASE CHAIN REACTION

The genetic heterogeneity of AML creates difficulties with establishing a singular approach to disease monitoring by sensitive molecular methodologies.[49–52] Subclonal genetic events occurring during expansion of the founding clone can further contribute to this challenge.[53] Among the different molecular assays, including RT-qPCR, droplet digital PCR (ddPCR), and NGS, the use of RT-qPCR has been recommended by the ELN MRD working party for MRD assessment because of its established high sensitivity.[9] RT-qPCR is used to measure molecular mutations and leukemia-associated fusion transcripts in a quantitative manner relative to a suitable housekeeper gene, usually $ABL1$.

RT-qPCR methods have been extensively used for MRD detection in patients with PML-$RARA$, $RUNX1$-$RUNXT1$, $CBFB$-$MYH11$ fusions, and $NPM1$ mutations, achieving high sensitivity of 10^{-4} to 10^{-6}. PML-$RARA$ fusion is one of the most established RT-qPCR assays for MRD detection, with an extensive standardization effort and indisputable impact on clinical outcomes.[54–60] Persistence of PML-$RARA$ transcripts (detected by RT-qPCR with a sensitivity of 10^{-4}) after treatment is associated with subsequent hematologic relapse.[57,58,60–64] Molecular positivity was the strongest predictor of disease relapse and RFS in multivariable analysis.[59] As a result, the 2003 international working group in AML recommended molecular remission, evaluated with at least 10^{-4} sensitivity, as a new surrogate end point in acute promyelocytic leukemia clinical trial response criteria.[65] In patients with AML with $RUNX1$-$RUNX1T1$ fusion, achieving a 3 log reduction in bone marrow fusion transcripts from baseline after consolidation was associated with significantly lower risk of relapse, and, importantly, MRD detection was more powerful for risk assessment in multivariable analysis than the presence of concurrent $FLT3$-ITD and KIT mutations.[66,67] $RUNX1$-$RUNX1T1$ patients who experience relapse after first CR, or fail to achieve a 3 log reduction in transcripts from baseline, seem to benefit from allogeneic HSCT.[68] For patients with $CBFB$-$MYH11$ fusion, detection of MRD by RT-qPCR (10^{-5} sensitivity) with less than 10 copies/10^5 $ABL1$ copies in peripheral blood at the end of consolidation was associated with decreased risk of relapse (78% vs

36%), whereas the OS showed no difference, likely because of good responses to salvage therapy.[69] NPM1 mutations can also be reliably followed by RT-qPCR by evaluating transcripts (sensitivity of 10^{-5} or 10^{-6} with locked nucleic acid, which suppresses amplification of wild-type[70]) or genomic DNA (sensitivity of 10^{-4}).[71] Several studies have confirmed that in $NPM1$ mutated AML postinduction MRD, detected by RT-qPCR, is associated with significantly higher risk of relapse and shorter OS.[34,70,72] In multivariable analysis, MRD status after 2 cycles of chemotherapy is the most powerful predictor of survival regardless of the presence of $FLT3$-ITD.[34] In addition, patients who failed to achieve greater than 4 log reduction in transcripts in peripheral blood showed improved outcome after allo-HSCT.[72] Furthermore, another study showed that an increase of greater than 10% mutated $NPM1/ABL1$ transcripts was most prognostic for relapse after allogeneic HSCT.[73]

A key advantage of fusion-based RT-qPCR is inherent specificity. Furthermore, the quantification of the independent housekeeping gene performed in parallel with the target under investigation, enabls identification of suboptimal samples that may contribute to false-negative results. In addition, locked nucleic acid RT-qPCR assays are ultrasensitive (10^{-5} to 10^{-7}) for detection of leukemia-associated alterations.[8] The theoretic advantage of such highly sensitive assays is the ability to detect very-low-level MRD and better identify patients at risk of relapse with the prospect of earlier initiation of therapy.[74] Furthermore, molecular assessment including RT-qPCR may be more amenable to standardization in comparison with MFC because of a greater operator dependence of the latter. A major effort at standardization of RT-qPCR was undertaken as part of the Europe Against Cancer Program and showed successful implementation across 26 laboratories by evaluating 9 of the most common fusions in AML, ALL, and CML.[75] However, a potential limitation of this method is that not all patients have a detectable marker available for molecular tracking. Relatedly, it is important to identify molecular markers that are stable at relapse and are not associated with preleukemic biology, which may give rise to false-negative and false-positive associations with relapse, respectively.

NEXT-GENERATION SEQUENCING

NGS technologies, which allow parallel and repeated sequencing of millions of small DNA fragments, can be used to evaluate a few genes or an entire genome. Increased understanding of the genomic landscape of AML and technical advances have now enabled the use of NGS-based panels to identify MRD. Klco and colleagues[76] applied NGS to risk stratify AML (n = 50). Although the mutational spectrum at diagnosis was not significantly associated with outcomes, patients (n = 24) with at least 1 persistent mutation (variant allele frequency [VAF] $\geq$2.5%) at day 30 postinduction had significantly inferior RFS and OS (HR, 3.67 and 2.86, respectively) compared with patients who cleared all mutations. The authors recently showed that mutations identified by a targeted 28-gene NGS panel (VAF $\geq$ 5%) in patients with AML achieving CR/CRi (CR with incomplete hematologic recovery) before allo-HSCT (n = 62) are associated with inferior RFS and OS (HR, 4.35 and 2.1, respectively) after HSCT.[48] These findings have been further confirmed by a large cohort (n = 428) from the HOVON/SAKK trials of patients with AML achieving CR/CRi after second induction.[77] Using a 54-gene panel capturing mutations frequently associated with AML, at least 1 mutation was identified in approximately 90% of diagnostic samples; persistent mutations in the CR or CRi setting were detected in approximately 50% these patients, with VAF ranging from 0.02% to 47%. Detection of mutations other than DNMT3A, TET2, and ASXL1, irrespective of the allele frequency (typically occurring at frequencies <2.5%), was strongly associated with increased relapse risk (55.4% vs 31.9% with no detection), as well as reduced RFS (36.6% vs 58.1%) and OS (41.9% vs 66.1%) at 4 years (P<.001 for all comparisons). These associations remained statistically significant after adjustment for age, WBC count, cytogenetic and/or molecular risk, and whether 1 or 2 induction cycles were required to enter CR or CRi.[77]

Conventional NGS assay has an intrinsic sequencing error rate that limits sensitivity for most single-nucleotide variants to ~1% to 2% of all reads. However, newer technology has significantly improved the sensitivity.[78] For example, a recent study showed that an error-corrected NGS assay decreased the lower limit of detection to 0.005% (eg, mutant IDH1) and showed a median background error of 0.0071% and a median sensitivity threshold of 0.015%.[79] NGS-based MRD assays will likely have limited role in a subset of patients with AML. As mentioned earlier, approximately 10% of sequenced AML cases did not show any mutations detected by a 54-gene panel.[77] Even a much larger gene panel is inadequate for some patients; for example, in a previous study, NGS of a panel of 264 genes recurrently mutated in AML was not informative in 5 of the 50 examined samples (10%).[76] Moreover, genetic clonal heterogeneity at diagnosis with evolution

over time and possibly emergence or selection of small subclones at relapse will complicate the NGS MRD detection. Distinction between pathogenic versus nonpathogenic, such as preleukemic, mutations is not always straightforward. Mutations in DNMT3A, TET2, and ASXL1 (collectively referred to as DTA mutations), the most common aberrations identified in people with age-related clonal hematopoiesis of indeterminate potential, often remained detectable during remission (in 78.7%, 54.2%, and 51.6% of cases, respectively) but with no associated increase in relapse risk or detriment in survival.[48,77] Technical advances and the increasing understanding of the clonal somatic mutation architecture in AML will likely resolve many of these limitations. NGS-based MRD approaches are also easy to standardize and to interpret compared with MFC.

CHALLENGES

WHAT IS THE SIGNIFICANCE OF MORPHOLOGIC COMPLETE REMISSION IN THE MINIMAL/MEASURABLE RESIDUAL DISEASE ERA?

Although morphologic CR has been used as the end point for evaluating chemotherapy efficacy in AML for 60 years, there are obvious limitations of defining CR by cytomorphology. One is imprecision in quantifying myeloblasts in bone marrow samples using light microscopy related to the survey of few (typically 200–500) nucleated bone marrow cells and intraobserver and interobserver variability in identifying myeloblasts.[8] Another issue is the imperfect ability to distinguish regenerating from leukemia myeloblasts by morphology. A few studies have shown that a positive MRD test was strongly associated with relapse risk, whereas myeloblast levels (<5% vs $\geq$5%) provided no additional prognostic information.[6,29,33] Data from children showed a substantial proportion (up to 30%) of subjects with greater than or equal to 5% myeloblasts but a negative MRD test by MFC and/or molecular assays and these patients had excellent outcomes, indicating that the increased blasts are a regenerating process. Similarly, approximately 10% of adult patients with AML with refractory disease or partial remission defined by morphology were MRD negative and their survival was similar to MRD-negative CR patients.[29] In contrast, outcomes of subjects with less than 5% myeloblasts but a positive MRD test were similar to those with greater than or equal to 5% myeloblasts. Patients with AML receiving myeloablative allotransplants in CR but with a positive MRD test had outcomes similar to patients not in morphologic CR.[7,30] These data suggest a need to move beyond morphologic CR, and that results of MRD testing could supplement or replace the current cytomorphology-based definition of remission. Such a change would have significant implications for therapy algorithms of persons with AML.

WHAT TESTS SHOULD BE CHOSEN FOR MINIMAL/MEASURABLE RESIDUAL DISEASE DETECTION?

RT-qPCR is usually of high sensitivity and therefore is currently considered the gold standard for patients with AML that harbor 1 or more suitable abnormalities, including *PML/RARA* fusions, *CBF* fusions, and mutant *NPM1*,[9] but this can only be applied to ~ 40% of patients with AML. In addition, *NPM1* mutated AML can relapse as *NPM1* wild-type, which prevents MRD detection by RT-qPCR.[80] For the patients who do not have these abnormalities, MFC is the choice, although a few recent studies suggest that NGS-based MRD testing is also complementary. The authors compared NGS testing (28-gene panel) and MFC (10-color, DfN approach) assay on MRD detection in patients with AML before allo-HSCT. Results of the 2 assays were concordant in ~70% of patients. Patients found to be MRD positive with both assays had the highest risk of relapse compared with patients who were negative by both assays; patients with discordant assay results had an intermediate outcome.[48] Jongen-Lavrencic and colleagues[77] analyzed samples from 340 patients with AML for MRD using both NGS (54-gene panel) and MFC (LAIP approach). Concordant results were obtained for most patients (~70%), and relapse rates were lowest in those without MRD detected by either method and highest in those with MRD detected in both assays; those with discordant results again had an intermediate outcome. The proportions of patients testing MRD positive and/or negative with NGS-based and MFC-based assays might change as methodologies evolve but, given the inherent limitations of each detection approach, combining both assays will provide maximal prognostic information. It remains unclear whether NGS assay will reach the sensitivity of RT-qPCR and therefore consolidate all the mutations including NPM1 in 1 single panel.[81] Newer droplet digital PCR (ddPCR) methods have emerged,[82,83] which provide an exact number of target molecules in the sample, without reference to standards or endogenous controls, and are becoming incorporated in routine clinical use. ddPCR for detection of *PML-RARA*

transcripts at diagnosis and for MRD evaluation showed comparable sensitivity with RT-qPCR and is therefore promising for future use.[84] Similar to RT-qPCR, a major disadvantage of ddPCR is that every single mutation/alteration needs a different primer set, which will restrict this application to disease-defining fusions and/or hotspot mutations.

STANDARDIZING THE MINIMAL/ MEASURABLE RESIDUAL DISEASE TEST: PARTICULARLY MULTICOLOR FLOW CYTOMETRY –BASED TESTING

The genetic and immunophenotypic heterogeneity of leukemic blasts increase the challenge of standardizing MRD detection protocols. Additional challenges to adopting MRD testing in routine clinical practice for patients with AML have included the absence of interlaboratory standardization; skill/expertise of personnel; or consensus regarding optimal key parameters, including type of specimen, the quality and number of viable cells used for analyses, MRD target, timing of MRD assessment, technology (eg, MFC vs RT-qPCR), testing protocols, and lack of established cutoff values. The ELN MRD working party recommendations address several of these issues. More multicenter and/or international collaborations will be needed for standardization of these MRD technologies, particularly the newer ones such as NGS-based methods and ddPCR. For MFC MRD testing, the ELN working party recommends the following markers: CD7, CD11b, CD13, CD15, CD19, CD33, CD34, CD45, CD56, CD117, and HLA-DR and, if necessary, monocytic markers CD64, CD14, and CD4. A minimum of an 8-color panel is suggested. Incorporating more markers aberrantly expressed by LSCs might improve the sensitivity and specificity of MFC MRD detection.[85,86] Because newer flow cytometers with more than 16 colors are available, and a marker cocktail (CLL-1/TIM-3/CD7/ CD11b/CD22/CD56) can be used for stem cell aberrancy, the concept of 1-tube MFC MRD assay with fixed antibody panel has been raised and is under investigation. Another potential novel approach is to measure blast to PDC ratio. In a small single-center study, blast to PDC ratio at an early postinduction time point was comparable with the DfN approach in predicting relapse.[47] Therefore, this approach, if confirmed in larger multicenter studies, could theoretically be easier to standardize because measurement of PDCs by MFC is highly reproducible and does not require high-level expertise.

WHAT SAMPLE TYPES SHOULD BE USED FOR MINIMAL/MEASURABLE RESIDUAL DISEASE?

Although bone marrow collection is an invasive procedure, can be traumatic, and in some cases the aspiration fails (dry tap), the ELN MRD working party recommends bone marrow sampling for MFC MRD testing because of the concern of a lower frequency of leukemia cells in peripheral blood.[9] Studies have shown that MRD levels in the peripheral blood are nearly 10 times lower, with a median of 29 days delayed conversion of negative RT-qPCR to positive than the corresponding bone marrow,[59] although peripheral blood MRD seemed to be more specific in a single study.[87] For molecular MRD testing, both bone marrow and peripheral blood are suggested. Balsat and colleagues[72] showed that the presence of mutant *NPM1* MRD in peripheral blood in first remission was a strong predictor of relapse, independent of cytogenetics and *FLT3-ITD* status, and might have application in selecting patients who would benefit from allo-HSCT. Peripheral blood sampling is less expensive and less painful for patients who may be unwilling to undergo the more frequent bone marrow sampling required to monitor MRD during various courses of treatment. MRD analysis of peripheral blood requires a minimum of 20 mL of blood; in patients with WBC counts less than 1×10^9/L, more blood may be necessary to improve sensitivity.

For molecular testing, the source of nucleic acid, genomic DNA (gDNA) or RNA, each has specific advantages and drawbacks that affect the ability to monitor the molecular target with high sensitivity and specificity. DNA is more stable than RNA in samples, providing greater flexibility in sample processing. An RNA-based approach first requires generation of complementary DNA by a reverse transcription reaction followed by qPCR. When RNA is used, the quality of the RNA template is a key determinant of the reproducibility and clinical significance of the results, and certain groups recommend to routinely use an RNA stabilizing solution when processing samples for MRD analysis.[88] RNA degradation, likely resulting from nuclease activity, reduces *BCR-ABL1* transcripts by 20% to 50% when peripheral blood anticoagulated with EDTA (ethylenediaminepentaacetic acid) is stored at ambient temperature for 24 to 48 hours.[88] In addition, RNA-based monitoring hinges on transcription, which can also be influenced by environmental selection and epigenetic factors, such as methylation. Furthermore, at the DNA level, leukemic fusions most commonly show unique breakpoints within introns, which theoretically provides a patient-specific and leukemia-specific marker when monitoring at the gDNA level and can be used to investigate any possibility of cross-contamination. Although this approach is feasible, as was shown for AML with the *RUNX1-RUNX1T1* fusion,[89] it is complex, requiring patient-specific primers, and may not be practical for routine clinical use. Another advantage of gDNA is that the molecular target, outside of amplification and loss of heterozygosity, is typically present on 1 allele per cell, allowing for a simplified absolute quantitation. In contrast, RNA transcripts are present in multiple copies per cell, and although this may aid with detection, it requires establishing a relative quantitation approach that can be standardized across laboratories. Nonetheless, use of RNA templates has been preferred because of their specificity and wide applicability (by targeting common postprocessing transcripts).

TIME POINTS, THRESHOLDS, AND REPORTING

During the treatment phase, MRD testing is commonly performed after induction, consolidation, pre-HSCT, and post-HSCT. No added value for MRD was seen at day 14.[90] During follow-up, not much is known about the optimal time intervals for clinically relevant sequential MFC measurements of MRD. The ELN working party recommends molecular MRD assessment every 3 months for 24 months after the end of treatment in bone marrow and peripheral blood for patients with *PML-RARA*, *CBF* fusion, and mutated *NPM1*. Monitoring beyond 2 years of follow-up should be based on the relapse risk of the patient.[9] More therapeutic agents, particularly differentiating agents, are being approved for the treatment of AML, and many of them achieve clinical response after multiple cycles. High-burden molecular alterations may remain despite remission,[91] and what time points and how to measure MRD remain to be clarified.

The threshold less than or greater than which patients should be considered MRD negative or MRD positive based on flow cytometric assessment of residual tumor amounts has been controversial. Different thresholds greater than the minimal detection limit as optimal cutoffs for the best segregation of patients into categories of relapse risk rather than using the technical detection limit of the MRD assay as threshold has been proposed. Therefore, cutoff levels of MFC MRD have been ranged from any detectable disease to 0.5% in various studies.[24,25] In many LAIP-based studies, a cutoff of 0.1% was used based on practical considerations and was found relevant in published work.[15–18,33] The cutoff minimum has also been adopted by the ELN MRD working party. However, several high-quality studies using DfN and LSC approaches showed that the risk of relapse and disease-related death among MRD-positive patients with a level less than 0.1%, but greater than the detection limit, was not reduced compared with higher levels of MRD.[31,86] This observation also holds true for molecular genetic–based approaches, suggesting that the 0.1% level is a poor representation of cure. These observations would not support using an artificial cutoff for MRD assay detection limit. It follows that any level of residual disease within the validated range of an assay should be defined as MRD positive as long as the assay is properly evaluated and powered to assess levels less than 0.1%. As a compromise, the ELN working party recommendation includes a category in the reporting as MFC MRD detectable and quantifiable but uncertain significance if MRD detected but less than 0.1%. For RT-qPCR, 10^{-4} is usually used as a cutoff. RT-qPCR analysis with a sensitivity of 10^{-5} continued to detect *RUNX1-RUNXT1* transcript in the marrow in a minority of patients (9%), who remained in long-term CR, suggesting an undetermined significance of less than 10^{-4} MRD level[67] and that technical sensitivity may not directly translate into clinical prognostic utility.

FALSE-POSITIVE AND FALSE-NEGATIVE OF MINIMAL/MEASURABLE RESIDUAL DISEASE TESTING

MRD is an independent prognostic factor in AML. However, in a subset of patients, the clinical outcome is different from that predicted by MRD testing. Up to 25% of patients without detectable MRD after induction therapy eventually relapse (false-negative). In contrast, a subset of patients with MRD positivity do not relapse and are cured (false-positive). False-negativity indicates that leukemic blasts are likely still present in these patients at a level less than the limit of detection by current techniques, are not detected because of clonal evolution, or were not present in the sample evaluated because of spatial distribution of the blasts and suboptimal sampling. Increasing sensitivity of MRD assays, better understanding of clonal architecture, and/or improving sampling accuracy may decrease false-negative cases. MRD test results can be falsely positive for various reasons, including damage to residual leukemic blasts that lead to delayed cell death, loss of leukemogenic potential through therapeutic

selection or differentiation, or further reductions in residual disease from the remaining therapy to be delivered. There may also be host mechanisms such as effective immune surveillance that keep low levels of residual disease in check. Important biological reasons to consider for false-positive MRD tests are the expression of the MRD markers on normal cells, preleukemia cells, or leukemia cells unable to cause relapse. Regardless of assay sensitivity, it is unrealistic to expect MRD to correlate perfectly with either outcome or relapse, particularly at early time points, as shown by the observation that, despite the theoretically greater sensitivity and specificity of single-gene MRD tests, both false-positive and false-negative results occur at similar rates.[70,92] The reasons for molecular genetic false-positives and false-negatives are overlapping, but not identical, to MFC, including identification of cells with no leukomogenic potential for false-positives, disease less than even the lower limit of detection, subclones of leukemic/preleukemic cells without the mutation being tested at the time but nonetheless leading to relapse, and possibly sampling for false-negatives. Existing data support the logical notion that both MFC and molecular approaches are complementary and that combining MFC and molecular MRD assessment leads to more powerful prognostication.[48,77]

Hourigan and colleagues[8] suggest sequential monitoring to increase the sensitivity of MRD testing, although the optimal interval and duration of sequential MRD testing is unknown and may depend on variables such as the type of AML or interval since achieving remission. Whether sequential MRD monitoring will necessarily improve specificity and therefore predictive power of the test is unclear. Given the potential risk of harm from unnecessary additional treatment prompted by a false-positive MRD test, some clinicians have advocated for a confirmatory second positive MRD test within 2 to 4 weeks of a positive MRD test before predicting relapse. It is by no means clear that such repetition will produce more accurate results if performed by the same methodology because of the intrinsic limitations of any given method. Of note, specificity limitations of either molecular genetic or MFC approaches do not seem to apply in posttransplant setting because all, or nearly all, patients with detectable MRD posttransplant had extremely poor outcomes.[81,93–95] This finding suggests that additional pretransplant/peritransplant therapy and the immune effect of transplant may be the primary drivers of MRD clearance in the few pretransplant MRD-positive patients who do not relapse. Another key point to consider is that not all MRD carries the same risk, and how to stratify low-risk versus high-risk MRD will be critical. Combining MFC MRD with NGS, LSC, and blast/PDC ratio may help stratify low-risk versus high-risk MRD and improve the predictive value.[47,48,77,86]

DOES KINETICS OF MINIMAL/MEASURABLE RESIDUAL DISEASE CLEARANCE MATTER?

Although the prognostic value of MRD test results in patients in CR for predicting subsequent leukemia relapse is convincing, the relevance of the rate of change in MRD levels during therapy is less clear. Many studies have shown that there is little difference in outcome between slower responders who only become MRD negative after second induction and patients who are MRD negative after just 1 course.[16,25,33,81] Achieving MRD negativity at day 15 after starting induction may not be as important as at late time points.[96] Rubnitz and colleagues[17] reported that pediatric patients with AML with MRD levels between 0.1% and 1% after first induction had similar prognosis to the patients with MRD less than 0.1%, but the same MRD levels after second induction had similar prognosis to MRD greater than 1%, suggesting that the early MRD is not as important because of late treatment strategy in abrogating the unfavorable prognosis typically associated with a slow clearance of leukemic cells. Whether the patients who converted to MRD negativity after consolidation therapy have similarly superior outcome is still controversial. A study from Buccisano and colleagues[25] showed that slow-responder patients, namely those entering MRD negativity only after consolidation, had the same outcome as those achieving early negativity. A prospective HOVON/SAKK study in 2013 suggests that patients with continuous MRD negativity have the best outcome, and patients with continuous MRD positivity have the worst. There were a limited number of patients who converted from MRD-positive to MRD-negative state after consolidation and these patients had an intermediate outcome.[16] In contrast, the patients who converted from MRD-negative to MRD-positive state at any time point had extremely poor outcomes.[16,29,93] In those followed by RUNX1-RUNX1T1 RT-qPCR, the most informative landmark for prediction of relapse and survival outcomes seems to be MRD test result in bone marrow samples after completing consolidation therapy,[97,98] whereas, for subjects followed by testing for mutated NPM1 by qPCR, it seems that assessing blood samples after the second cycle of chemotherapy is most accurate.[34] In the setting of HSCT, patients with pretransplant MRD had inferior outcome regardless of day 28 posttransplant MRD. If pretransplant MRD-positive patients became negative at day 28 posttransplant, approximately 30% of the patients had achieved long-term survival. However, all the patients who were pretransplant MRD negative but became posttransplant MRD positive died shortly.[93] There is still much need to understand how the kinetics of MRD are best used in specific subtype and therapy contexts to predict clinical outcomes and perhaps for therapy decision making in AML.

MINIMAL/MEASURABLE RESIDUAL DISEASE–DIRECTED THERAPY

An attractive but still unaddressed question is whether MRD results should be used to routinely guide therapy in AML. There are no data from large randomized studies on the efficacy of MRD test–directed therapy in AML. In APL, studies suggest that therapy based on results of MRD testing can prevent clinical relapse.[57,62,63] In NPM1 mutated AML, postinduction MRD-positive patients had a significantly better outcome if selected to receive HSCT.[72] In patients with RUNX1-RUNXT1, postconsolidation MRD was used for risk stratification. MRD-positive patients (defined by <3 log reduction RT-qPCR) benefited from HSCT (cumulative incidence of relapse, 22.1% vs 78.9% compared with chemotherapy), whereas chemotherapy alone achieved a low relapse rate in the MRD-negative group. These results indicate that MRD-directed risk stratification treatment may improve the outcome of RUNX1-RUNXT1 AML.[68] There are a few additional single-center studies in which therapy was directed by results of MRD testing.[95,99,100] A recent multicenter phase 2 trial studied the role of preemptive azacitidine therapy in AML MRD-positive patients after consolidation or HSCT. Thirty-one out of 53 patients remained relapse free and 19 patients achieved major response (MRD negative) 6 months after azacitidine therapy.[101] Although data suggest the possibility that MRD-directed therapy could decrease or delay relapse, these data should be interpreted cautiously because the studies were uncontrolled. Even if relapses can be delayed or avoided in some patients, MRD-directed therapy may not result in better survival because some patients who relapse can be rescued with chemotherapy and/or an allotransplant. A multicenter randomized controlled trial is needed to address this question. Notably, the optimal type of therapy to convert a patient from MRD positive to negative remains unclear, particularly in the era of emerging agents such as immunotherapy; targeted therapy, including tyrosine kinase inhibitors; and BCL-2 inhibitors. It is possible that MRD-directed therapy should differ depending on the underlying molecular and cytogenetic background and clonal architecture of AML in individual patients.

SURROGATE OF END POINT

An efficacy-response biomarker could be a surrogate end point. A surrogate end point predicts a specific clinical outcome of the patient at some later time and can be used as the basis of marketing application approval decisions. MRD test results are an indirect measure of numbers of residual leukemia cells and becoming MRD test negative may be a plausible indicator of reduced (or delayed) relapse risk. However, a surrogate end point does not measure the clinical benefit of primary interest but instead predicts the clinical benefit based on epidemiologic, therapeutic, pathophysiologic, or other scientific evidence. The question arises whether becoming MRD test negative is a biologically plausible surrogate for improved survival. For regulatory purposes, and specifically the qualification or acceptance of a surrogate, MRD would need to be proved with statistical rigor to be a valid surrogate for survival.[37]

SUMMARY AND PROSPECTS

The importance of MRD in AML has been firmly established. The recent ELN recommendation to establish CR-MRD negativity as a separate category of treatment response represents a major step in integrating MRD research into clinical practice. The slow acceptance of MRD as standard care is in part caused by a lack of standardization in methodology and guidelines for MRD assessment, especially regarding the clinically relevant detection sensitivity, optimal methods for evaluation, and the timing of MRD testing. Thinly distributed resources and expertise in interpreting MRD testing is clearly another reason. It is hoped that the recently published guidelines by the ELN working party will resolve some of these issues and promote widespread adoption of MRD testing for monitoring of therapeutic efficacy and/or the prognosis of patients with AML. Assessment of treatment response focused on MRD likely will require an integrated approach combining immunophenotyping and molecular detection techniques beyond evaluation at the time of hematologic recovery as recommended by current guidelines.[1,35] Future approaches will require more uniform disease-specific and treatment-specific protocols that include a schedule for MRD monitoring using appropriate targets, standard procedures, and clinically validated thresholds that are applied in all laboratories. This approach will ensure optimal and consistent results for risk assessment and personalized therapy. In addition, prospective studies using standardized protocols in randomized trials are necessary to prove the efficacy of MRD-directed therapeutic interventions.

ACKNOWLEDGMENTS

The authors thank Dr Aaron Goldberg at the MSKCC Leukemia Service for critical reading. W.X. prepared the first draft. W.X., K.P., and M.R. cowrote and approved the article.

REFERENCES

1. O'Donnell MR, Tallman MS, Abboud CN, et al. Acute myeloid leukemia, version 3.2017, NCCN clinical practice guidelines in oncology. J Natl Compr Canc Netw 2017;15(7):926–57.
2. Schlenk RF, Benner A, Hartmann F, et al. Risk-adapted postremission therapy in acute myeloid leukemia: results of the German multicenter AML HD93 treatment trial. Leukemia 2003;17(8):1521–8.
3. Wheatley K, Burnett AK, Goldstone AH, et al. A simple, robust, validated and highly predictive index for the determination of risk-directed therapy in acute myeloid leukaemia derived from the MRC AML 10 trial. United Kingdom Medical Research Council's Adult and Childhood Leukaemia Working Parties. Br J Haematol 1999;107(1):69–79.
4. Kern W, Haferlach T, Schoch C, et al. Early blast clearance by remission induction therapy is a major independent prognostic factor for both achievement of complete remission and long-term outcome in acute myeloid leukemia: data from the German AML Cooperative Group (AMLCG) 1992 Trial. Blood 2003;101(1):64–70.
5. Hagenbeek A, Martens AC. Minimal residual disease in acute leukemia: from experimental models to man. Bone Marrow Transplant 1989;4(Suppl 3): 68–9.
6. Inaba H, Coustan-Smith E, Cao X, et al. Comparative analysis of different approaches to measure treatment response in acute myeloid leukemia. J Clin Oncol 2012;30(29):3625–32.
7. Araki D, Wood BL, Othus M, et al. Allogeneic hematopoietic cell transplantation for acute myeloid leukemia: time to move toward a minimal residual disease-based definition of complete remission? J Clin Oncol 2016;34(4):329–36.
8. Hourigan CS, Gale RP, Gormley NJ, et al. Measurable residual disease testing in acute myeloid leukaemia. Leukemia 2017;31(7):1482–90.
9. Schuurhuis GJ, Heuser M, Freeman S, et al. Minimal/measurable residual disease in AML: a

consensus document from the European Leuke-miaNet MRD Working Party. Blood 2018;131(12): 1275–91.

10. Chen X, Wood BL. Monitoring minimal residual disease in acute leukemia: Technical challenges and interpretive complexities. Blood Rev 2017;31(2): 63–75.

11. Bloomfield CD, Estey E, Pleyer L, et al. Time to repeal and replace response criteria for acute myeloid leukemia? Blood Rev 2018;32(5):416–25.

12. Ossenkoppele G, Schuurhuis GJ. MRD in AML: does it already guide therapy decision-making? Hematology Am Soc Hematol Educ Program 2016;2016(1):356–65.

13. Kohnke T, Sauter D, Ringel K, et al. Early assessment of minimal residual disease in AML by flow cytometry during aplasia identifies patients at increased risk of relapse. Leukemia 2015;29(2): 377–86.

14. Tierens A, Bjørklund E, Siitonen S, et al. Residual disease detected by flow cytometry is an independent predictor of survival in childhood acute myeloid leukaemia; results of the NOPHO-AML 2004 study. Br J Haematol 2016;174(4):600–9.

15. Freeman SD, Virgo P, Couzens S, et al. Prognostic relevance of treatment response measured by flow cytometric residual disease detection in older patients with acute myeloid leukemia. J Clin Oncol 2013;31(32):4123–31.

16. Terwijn M, van Putten WL, Kelder A, et al. High prognostic impact of flow cytometric minimal residual disease detection in acute myeloid leukemia: data from the HOVON/SAKK AML 42A study. J Clin Oncol 2013;31(31):3889–97.

17. Rubnitz JE, Inaba H, Dahl G, et al. Minimal residual disease-directed therapy for childhood acute myeloid leukaemia: results of the AML02 multicentre trial. Lancet Oncol 2010;11(6):543–52.

18. San Miguel JF, Vidriales MB, Lopez-Berges C, et al. Early immunophenotypical evaluation of minimal residual disease in acute myeloid leukemia identifies different patient risk groups and may contribute to postinduction treatment stratification. Blood 2001;98(6):1746–51.

19. Chen X, Xie H, Wood BL, et al. Relation of clinical response and minimal residual disease and their prognostic impact on outcome in acute myeloid leukemia. J Clin Oncol 2015;33(11):1258–64.

20. Othus M, Wood BL, Stirewalt DL, et al. Effect of measurable ('minimal') residual disease (MRD) information on prediction of relapse and survival in adult acute myeloid leukemia. Leukemia 2016;30: 2080.

21. Venditti A, Buccisano F, Del Poeta G, et al. Level of minimal residual disease after consolidation therapy predicts outcome in acute myeloid leukemia. Blood 2000;96(12):3948–52.

22. Kern W, Voskova D, Schoch C, et al. Determination of relapse risk based on assessment of minimal residual disease during complete remission by multiparameter flow cytometry in unselected patients with acute myeloid leukemia. Blood 2004;104(10): 3078–85.

23. Buccisano F, Maurillo L, Spagnoli A, et al. Cytogenetic and molecular diagnostic characterization combined to postconsolidation minimal residual disease assessment by flow cytometry improves risk stratification in adult acute myeloid leukemia. Blood 2010;116(13):2295–303.

24. San Miguel JF, Martinez A, Macedo A, et al. Immunophenotyping investigation of minimal residual disease is a useful approach for predicting relapse in acute myeloid leukemia patients. Blood 1997; 90(6):2465–70.

25. Buccisano F, Maurillo L, Gattei V, et al. The kinetics of reduction of minimal residual disease impacts on duration of response and survival of patients with acute myeloid leukemia. Leukemia 2006;20(10): 1783–9.

26. Al-Mawali A, Gillis D, Hissaria P, et al. Incidence, sensitivity, and specificity of leukemia-associated phenotypes in acute myeloid leukemia using specific five-color multiparameter flow cytometry. Am J Clin Pathol 2008;129(6):934–45.

27. van der Velden VHJ, van der Sluijs-Geling A, Gibson BES, et al. Clinical significance of flowcytometric minimal residual disease detection in pediatric acute myeloid leukemia patients treated according to the DCOG ANLL97/MRC AML12 protocol. Leukemia 2010;24:1599.

28. Vidriales M-B, Pérez-López E, Pegenaute C, et al. Minimal residual disease evaluation by flow cytometry is a complementary tool to cytogenetics for treatment decisions in acute myeloid leukaemia. Leuk Res 2016;40:1–9.

29. Freeman SD, Hills RK, Virgo P, et al. Measurable residual disease at induction redefines partial response in acute myeloid leukemia and stratifies outcomes in patients at standard risk without NPM1 mutations. J Clin Oncol 2018;36(15): 1486–97.

30. Walter RB, Gooley TA, Wood BL, et al. Impact of pretransplantation minimal residual disease, as detected by multiparametric flow cytometry, on outcome of myeloablative hematopoietic cell transplantation for acute myeloid leukemia. J Clin Oncol 2011;29(9):1190–7.

31. Walter RB, Buckley SA, Pagel JM, et al. Significance of minimal residual disease before myeloablative allogeneic hematopoietic cell transplantation for AML in first and second complete remission. Blood 2013;122(10):1813–21.

32. Walter RB, Gyurkocza B, Storer BE, et al. Comparison of minimal residual disease as outcome

predictor for AML patients in first complete remission undergoing myeloablative or nonmyeloablative allogeneic hematopoietic cell transplantation. Leukemia 2015;29(1):137–44.

33. Loken MR, Alonzo TA, Pardo L, et al. Residual disease detected by multidimensional flow cytometry signifies high relapse risk in patients with de novo acute myeloid leukemia: a report from Children's Oncology Group. Blood 2012;120(8):1581–8.

34. Ivey A, Hills RK, Simpson MA, et al. Assessment of minimal residual disease in standard-risk AML. N Engl J Med 2016;374(5):422–33.

35. Dohner H, Estey E, Grimwade D, et al. Diagnosis and management of AML in adults: 2017 ELN recommendations from an international expert panel. Blood 2017;129(4):424–47.

36. Epstein-Peterson ZD, Devlin SM, Stein EM, et al. Widespread use of measurable residual disease in acute myeloid leukemia practice. Leuk Res 2018;67:92–8.

37. Hematologic malignancies: regulatory considerations for use of minimal residual disease in development of drug and biological products for treatment guidance for Industry. 2018. Available at: https://www.fda.gov/downloads/Drugs/GuidanceComplianceRegulatoryInformation/Guidances/UCM623333.pdf.

38. Langebrake C, Creutzig U, Dworzak M, et al. Residual disease monitoring in childhood acute myeloid leukemia by multiparameter flow cytometry: the MRD-AML-BFM Study Group. J Clin Oncol 2006;24(22):3686–92.

39. Baer MR, Stewart CC, Dodge RK, et al. High frequency of immunophenotype changes in acute myeloid leukemia at relapse: implications for residual disease detection (Cancer and Leukemia Group B Study 8361). Blood 2001;97(11):3574–80.

40. Zhou Y, Wood BL. Methods of detection of measurable residual disease in AML. Curr Hematol Malig Rep 2017;12(6):557–67.

41. Zeijlemaker W, Gratama JW, Schuurhuis GJ. Tumor heterogeneity makes AML a "moving target" for detection of residual disease. Cytometry B Clin Cytom 2014;86(1):3–14.

42. Wood BL, Arroz M, Barnett D, et al. 2006 Bethesda International Consensus recommendations on the immunophenotypic analysis of hematolymphoid neoplasia by flow cytometry: optimal reagents and reporting for the flow cytometric diagnosis of hematopoietic neoplasia. Cytometry B Clin Cytom 2007;72(Suppl 1):S14–22.

43. Kalina T, Flores-Montero J, van der Velden VH, et al. EuroFlow standardization of flow cytometer instrument settings and immunophenotyping protocols. Leukemia 2012;26(9):1986–2010.

44. van Dongen JJ, Lhermitte L, Bottcher S, et al. EuroFlow antibody panels for standardized n-dimensional flow cytometric immunophenotyping of normal, reactive and malignant leukocytes. Leukemia 2012;26(9):1908–75.

45. Wood BL. Ten-color immunophenotyping of hematopoietic cells. Curr Protoc Cytom 2005;Chapter 6:Unit6.21.

46. Zeijlemaker W, Kelder A, Oussoren-Brockhoff YJ, et al. A simple one-tube assay for immunophenotypical quantification of leukemic stem cells in acute myeloid leukemia. Leukemia 2016;30(2):439–46.

47. Xiao W, Goldberg AD, Famulare C, et al. Loss of plasmacytoid dendritic cell differentiation is highly predictive for post-induction measurable residual disease and inferior outcomes in acute myeloid leukemia. Haematologica 2018, [Epub ahead of print].

48. Getta BM, Devlin SM, Levine RL, et al. Multicolor flow cytometry and multigene next-generation sequencing are complementary and highly predictive for relapse in acute myeloid leukemia after allogeneic transplantation. Biol Blood Marrow Transplant 2017;23(7):1064–71.

49. Ley TJ, Miller C, Ding L, et al. Genomic and epigenomic landscapes of adult de novo acute myeloid leukemia. N Engl J Med 2013;368(22):2059–74.

50. Grimwade D, Ivey A, Huntly BJP. Molecular landscape of acute myeloid leukemia in younger adults and its clinical relevance. Blood 2016;127(1):29–41.

51. Tarlock K, Zhong S, He Y, et al. Distinct age-associated molecular profiles in acute myeloid leukemia defined by comprehensive clinical genomic profiling. Oncotarget 2018;9(41):26417–30.

52. Arber DA, Brunning RD, Le Beau MM, et al. Acute myeloid leukemia with recurrent genetic abnormalities. In: Swerdlow SH, Campo E, Harris NL, et al, editors. WHO classification of tumours of haematopoietic and lymphoid tissues revised. 4th edition. Lyon (France): IARC Press; 2017. p. 130–45.

53. Welch JS, Ley TJ, Link DC, et al. The origin and evolution of mutations in acute myeloid leukemia. Cell 2012;150(2):264–78.

54. Cicconi L, Fenaux P, Kantarjian H, et al. Molecular remission as a therapeutic objective in acute promyelocytic leukemia. Leukemia 2018;32(8):1671–8.

55. Santamaria C, Chillon MC, Fernandez C, et al. Using quantification of the PML-RARalpha transcript to stratify the risk of relapse in patients with acute promyelocytic leukemia. Haematologica 2007;92(3):315–22.

56. Sanz MA, Grimwade D, Tallman MS, et al. Management of acute promyelocytic leukemia: recommendations from an expert panel on behalf of the European LeukemiaNet. Blood 2009;113(9):1875–91.

57. Diverio D, Rossi V, Avvisati G, et al. Early detection of relapse by prospective reverse transcriptase-

polymerase chain reaction analysis of the PML/RARalpha fusion gene in patients with acute promyelocytic leukemia enrolled in the GIMEMA-AIEOP multicenter "AIDA" trial. GIMEMA-AIEOP Multicenter "AIDA" Trial. Blood 1998;92(3):784–9.

58. Martinelli G, Remiddi C, Visani G, et al. Molecular analysis of PML-RAR alpha fusion mRNA detected by reverse transcription-polymerase chain reaction assay in long-term disease-free acute promyelocytic leukaemia patients. Br J Haematol 1995;90(4):966–8.

59. Grimwade D, Jovanovic JV, Hills RK, et al. Prospective minimal residual disease monitoring to predict relapse of acute promyelocytic leukemia and to direct pre-emptive arsenic trioxide therapy. J Clin Oncol 2009;27(22):3650–8.

60. Lo-Coco F, Avvisati G, Vignetti M, et al. Retinoic acid and arsenic trioxide for acute promyelocytic leukemia. N Engl J Med 2013;369(2):111–21.

61. Burnett AK, Grimwade D, Solomon E, et al. Presenting white blood cell count and kinetics of molecular remission predict prognosis in acute promyelocytic leukemia treated with all-trans retinoic acid: result of the Randomized MRC Trial. Blood 1999;93(12):4131–43.

62. Lo Coco F, Diverio D, Avvisati G, et al. Therapy of molecular relapse in acute promyelocytic leukemia. Blood 1999;94(7):2225–9.

63. Esteve J, Escoda L, Martin G, et al. Outcome of patients with acute promyelocytic leukemia failing to front-line treatment with all-trans retinoic acid and anthracycline-based chemotherapy (PETHEMA protocols LPA96 and LPA99): benefit of an early intervention. Leukemia 2007;21(3):446–52.

64. Platzbecker U, Avvisati G, Cicconi L, et al. Improved outcomes with retinoic acid and arsenic trioxide compared with retinoic acid and chemotherapy in non-high-risk acute promyelocytic leukemia: final results of the randomized Italian-German APL0406 trial. J Clin Oncol 2017;35(6):605–12.

65. Cheson BD, Bennett JM, Kopecky KJ, et al. Revised recommendations of the international working group for diagnosis, standardization of response criteria, treatment outcomes, and reporting standards for therapeutic trials in acute myeloid leukemia. J Clin Oncol 2003;21(24):4642–9.

66. Jourdan E, Boissel N, Chevret S, et al. Prospective evaluation of gene mutations and minimal residual disease in patients with core binding factor acute myeloid leukemia. Blood 2013;121(12):2213–23.

67. Willekens C, Blanchet O, Renneville A, et al. Prospective long-term minimal residual disease monitoring using RQ-PCR in RUNX1-RUNX1T1-positive acute myeloid leukemia: results of the French CBF-2006 trial. Haematologica 2016;101(3):328–35.

68. Zhu HH, Zhang XH, Qin YZ, et al. MRD-directed risk stratification treatment may improve outcomes of t(8;21) AML in the first complete remission: results from the AML05 multicenter trial. Blood 2013;121(20):4056–62.

69. Yin JA, O'Brien MA, Hills RK, et al. Minimal residual disease monitoring by quantitative RT-PCR in core binding factor AML allows risk stratification and predicts relapse: results of the United Kingdom MRC AML-15 trial. Blood 2012;120(14):2826–35.

70. Kronke J, Schlenk RF, Jensen KO, et al. Monitoring of minimal residual disease in NPM1-mutated acute myeloid leukemia: a study from the German-Austrian acute myeloid leukemia study group. J Clin Oncol 2011;29(19):2709–16.

71. Gorello P, Cazzaniga G, Alberti F, et al. Quantitative assessment of minimal residual disease in acute myeloid leukemia carrying nucleophosmin (NPM1) gene mutations. Leukemia 2006;20(6):1103–8.

72. Balsat M, Renneville A, Thomas X, et al. Postinduction minimal residual disease predicts outcome and benefit from allogeneic stem cell transplantation in acute myeloid leukemia with NPM1 mutation: a study by the acute leukemia French Association Group. J Clin Oncol 2017;35(2):185–93.

73. Shayegi N, Kramer M, Bornhauser M, et al. The level of residual disease based on mutant NPM1 is an independent prognostic factor for relapse and survival in AML. Blood 2013;122(1):83–92.

74. Selim AG, Moore AS. Molecular minimal residual disease monitoring in acute myeloid leukemia: challenges and future directions. J Mol Diagn 2018;20(4):389–97.

75. Gabert J, Beillard E, van der Velden VH, et al. Standardization and quality control studies of 'real-time' quantitative reverse transcriptase polymerase chain reaction of fusion gene transcripts for residual disease detection in leukemia - a Europe Against Cancer program. Leukemia 2003;17(12):2318–57.

76. Klco JM, Miller CA, Griffith M, et al. Association between mutation clearance after induction therapy and outcomes in acute myeloid leukemia. JAMA 2015;314(8):811–22.

77. Jongen-Lavrencic M, Grob T, Hanekamp D, et al. Molecular minimal residual disease in acute myeloid leukemia. N Engl J Med 2018;378(13):1189–99.

78. Young AL, Wong TN, Hughes AE, et al. Quantifying ultra-rare pre-leukemic clones via targeted error-corrected sequencing. Leukemia 2015;29(7):1608–11.

79. Thol F, Gabdoulline R, Liebich A, et al. Measurable residual disease monitoring by NGS before allogeneic hematopoietic cell transplantation in AML. Blood 2018;132(16):1703–13.

80. Höllein A, Meggendorfer M, Dicker F, et al. *NPM1* mutated AML can relapse with wild-type *NPM1*: persistent clonal hematopoiesis can drive relapse. Blood Adv 2018;2(22):3118–25.

81. Zhou Y, Othus M, Walter RB, et al. Deep NPM1 sequencing following allogeneic hematopoietic cell transplantation improves risk assessment in adults with NPM1-mutated AML. Biol Blood Marrow Transplant 2018;24(8):1615–20.

82. Jennings LJ, George D, Czech J, et al. Detection and quantification of BCR-ABL1 fusion transcripts by droplet digital PCR. J Mol Diagn 2014;16(2): 174–9.

83. Wang WJ, Zheng CF, Liu Z, et al. Droplet digital PCR for BCR/ABL(P210) detection of chronic myeloid leukemia: a high sensitive method of the minimal residual disease and disease progression. Eur J Haematol 2018;101(3):291–6.

84. Brunetti C, Anelli L, Zagaria A, et al. Droplet digital PCR is a reliable tool for monitoring minimal residual disease in acute promyelocytic leukemia. J Mol Diagn 2017;19(3):437–44.

85. Coustan-Smith E, Song G, Shurtleff S, et al. Universal monitoring of minimal residual disease in acute myeloid leukemia. JCI Insight 2018;3(9), [pii: 98561].

86. Zeijlemaker W, Grob T, Meijer R, et al. CD34+CD38− leukemic stem cell frequency to predict outcome in acute myeloid leukemia. Leukemia 2018, [Epub ahead of print].

87. Zeijlemaker W, Kelder A, Oussoren-Brockhoff YJ, et al. Peripheral blood minimal residual disease may replace bone marrow minimal residual disease as an immunophenotypic biomarker for impending relapse in acute myeloid leukemia. Leukemia 2016; 30(3):708–15.

88. Branford S, Cross NC, Hochhaus A, et al. Rationale for the recommendations for harmonizing current methodology for detecting BCR-ABL transcripts in patients with chronic myeloid leukaemia. Leukemia 2006;20(11):1925–30.

89. Duployez N, Nibourel O, Marceau-Renaut A, et al. Minimal residual disease monitoring in t(8;21) acute myeloid leukemia based on RUNX1-RUNX1T1 fusion quantification on genomic DNA. Am J Hematol 2014;89(6):610–5.

90. Chen X, Othus M, Wood BL, et al. Flow cytometric demonstration of decrease in bone marrow leukemic blasts after 'Day 14' without further therapy in acute myeloid leukemia. Leuk Lymphoma 2017;58(11):2717–9.

91. Amatangelo MD, Quek L, Shih A, et al. Enasidenib induces acute myeloid leukemia cell differentiation to promote clinical response. Blood 2017;130(6): 732–41.

92. Corbacioglu A, Scholl C, Schlenk RF, et al. Prognostic impact of minimal residual disease in CBFB-MYH11-positive acute myeloid leukemia. J Clin Oncol 2010;28(23):3724–9.

93. Zhou Y, Othus M, Araki D, et al. Pre- and post-transplant quantification of measurable ('minimal') residual disease via multiparameter flow cytometry in adult acute myeloid leukemia. Leukemia 2016; 30(7):1456–64.

94. Shah MV, Jorgensen JL, Saliba RM, et al. Early post-transplant minimal residual disease assessment improves risk stratification in acute myeloid leukemia. Biol Blood Marrow Transplant 2018; 24(7):1514–20.

95. Wang Y, Wu DP, Liu QF, et al. In adults with t(8;21) AML, posttransplant RUNX1/RUNX1T1-based MRD monitoring, rather than c-KIT mutations, allows further risk stratification. Blood 2014;124(12): 1880–6.

96. Tierens A, Bjorklund E, Siitonen S, et al. Residual disease detected by flow cytometry is an independent predictor of survival in childhood acute myeloid leukaemia; results of the NOPHO-AML 2004 study. Br J Haematol 2016; 174(4):600–9.

97. Agrawal M, Corbacioglu A, Paschka P, et al. Minimal residual disease monitoring in acute myeloid leukemia (AML) with translocation t(8;21)(q22;q22): results of the AML Study Group (AMLSG). Blood 2016;128(22):1207.

98. Weisser M, Haferlach C, Hiddemann W, et al. The quality of molecular response to chemotherapy is predictive for the outcome of AML1-ETO-positive AML and is independent of pretreatment risk factors. Leukemia 2007;21(6):1177–82.

99. Sockel K, Wermke M, Radke J, et al. Minimal residual disease-directed preemptive treatment with azacitidine in patients with NPM1-mutant acute myeloid leukemia and molecular relapse. Haematologica 2011;96(10):1568–70.

100. Platzbecker U, Wermke M, Radke J, et al. Azacitidine for treatment of imminent relapse in MDS or AML patients after allogeneic HSCT: results of the RELAZA trial. Leukemia 2012;26(3):381–9.

101. Platzbecker U, Middeke JM, Sockel K, et al. Measurable residual disease-guided treatment with azacitidine to prevent haematological relapse in patients with myelodysplastic syndrome and acute myeloid leukaemia (RELAZA2): an open-label, multicentre, phase 2 trial. Lancet Oncol 2018;19(12):1668–79.

Acute Leukemias of Ambiguous Lineage
Clarification on Lineage Specificity

Jason H. Kurzer, MD, PhD[a],*, Olga K. Weinberg, MD[b]

KEYWORDS

- Mixed phenotype acute leukemia • Acute undifferentiated leukemia • KMT2A • Lineage

Key Points

- Acute leukemias of ambiguous lineage are rare and include acute leukemias that show no evidence of myeloid, B-, or T-lymphoid lineage commitment (acute undifferentiated leukemia) or show evidence of commitment to more than one lineage (mixed-phenotype acute leukemia [MPAL]).

- Current criteria have reduced the reported incidence of mixed lineage leukemias via emphasizing fewer markers and categorizing some biphenotypic leukemias with recurrent cytogenetic abnormalities or complex karyotypes as other entities.

- Genomic and expression profile data for MPAL reveal mutations and transcripts commonly seen in both acute myeloid leukemia and acute lymphoblastic leukemia (ALL), with T/myeloid MPAL showing overlapping features with early T-cell precursor lymphoblastic leukemia.

- Acute leukemias of ambiguous lineage generally show a poor prognosis, with ALL-like therapy as a common approach to treatment.

ABSTRACT

Acute leukemias of ambiguous lineage (ALAL) include acute undifferentiated leukemia and mixed-phenotype acute leukemia (MPAL). This article provides an overview of the diagnosis of ALAL and focuses on the data accounting for the current lineage-assignment criteria for blasts harboring more than one lineage-associated marker. In addition, the currently known molecular data are reviewed, which show that MPAL-associated gene mutations, methylation signatures, and expression profiles are a mixture of those seen in both acute myeloid leukemia and acute lymphoblastic leukemia. Finally, the prognosis and current treatments of MPAL are briefly discussed.

OVERVIEW

Acute leukemias of ambiguous lineage (ALAL) are those leukemias that either fail to show evidence of myeloid, B-, or T-lymphoid lineage commitment or show evidence of commitment to more than one lineage.[1-5] These leukemias include acute undifferentiated leukemia and mixed-phenotype acute leukemia (MPAL). MPAL includes both biphenotypic leukemia (a leukemia with more than one lineage-defining marker on a single blast population) and bilineal leukemia (a leukemia composed of 2 or more single lineage leukemia populations).[6,7]

ALAL represents a heterogeneous group of orphan diseases, with the World Health Organization (WHO) listing 4 basic categories (**Box 1**).[6] MPAL accounts for ~2% to 3% of acute leukemia and 0.35 cases/1,000,000 person-years and has a male predominance (~1:1.6).[4,8-11] Amongst cases of MPAL, the B/myeloid subtype accounts for 59%, whereas the T/myeloid, B/T, and trilineage subtypes account for 35%, 4%, and 2%, respectively.[10] Acute undifferentiated leukemia is

Disclosure Statement: The authors have nothing to disclose.
a Department of Pathology, Stanford University School of Medicine, 300 Pasteur Drive, Room 1401K, Stanford, CA 94305, USA; b Department of Pathology, Boston Children's Hospital, BCH 3027, 300 Longwood Avenue Bader 126.2, Boston, MA 02115, USA
* Corresponding author.
E-mail address: kurzer@stanford.edu

Surgical Pathology 12 (2019) 687–697
https://doi.org/10.1016/j.path.2019.03.008

rarer still, occurring at a frequency not currently established.

The different treatment regimens for acute myeloid leukemia (AML) and acute lymphoblastic leukemia (ALL) make ALAL a challenge both diagnostically and therapeutically. Thus, a fundamental task has been to develop a classification system that most effectively enables appropriate therapeutic decisions. Herein, in addition to providing an overview of the microscopic, diagnostic, and prognostic features of ALAL, the authors discuss the historical data accounting for the current classification system. Furthermore, recent molecular studies that cast new light on the nature of these leukemias are also reviewed.

MICROSCOPIC FEATURES

The blasts from ALAL are morphologically diverse. Acute undifferentiated leukemia (AUL) blasts usually lack standard myeloid features (eg, azurophilic granules in the cytoplasm). They are frequently small to intermediate in size; show high nuclear:-cytoplasmic ratios; have nuclei with round nuclear contours, prominent nucleoli, and minimal cytoplasm; and do not show diagnostic features, such as Auer rods.[6] However, atypical morphologies, including moderate amounts of cytoplasm with cytoplasmic vacuoles have also been described, and rarely, the hand-mirror morphology sometimes seen in lymphoblastic leukemias may be present.[12]

Generally speaking, MPAL blasts may resemble myeloblasts or monoblasts and occasionally lymphoblasts; there may be dual/dimorphic populations, or blasts may seem similar to

undifferentiated leukemias.[10,13] MPAL with t(9;22)(q34.1;q11.2) typically shows a dimorphic population of myeloblasts and lymphoblasts and not much myeloid maturation.[6] Similarly, MPAL with t(v;11q23.3) also usually shows dimorphic blast populations, with blasts resembling monoblasts and lymphoblasts (**Fig. 1**).[6]

DIAGNOSIS

MIXED-PHENOTYPE ACUTE LEUKEMIA

It has been recognized for decades that certain acute leukemias fail to conform to single lineage assignment; thus, various classification systems were proposed in the 1990s to diagnose biphenotypic leukemias.[14–18] Acknowledging that unilineage leukemias occasionally exhibit aberrant marker expression; groups attempted to exclude these entities by developing score-based systems, thereby requiring multiple lineage-specific markers to diagnose biphenotypic leukemia.[14–16]

In 1991, Catovsky and colleagues[15] put forth one of the first prominent scoring classification systems (**Table 1**). In a series of 166 acute leukemias, they showed 13% of AML cases and 3% of ALL cases constituted biphenotypic leukemias under their system.[15] In 1995 and 1998, the European Group for the Immunologic Characterization of Leukemias (EGIL) further modified the Catovsky system, primarily by increasing the weight of certain markers and adding and subtracting others (**Table 2**).[16,19] Subsequently, the third edition of the WHO Classification of Tumors and Lymphoid Tissues adopted the EGIL system.[20]

Despite the aim of increasing diagnostic specificity, concern persisted that biphenotypic leukemia was overdiagnosed.[21] The high weight of certain markers (eg, CD79a and CD2), incorrect application of EGIL criteria, and the inclusion of cases with recurrent cytogenetic abnormalities likely explain the excess.[2,15] The fourth edition of the WHO Classification of Tumours of Haematopoietic and Lymphoid Tissues therefore revised the biphenotypic criteria, using fewer and more specific markers and abandoned scoring altogether (**Table 3**).[21] The 2016/2017 revisions essentially reaffirmed this decision.[6,22]

The WHO definition of MPAL does not differentiate between biphenotypic and bilineal acute leukemias. The total sum of MPAL blasts must be greater than or equal to 20%; with the individual populations of bilineal MPAL classified according to standard AML and ALL criteria.[6] In contrast, biphenotypic MPAL requires the use of lineage-assignment criteria (see **Table 3**). For biphenotypic MPAL, the WHO classification system

Fig. 1. Case from 7-week-old infant with MPAL with t(4;11)(q21;q23). (*A*) Peripheral blood smear revealing both lymphoblast- and monoblast-appearing immature cells. (*B*) Flow cytometry reveals a B-lymphoblastic (*green*) and a monocytic (*yellow*) population, which are contiguous on the CD45 versus SSC plot but separable by lineage-specific markers. SSC, side scatter.

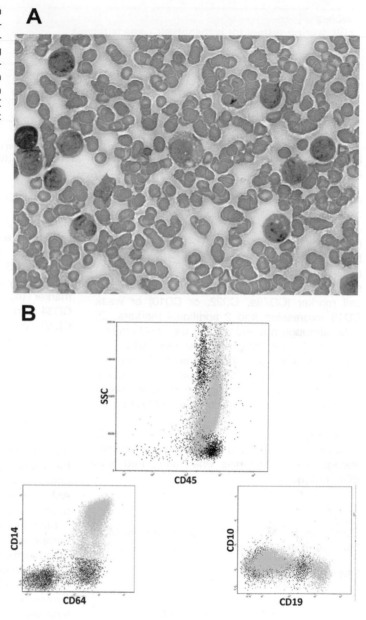

Table 1
Catovsky scoring system for biphenotypic acute leukemia

Points	B-Lineage	T-Lineage	Myeloid Lineage
2	cCD22, cμ chain	cCD3	MPO
1	CD10, CD19, CD24	CD2, CD5, TCR rearr. (β or δ chain)	CD33, CD13 m/c, CD14 m/c, AML morphology or cytochemistry (other than MPO)
0.5	TdT; IgH rearr.	TdT, CD7	CD11b, CD11c, CD15

Adapted from Catovsky D, Matutes E, Buccheri V, et al. A classification of acute leukemia for the 1990s. Ann Hematol 1991;62(1):16–21; with permission.

Table 2
EGIL scoring system for biphenotypic acute leukemia

Points	B Lineage	T Lineage	Myeloid Lineage
2	CD79a, cIgM, cCD22	CD3, TCR-α/β, TCR-γδ	MPO, lysozyme
1	CD19, CD10, CD20	CD2, CD5, CD8, CD10	CD13, CD33, CDw65, CD117[a]
0.5	TdT, CD24	TdT, CD7, CD1a	CD14, CD15, CD64,

[a] CD117 was initially assigned a weight of 0.5 but was upgraded to 1.[19]
Adapted from Bene MC, Castoldi G, Knapp W, et al. Proposals for the immunologic classification of acute leukemias. European Group for the Immunologic Characterization of Leukemias (EGIL). Leukemia 1995;9(10):1783–6; with permission.

assigns T-lineage to blasts expressing cytoplasmic or surface CD3. Expression of myeloperoxidase (MPO) or at least 2 monocytic markers (nonspecific esterase, CD11c, CD14, CD64, or lysozyme) denotes myeloid lineage. Assignment of B-lineage requires multiple lines of evidence: strong expression of CD19 plus one additional B-cell marker (CD79a, CD22, or CD10) or weak CD19 expression and 2 additional markers. Of note, although not endorsed in the WHO criteria, Béné and Porwit[2] have advocated using additional B-cell antigens (eg, CD24, intracytoplasmic mu chains, CD20, and CD21) to assist in assigning B-lineage. Importantly, cases that meet criteria for other WHO-defined entities are excluded from a diagnosis of MPAL.

As expected, use of the WHO criteria reduced the reported incidence of mixed-lineage acute leukemias when compared with EGIL criteria.[23,24]

Table 3
WHO requirements for lineage assignment in biphenotypic acute leukemia

Myeloid	MPO Or Evidence of monocytic differentiation: ≥2 of NSE, CD11c, CD14, and CD64
B-lineage	Strong CD19 and ≥1 strongly expressed marker: CD79a, cCD22, or CD10 Or Weak CD19 and ≥2 strongly expressed marker: CD79a, cCD22, or CD10
T-lineage	cCD3 (at level of expression of background T cells) or surface CD3

Adapted from Swerdlow SH, Campo E, Harris NL, et al., eds. WHO classification of tumors of haematopoietic and lymphoid tissues. Revised 4th edition. Lyon: International Agency for Research on Cancer; 2017; with permission.

ACUTE UNDIFFERENTIATED LEUKEMIA

Historically, criteria for AUL have remained consistent in that a diagnosis of AUL requires the lack of expression of lineage-specific markers.[6] AUL lacks cCD3, MPO, CD19, cCD22, and CD79a and usually expresses only one surface lineage marker (eg, CD13, CD33, or CD7). As such, CD34 and HLA-DR expression with or without CD38 or terminal deoxynucleotidyl transferase (TdT) is common.[2]

LINEAGE MARKERS

T-Lineage

In the past, T-lineage was frequently assessed by CD2, CD7, TdT, CD5, CD1a, CD4, CD8, and TCR α/β expression.[25–27] However, CD2 and CD7 had been found in many leukemias with morphologic and immunophenotypic findings consistent with AML, arguing against the specificity of these markers for T-lineage.[27–31]

Studying the T-cell receptor (TCR) complex component, CD3, resulted in the recognition of cytoplasmic CD3 expression as an early event in T-cell development, and thus its use as a lineage marker of T-ALL was investigated.[25–27,32–34] Using fluorescence microscopy, Campana and colleagues,[25] van Dongen and colleagues,[26] and Janossy and colleagues[27] showed cCD3 expression in 100% of cases of T-ALL and no cases of B-ALL or AML. Janossy and colleagues[27] further showed that amongst 500 cases of acute leukemia, cCD3 staining was the most reliable and predictive of T-ALL (expressed in all 59 cases of T-ALL), in contrast to CD2 (expressed in only 71.2% of T-ALL cases).

Consequently, cCD3 became regarded as the most T-lineage–specific marker, with both the Catovsky and EGIL systems designating the highest weight to CD3 for T-lineage assignment (see **Tables 1** and **2**).[15,16] Nevertheless, using multiparameter flow cytometry, cCD3 can rarely be detected in leukemias that are otherwise consistent with AML.[28,35,36] As such, per the WHO classification system, T-lineage assignment requires a fraction of blasts to show strong cCD3 expression, with the brightest expression comparable to background T cells.[6,21] Despite this requirement, the negative predictive value of dim, rather than strong, CD3 expression for T-lineage is unknown.

B-Lineage

CD19 was first identified using the anti-B4 antibody and noted to be expressed exclusively in B cells.[37] Anderson and colleagues[38] found CD19 present in 94% of 117 cases of non-T-ALL and absent in cases of T-ALL and AML (15 and 148 cases, respectively) and detected CD10 expression in 88% of non-T-ALL, 8% of T-ALL, and no cases of AML. These data implicated CD19 as a specific B-lineage marker, with CD10 expression at least favoring B-lineage. Nevertheless, CD19 can be detected in AML, particularly t(8;21)(q22;q22)-associated AML.[39] The EGIL scoring system consequently assigned intermediate weight to CD19 as a B-lineage marker, whereas CD19 is necessary but not sufficient for B-lineage assignment for the WHO classification system.[6,16] CD10 is used only as confirmatory evidence of B-lineage but cannot be used to define B/T MPAL.[6]

Because CD22, an inhibitory coreceptor for the B-cell receptor (BCR), is originally localized in the cytoplasm of maturing precursor B cells,[40] Janossy and colleagues[27] investigated the use of cytoplasmic CD22 as a lineage-specific marker in B-ALL. In an initial study of 100 leukemias, they detected cCD22 in all 42 cases of B-ALL, and in an expanded study cCD22 was found in 224 or 227 cases of B-ALL.[27] In contrast, neither cCD22 nor mCD22 was seen in 40 cases of AML or 19 cases of T-ALL.[27] Thus, experts weighted cCD22 heavily in B-lineage scoring systems.[15,16] Nevertheless, basophils and AML with basophilic, mast cell, or dendritic differentiation can express CD22, and certain anti-CD22 clones historically recognized dendritic and columnar epithelial cells.[41,42] For these reasons, the WHO only uses CD22 as confirmatory evidence of B-lineage, although its expression precludes a diagnosis of AUL.[6]

CD79a is a protein within the membranes of B cells and complexes with CD79b and immunoglobulin mu to form the BCR complex.[43] Cytoplasmic expression of CD79a is one of the earliest events detected in B-lineage commitment, and its expression remains until full plasma cell differentiation.[44,45] Nevertheless, CD79a expression can be present in cases of both T-ALL[46,47] and AML[48,49] and has been found on circulating myeloid cells from patients with lung cancer.[50] Thus, like CD22, CD79a is used as confirmatory rather than required evidence of B-lineage and cannot be used to define B/T MPAL.[6]

TdT is a DNA polymerase that adds random nucleotides to DNA during V(D)J recombination.[51] TdT is almost always present in immature B and T neoplasms but can be seen in AML as well, making it only minimally specific for lymphoblasts.[52,53] As such, TdT is weighted low in the EGIL scoring system and is omitted entirely from the WHO system.[6,16]

Myeloid

MPO, an enzyme localized to primary granules and membranes of granulocytes, has been considered the most specific marker for the myeloid lineage.[54] The original French–American–British (FAB) classification of leukemias recommended using cytochemical stains for MPO, or alternatively Sudan Black B, to aid in classifying blasts as myeloid and required at least 3% of blasts to express MPO.[55] Using monoclonal antibodies, Buccheri and colleagues[54] detected MPO in 92% of 103 AML cases versus 2 of 77 ALL cases, further supporting MPO as a myeloid-specific marker. MPO was thus given the highest weight in the EGIL scoring system (10% cutoff) and is sufficient for assignment of myeloid lineage in the WHO classification system.[6,16]

Of note, the WHO has set no threshold for MPO positivity; however, extra care should be taken to discriminate small MPO populations from background nonneoplastic myeloid blasts.[56] Moreover, cases with an otherwise B-ALL immunophenotype with MPO as the sole aberrancy present a unique challenge, particularly as some reagents show nonspecific binding to MPO, and MPO mRNA can frequently be detected in B-ALL.[57–60] It has been argued that these cases (at least with dim MPO expression) may be best classified as B-ALL,[3,6,56] with the caveat that these leukemias may represent a higher-risk group.[59,61]

The multifunctional enzyme, CD13 (aka aminopeptidase N); the sialic acid–binding immunoglobulin-like protein, CD33; and the c-Kit receptor, CD117, are additional markers associated with myeloid lineage.[19,62,63] Nevertheless, both CD13 and CD33 have long been detected in lymphoblastic leukemias,[31] with Janossy and colleagues[27] showing aberrant expression of CD13 and CD33 in 9.4% of 180 and 9.3% of 150 cases of B-ALL, respectively. As such, CD13 and CD33 are weighted intermediately in scoring systems and are irrelevant for the diagnosis of biphenotypic MPALs according to the WHO.[6,15,16,19]

In 1998, the EGIL performed an extensive review of CD117 reactivity in 1937 leukemias and found it to be positive in 67% of AMLs and 4% of ALLs, indicating more specificity for AML than CD13 and CD33.[19] They additionally found CD117 in leukemias without other myeloid or lymphoid markers (ie, AUL).[19] These data caused the EGIL to weight CD117 at an intermediate weight; however, like CD13 and CD33, it is not used by the current WHO criteria, which prefers fewer, more specific markers for lineage assignment.

DIFFERENTIAL DIAGNOSIS

MIXED-PHENOTYPE ACUTE LEUKEMIA

The primary challenge in diagnosing MPAL is ruling out cytogenetically defined neoplasms that demonstrate an MPAL-like immunophenotype. Making these distinctions is often critical due to the different therapies involved. However, the delay between immunophenotyping and receipt of additional data frequently necessitates pathologists to rely on morphologic and immunophenotypic clues.

AML with t(8;21)(q22;q22.1) is an AML that is notorious for expressing B-lineage markers, including CD19, PAX5, and CD79a, and could potentially seem consistent with B/myeloid MPAL. However, unlike MPAL, the blasts of t(8;21) AML tend to be large, have perinuclear clearing, and contain abundant cytoplasm, which may possess characteristic "salmon pink" granules or Auer rods.

AML with myelodysplasia-related changes (AML-MRC) is defined by a history of myelodysplastic syndrome, myelodysplasia-related cytogenetic abnormalities, and/or multilineage dysplasia. Morphologic identification of multilineage dysplasia may aid in favoring AML-MRC until receipt of ancillary results. Importantly, lymphoid marker expression does not exclude AML-MRC, and consequently AML-MRC trumps MPAL in the WHO classification system.[6] Because complex karyotypes, del(7q) and del(5q), are sufficient to diagnose AML-MRC, confusion exists due to these aberrancies having been reported in association with MPAL, both in the literature and the current WHO "blue book."[6,64] Until further research clarifies the genetic boundaries between these neoplasms, it is advised to classify these MPAL-like leukemias as AML-MRC.

Acute leukemias presenting de novo with t(9;22) translocations are consistent with MPAL with t(9;22), whereas patients with a history of CML that develop blast crisis with mixed phenotype are not. Similarly, patients with CML in blast crisis with lineage switch are also excluded. A careful review of patient history is thus essential.

Myeloid/lymphoid neoplasms with FGFR1 rearrangement are a group of hematopoietic neoplasms that can present as acute leukemias expressing mixed lineage markers. As the FGFR1 rearrangement is definitional, they may not be diagnosed as MPAL. Morphologic clues to the possible presence of an FGFR1 rearrangement include prominent eosinophilia, which is frequently associated with this disease.

The newly described early T-cell precursor lymphoblastic leukemia is characterized by expression of CD7, one or more myeloid/stem cell markers (CD117, CD34, CD117, HLA-DR, CD13, CD33, CD11b, and CD65), and cytoplasmic CD3.[6,22,65] The coexpression of myeloid markers and CD3 makes distinguishing early T-cell precursor (ETP)-ALL from T/myeloid MPAL problematic. To this end, blasts with an ETP immunophenotype but with coexpression of MPO are classified as T/myeloid MPAL, as MPO expression is, by definition, negative in ETP-ALL. As described later, molecular data blur the distinction between these entities, and whether ETP-ALL is a special type of T-ALL or a special type of T/myeloid MPAL remains to be seen.[11,66]

ACUTE UNDIFFERENTIATED LEUKEMIA

The chief entity within the differential of AUL is AML with minimal differentiation. It is important to remember that the EGIL scoring systems and WHO lineage assignment rules for biphenotypic leukemias are not required for assigning lineage to single lineage leukemias. As such, AML with minimal differentiation typically lacks MPO and monocytic markers but are myeloid leukemias due to the expression of at least 2 myeloid-associated markers, including CD13, CD33, and CD117. Before diagnosing AUL, one should exclude rare entities, such as blastic plasmacytoid dendritic cell neoplasms, natural killer cell neoplasms, and basophilic neoplasms. The presence of a complex karyotype or other myelodysplasia-related cytogenetic abnormalities favors a diagnosis of AML-MRC.

GENETICS

Comparing the underlying chromosomal, genetic, epigenetic, and expression profiles of ALAL with single lineage leukemias provides an opportunity to determine if these entities cluster with their myeloid or lymphoid counterparts and offers the possibility of 1 day refining diagnostic algorithms.

MIXED-PHENOTYPE ACUTE LEUKEMIA

The majority (64%–87%) of MPAL have an abnormal karyotype.[8–10,64,67] The most common abnormalities are rearrangements of t(9;22) and t(v;11q23), which are more commonly B/myeloid.[6,15,21,68] In addition to these 2 widely recognized aberrancies, other cytogenetic abnormalities, particularly observed in the B/myeloid subtype, include del(1)(p32), trisomy 4, del(6q), 12p11.2 abnormalities, and near-tetraplooidy.[10,16,64,69,70] It has been reported that about one-third of biphenotypic leukemias demonstrate a complex karyotype; however, most, if not all, of these leukemias would currently meet the WHO criteria for AML with myelodysplasia-related changes.[8,10,64,67]

The t(9;22) rearrangement occurs in ~15% to 20% of cases and is more common in adults.[4,8,10,69] The p190 transcript, more commonly seen in ALL, is the most frequent fusion product, whereas it has been argued that the presence of the p210 transcript should raise suspicion for the blast crisis of CML.[6,71] Cases of MPAL with t(9;22) can harbor additional cytogenetic abnormalities, but at a lower frequency than t(9;22)-ALL.[71]

MPAL with KMT2A rearrangements accounts for ~10% of cases of ALAL and occurs more frequently in infants.[10,11,13] The fusion partner for KMT2A is often AFF1, although other rearrangements include MLLT3 and MLLT1.[11,69,70] KMT2A rearrangements are associated with a low mutation burden, copy number alterations, and single nucleotide variants or insertions/deletions when compared with B and T/myeloid MPAL, not otherwise specified, which may explain the earlier age of onset.[11]

Regarding the general mutational spectrum of MPAL, it has been suggested that the founding lesions in the cell of origin, rather than accumulation of further hits promote lineage promiscuity, although the debate is far from settled.[11] Recent studies show that epigenetic and transcription factor gene alterations seem to occur early in leukemogenesis, likely in progenitors primed for lineage aberrancy, whereas signaling mutations occur later.[11,67]

MPAL-associated gene mutations are a mixture of those commonly seen in both AML and ALL. In 2012, Yan and colleagues[8] reported deletions of the ALL-associated gene, IKZF1, as well as mutations of AML-associated epigenetic modifiers, TET2, EZH2, and ASXL1in B/myeloid leukemias. In 2016, Eckstein and colleagues[72] found similar

mutations and identified mutations of the AML-associated gene, DNMT3A, occurring primarily in older patients. In 2018, Takahashi and colleagues[67] studied 31 adult patients with MPAL and found 38 recurrently mutated genes, including NOTCH1, RUNX1, DNMT3A, and IDH2. Alexander and colleagues[11] performed an extensive study of the genetics of childhood MPAL on 115 cases of ALAL. They identified 158 recurrently mutated genes, including the AML-associated genes, FLT3, RUNX1, CUX1, and CEBPA, and the ALL-associated genes CDKN2A/CDKN2B, ETV6, and VPREB1.[11] Most of the MPAL cases harbored mutually exclusive mutations of either WT1, ETV6, RUNX1, or CEBPA.[11] Also in 2018, in a study of 29 cases, Xiao and colleagues[73] reported similar common gene mutations, including PHF6, DNMT3A, TET2, WT1, RUNX1, KRAS, FLT3, ETV6, ASXL1, IDH2, and NRAS.

T/myeloid MPAL is reported to have a higher mutational burden than B/myeloid MPAL and commonly shows mutations in epigenetic regulators (eg, EZH2, PHF6, and DNMT3A) and JAK/STAT signaling proteins.[11,67,73–75] Of note, Xiao and colleagues[73] found PHF6 mutations and DNMT3A mutations to be mutually exclusive, occurring in younger and older patients, respectively.

As mentioned earlier, T/myeloid MPAL shares many similarities in its molecular profile with ETP ALL.[11,66,76] Alexander and colleagues[11] showed that MYB amplification, LEF1 deletion, CDKN2A/B deletions, and amplification of the NOTCH1-driven MYC enhancer were common in T-ALL and rare in T/myeloid MPAL and ETP-ALL. Similarly, compared with T-ALL, T/myeloid and ETP ALL less frequently show alterations in the transcription factors, TAL1/2, TLX1/3, LMO1/2, NKX2-1, HOXA10, and LYL1.[11] Furthermore, although T-ALL associated mutations in NOTCH1 are present in T/myeloid MPAL, they are less common in T/myeloid MPAL and ETP ALL.[8,11,67,77] Moreover, as opposed to T-ALL, both T/myeloid MPAL and ETP ALL often show biallelic WT1 alterations and similar frequencies of mutations of WT1, ETV6, EZH2, and FLT3.[11] Both ETP-ALL and T/myeloid MPAL show similar alterations in signaling pathways, including Ras and JAK-STAT pathways, whereas PI3K signaling is more common in T-ALL.[11,66] Arguing, perhaps, for a difference between T/myeloid MPAL and ETP ALL is that T/myeloid MPAL frequently shows mutations of CUX1 and CEBPA, whereas ETP and T-ALL do not.[11]

The high resolution of modern molecular techniques allowed Alexander and colleagues[11] to identify rearrangements of ZNF384 as a common alteration in pediatric B/myeloid leukemia; however, this rearrangement has not yet been reported in adult patients.[67] In their study, ZNF384 rearrangements were present in 48% of B/myeloid MPAL and involved TCF3, EP300, TAF15, and CREBBP, with various portions of ZNF384 being involved.[11] ZNF384 rearrangements are also seen in B-ALL that does not meet criteria for MPAL.[78] Compared with B-ALL with ZNF384 rearrangements, B/myeloid MPAL shows similar genomic mutations except B/myeloid MPAL may contain KDM6A mutations.[11]

B/T MPAL is rare, and few studies of its mutational landscape exist. A recent case series has revealed common mutations in PHF6, followed by WT1, JAK3, MED12, CTCF, IL7R, NOTCH1, SF3B1, PTPN11,EZH2, DNMT3A, and TP53.[72,79,80]

T/myeloid and B/myeloid leukemia cluster with different methylation signatures, with T/myeloid MPAL showing more hypermethylated CpG islands.[67] T/myeloid MPAL tends to have hypomethylation of TCR-associated signaling genes, suggesting the possibility that CD3 expression in T/myeloid MPAL is due to promoter hypomethylation.[67] In B/myeloid MPAL, IRF8- and IRF4-binding motifs tend to be hypomethylated.[67]

Gene expression data indicate that MPAL has a unique transcription profile that usually lies somewhere between ALL and AML.[81] B/myeloid MPAL expression profiles show upregulation of IRF4/IRF8 targets, BCR signaling, and nuclear factor κB pathways.[67] In pediatric ZNF384-rearranged B/myeloid MPAL, the expression profiles resemble B-ALL, with gene set enrichment analysis indicating an arrest at a more mature stage of development compared with other B/myeloid MPAL, but at an earlier stage compared with B-ALL.[11] FLT3 expression is higher in ZNF384r MPAL compared with other MPAL. T/myeloid MPAL tends to express a TCR profile similar to ETP, which is more consistent with the profile of a hematopoietic stem cell (HSC) than a T-cell precursor.[11,66,67]

ACUTE UNDIFFERENTIATED LEUKEMIA

Because of its rarity, little is known about the genomic landscape of acute undifferentiated leukemia. Cuneo and colleagues[82] studied 9 cases of AUL in the late 1990s using FAB criteria and found that three harbored del(5q), three others possessed trisomy(13), another showed isolated trisomy(12), and a complex karyotype was found in one patient. In addition, overexpression of the poor prognostic markers, BAALC, ERG, and MN1, has been shown in AUL compared with other leukemias, but commonly mutated genes have not yet been reported.[79]

PROGNOSIS

The prognosis of ALAL has generally been poor, with MPAL remission rates between 61% and 85% and a median overall survival (OS) of 15 to 18 months.[4,7] Retrospective studies indicate inferior outcome for patients with MPAL compared with AML and ALL; however, a study that excluded MPAL-like leukemias with complex karyotypes found MPAL outcomes to be similar to ALL.[4,9,24] Recent studies indicate that HSC transplantation (HSCT) for patients in remission might improve outcome to levels similar to patients with AML and ALL.[83,84] Most studies do not find a survival impact based on immunophenotype; however, a higher relapse incidence has been observed in T-Myeloid MPAL.[4,11,73,85] KMT2A rearrangement is associated with poor prognosis (21.2% five-year OS).[11] Small studies suggest that bilineal MPAL may have a poorer outcome than biphenotypic leukemia.[86]

Because of the rarity of the disease, there is a dearth of data to inform treatment regimens for MPAL. There is no consensus with respect to AML- or ALL-based therapy for MPAL, but most retrospective trials suggest better remission rates for ALL-like therapy as opposed to AML-like therapy.[4,7,10,87] Moreover, combined AML-/ALL-therapy does not show obvious benefits over ALL-like therapy alone.[4] As mentioned earlier, studies of HSCT use in first remission seem promising, and therefore, Wolach and Stone have advocated for the use of ALL-like regimens to achieve first remission, followed by allogeneic stem-cell transplant, with the addition of tyrosine kinase inhibitors for patients with t(9;22).[7] In a relatively small study, it was shown that patients with an ALL-like methylation pattern who received an ALL-like therapy or patients with an AML-like pattern who received AML therapy were more likely to achieve complete remission, as opposed to those who received unmatched therapy.[67]

REFERENCES

1. Weinberg OK, Arber DA. Mixed-phenotype acute leukemia: historical overview and a new definition. Leukemia 2010;24(11):1844–51.
2. Béné MC, Porwit A. Acute leukemias of ambiguous lineage. Semin Diagn Pathol 2012;29(1):12–8.
3. Porwit A, Béné MC. Acute leukemias of ambiguous origin. Am J Clin Pathol 2015;144(3):361–76.
4. Wolach O, Stone RM. Mixed-phenotype acute leukemia: current challenges in diagnosis and therapy. Curr Opin Hematol 2017;24(2):139.
5. Charles NJ, Boyer DF. Mixed-phenotype acute leukemia: diagnostic criteria and pitfalls. Arch Pathol Lab Med 2017;141(11):1462–8.

6. Swerdlow SH, Campo E, Harris NL, et al, editors. WHO classification of tumours of haematopoietic and lymphoid tissues. Revised 4th edition. Lyon (France): International Agency for Research on Cancer; 2017.

7. Wolach O, Stone RM. How I treat mixed-phenotype acute leukemia. Blood 2015;125(16):2477–85.

8. Yan L, Ping N, Zhu M, et al. Clinical, immunophenotypic, cytogenetic, and molecular genetic features in 117 adult patients with mixed-phenotype acute leukemia defined by WHO-2008 classification. Haematologica 2012;97(11):1708–12.

9. Shi R, Munker R. Survival of patients with mixed phenotype acute leukemias: a large population-based study. Leuk Res 2015;39(6):606–16.

10. Matutes E, Pickl WF, van't Veer M, et al. Mixed-phenotype acute leukemia: clinical and laboratory features and outcome in 100 patients defined according to the WHO 2008 classification. Blood 2011;117(11):3163–71.

11. Alexander TB, Gu Z, Iacobucci I, et al. The genetic basis and cell of origin of mixed phenotype acute leukaemia. Nature 2018;562(7727):373–9.

12. Bassan R, Biondi A, Benvestito S, et al. Acute undifferentiated leukemia with CD7+ and CD13+ immunophenotype. Lack of molecular lineage commitment and association with poor prognostic features. Cancer 1992;69(2):396–404.

13. Gerr H, Zimmermann M, Schrappe M, et al. Acute leukaemias of ambiguous lineage in children: characterization, prognosis and therapy recommendations. Br J Haematol 2010;149(1):84–92.

14. Mirro J, Kitchingman G. The morphology, cytochemistry, molecular characteristics and clinical significance of acute mixed-lineage leukaemia. In: Scott C, editor. Leukaemia cytochemistry: principles and practice. Chichester (England): Ellis Horwood; 1989. p. 155–79.

15. Catovsky D, Matutes E, Buccheri V, et al. A classification of acute leukaemia for the 1990s. Ann Hematol 1991;62(1):16–21.

16. Bene MC, Castoldi G, Knapp W, et al. Proposals for the immunological classification of acute leukemias. European Group for the Immunological Characterization of Leukemias (EGIL). Leukemia 1995;9(10):1783–6.

17. Matutes E, Buccheri V, Morilla R, et al. Immunological, ultrastructural and molecular features of unclassifiable acute leukaemia. In: Ludwig W-D, Thiel E, editors. Recent advances in cell biology of acute leukemia. Recent results in cancer research. Berlin: Springer; 1993. p. 41–52.

18. Garand R, Béné MC. A new approach of acute lymphoblastic leukemia immunophenotypic classification: 1984-1994 the GEIL experience. Groupe d'Etude Immunologique des Leucémies. Leuk Lymphoma 1994;13(Suppl 1):1–5.

19. Bene MC, Bernier M, Casasnovas RO, et al. The reliability and specificity of c-kit for the diagnosis of acute myeloid leukemias and undifferentiated leukemias. The European Group for the Immunological Classification of Leukemias (EGIL). Blood 1998;92(2):596–9.

20. Jaffe ES, Harris NL, Stein H, et al, editors. WHO classification of tumours of haematopoietic and lymphoid tissues. 3rd edition. Lyon (France): International Agency for Research on Cancer Press; 2001.

21. Swerdlow SH, Campo E, Harris NL, et al, editors. WHO classification of tumours of haematopoietic and lymphoid tissues. 4th edition. Lyon (France): International Agency for Research on Cancer; 2008.

22. Arber DA, Orazi A, Hasserjian R, et al. The 2016 revision to the World Health Organization classification of myeloid neoplasms and acute leukemia. Blood 2016;127(20):2391–405.

23. van den Ancker W, Terwijn M, Westers TM, et al. Acute leukemias of ambiguous lineage: diagnostic consequences of the WHO2008 classification. Leukemia 2010;24(7):1392–6.

24. Weinberg OK, Seetharam M, Ren L, et al. Mixed phenotype acute leukemia: a study of 61 cases using World Health Organization and European Group for the Immunological Classification of Leukaemias criteria. Am J Clin Pathol 2014;142(6):803–8.

25. Campana D, Thompson JS, Amlot P, et al. The cytoplasmic expression of CD3 antigens in normal and malignant cells of the T lymphoid lineage. J Immunol 1987;138(2):648–55.

26. van Dongen JJ, Krissansen GW, Wolvers-Tettero IL, et al. Cytoplasmic expression of the CD3 antigen as a diagnostic marker for immature T-cell malignancies. Blood 1988;71(3):603–12.

27. Janossy G, Coustan-Smith E, Campana D. The reliability of cytoplasmic CD3 and CD22 antigen expression in the immunodiagnosis of acute leukemia: a study of 500 cases. Leukemia 1989;3(3):170–81.

28. Bradstock K, Matthews J, Benson E, et al. Prognostic value of immunophenotyping in acute myeloid leukemia. Australian Leukaemia Study Group. Blood 1994;84(4):1220–5.

29. Vodinelich L, Tax W, Bai Y, et al. A monoclonal antibody (WT1) for detecting leukemias of T-cell precursors (T-ALL). Blood 1983;62(5):1108–13.

30. Haynes BF, Eisenbarth GS, Fauci AS. Human lymphocyte antigens: production of a monoclonal antibody that defines functional thymus-derived lymphocyte subsets. Proc Natl Acad Sci U S A 1979;76(11):5829–33.

31. Drexler HG, Thiel E, Ludwig WD. Acute myeloid leukemias expressing lymphoid-associated antigens: diagnostic incidence and prognostic significance. Leukemia 1993;7(4):489–98.

32. Link MP, Stewart SJ, Warnke RA, et al. Discordance between surface and cytoplasmic expression of the Leu-4 (T3) antigen in thymocytes and in blast cells from childhood T lymphoblastic malignancies. J Clin Invest 1985;76(1):248–53.

33. Furley AJ, Mizutani S, Weilbaecher K, et al. Developmentally regulated rearrangement and expression of genes encoding the T cell receptor-T3 complex. Cell 1986;46(1):75–87.

34. Campana D, Janossy G, Coustan-Smith E, et al. The expression of T cell receptor-associated proteins during T cell ontogeny in man. J Immunol 1989; 142(1):57–66.

35. Legrand O, Perrot J-Y, Baudard M, et al. The immunophenotype of 177 adults with acute myeloid leukemia: proposal of a prognostic score. Blood 2000; 96(3):870–7.

36. Lewis RE, Cruse JM, Sanders CM, et al. Aberrant expression of T-cell markers in acute myeloid leukemia. Exp Mol Pathol 2007;83(3):462–3.

37. Nadler LM, Anderson KC, Marti G, et al. B4, a human B lymphocyte-associated antigen expressed on normal, mitogen-activated, and malignant B lymphocytes. J Immunol 1983;131(1):244–50.

38. Anderson KC, Bates MP, Slaughenhoupt BL, et al. Expression of human B cell-associated antigens on leukemias and lymphomas: a model of human B cell differentiation. Blood 1984;63(6):1424–33.

39. Ball ED, Davis RB, Griffin JD, et al. Prognostic value of lymphocyte surface markers in acute myeloid leukemia [see comments]. Blood 1991; 77(10):2242–50.

40. Campana D, Janossy G, Bofill M, et al. Human B cell development. I. Phenotypic differences of B lymphocytes in the bone marrow and peripheral lymphoid tissue. J Immunol 1985;134(3):1524–30.

41. Toba K, Hanawa H, Fuse I, et al. Difference in CD22 molecules in human B cells and basophils. Exp Hematol 2002;30(3):205–11.

42. Sato N, Kishi K, Toba K, et al. Simultaneous expression of CD13, CD22 and CD25 is related to the expression of Fc epsilon R1 in non-lymphoid leukemia. Leuk Res 2004;28(7):691–8.

43. Weiss A, Littman DR. Signal transduction by lymphocyte antigen receptors. Cell 1994;76(2): 263–74.

44. Patterson HC, Kraus M, Wang D, et al. Cytoplasmic Ig alpha serine/threonines fine-tune Ig alpha tyrosine phosphorylation and limit bone marrow plasma cell formation. J Immunol 2011;187(6):2853–8.

45. Leduc I, Preud'homme JL, Cogné M. Structure and expression of the mb-1 transcript in human lymphoid cells. Clin Exp Immunol 1992;90(1):141–6.

46. Hashimoto M, Yamashita Y, Mori N. Immunohistochemical detection of CD79a expression in precursor T cell lymphoblastic lymphoma/leukaemias. J Pathol 2002;197(3):341–7.

47. Pilozzi E, Pulford K, Jones M, et al. Co-expression of CD79a (JCB117) and CD3 by lymphoblastic lymphoma. J Pathol 1998;186(2):140–3.

48. Arber DA, Jenkins KA, Slovak ML. CD79 alpha expression in acute myeloid leukemia. High frequency of expression in acute promyelocytic leukemia. Am J Pathol 1996;149(4):1105–10.

49. Bhargava P, Kallakury BVS, Ross JS, et al. CD79a is heterogeneously expressed in neoplastic and normal myeloid precursors and megakaryocytes in an antibody clone-dependent manner. Am J Clin Pathol 2007;128(2):306–13.

50. Luger D, Yang Y, Raviv A, et al. Expression of the B-cell receptor component CD79a on immature myeloid cells contributes to their tumor promoting effects. PLoS One 2013;8(10):e76115.

51. Desiderio SV, Yancopoulos GD, Paskind M, et al. Insertion of N regions into heavy-chain genes is correlated with expression of terminal deoxytransferase in B cells. Nature 1984;311(5988):752–5.

52. Borowitz MJ, Lynn Guenther K, Shults KE, et al. Immunophenotyping of acute leukemia by flow cytometric analysis: use of CD45 and right-angle light scatter to gate on leukemic blasts in three-color analysis. Am J Clin Pathol 1993;100(5): 534–40.

53. Paietta E, Racevskis J, Bennett JM, et al. Differential expression of terminal transferase (TdT) in acute lymphocytic leukaemia expressing myeloid antigens and TdT positive acute myeloid leukaemia as compared to myeloid antigen negative acute lymphocytic leukaemia. Br J Haematol 1993;84(3): 416–22.

54. Buccheri V, Shetty V, Yoshida N, et al. The role of an anti-myeloperoxidase antibody in the diagnosis and classification of acute leukaemia: a comparison with light and electron microscopy cytochemistry. Br J Haematol 1992;80(1):62–8.

55. Bennett JM, Catovsky D, Daniel MT, et al. Proposals for the classification of the acute leukaemias. French-American-British (FAB) co-operative group. Br J Haematol 1976;33(4):451–8.

56. Borowitz MJ. Mixed phenotype acute leukemia. Cytometry B Clin Cytom 2014;86(3):152–3.

57. Arber DA, Snyder DS, Fine M, et al. Myeloperoxidase immunoreactivity in adult acute lymphoblastic leukemia. Am J Clin Pathol 2001;116(1):25–33.

58. Zhou M, Findley HW, Zaki SR, et al. Expression of myeloperoxidase mRNA by leukemic cells from childhood acute lymphoblastic leukemia. Leukemia 1993;7(8):1180–3.

59. Oberley MJ, Li S, Orgel E, et al. Clinical significance of isolated myeloperoxidase expression in pediatric B-lymphoblastic leukemia. Am J Clin Pathol 2017; 147(4):374–81.

60. Leong CF, Kalaichelvi AVM, Cheong SK, et al. Comparison of myeloperoxidase detection by flow

cytometry using two different clones of monoclonal antibodies. Malays J Pathol 2004;26(2):111–6.

61. Kang H, Chen I-M, Wilson CS, et al. Gene expression classifiers for relapse-free survival and minimal residual disease improve risk classification and outcome prediction in pediatric B-precursor acute lymphoblastic leukemia. Blood 2010;115(7): 1394–405.

62. Mina-Osorio P. The moonlighting enzyme CD13: old and new functions to target. Trends Mol Med 2008; 14(8):361–71.

63. Laszlo GS, Estey EH, Walter RB. The past and future of CD33 as therapeutic target in acute myeloid leukemia. Blood Rev 2014;28(4):143–53.

64. Manola KN. Cytogenetic abnormalities in acute leukaemia of ambiguous lineage: an overview. Br J Haematol 2013;163(1):24–39.

65. Coustan-Smith E, Mullighan CG, Onciu M, et al. Early T-cell precursor leukaemia: a subtype of very high-risk acute lymphoblastic leukaemia. Lancet Oncol 2009;10(2):147–56.

66. Zhang J, Ding L, Holmfeldt L, et al. The genetic basis of early T-cell precursor acute lymphoblastic leukaemia. Nature 2012;481(7380):157–63.

67. Takahashi K, Wang F, Morita K, et al. Integrative genomic analysis of adult mixed phenotype acute leukemia delineates lineage associated molecular subtypes. Nat Commun 2018;9(1):2670.

68. Chen SJ, Flandrin G, Daniel MT, et al. Philadelphia-positive acute leukemia: lineage promiscuity and inconsistently rearranged breakpoint cluster region. Leukemia 1988;2(5):261–73.

69. Carbonell F, Swansbury J, Min T, et al. Cytogenetic findings in acute biphenotypic leukaemia. Leukemia 1996;10(8):1283–7.

70. Owaidah TM, Al Beihany A, Iqbal MA, et al. Cytogenetics, molecular and ultrastructural characteristics of biphenotypic acute leukemia identified by the EGIL scoring system. Leukemia 2006;20(4):620–6.

71. Wang Y, Gu M, Mi Y, et al. Clinical characteristics and outcomes of mixed phenotype acute leukemia with Philadelphia chromosome positive and/or bcr-abl positive in adult. Int J Hematol 2011;94(6):552–5.

72. Eckstein OS, Wang L, Punia JN, et al. Mixed-phenotype acute leukemia (MPAL) exhibits frequent mutations in DNMT3A and activated signaling genes. Exp Hematol 2016;44(8):740–4.

73. Xiao W, Bharadwaj M, Levine M, et al. PHF6 and DNMT3A mutations are enriched in distinct subgroups of mixed phenotype acute leukemia with T-lineage differentiation. Blood Adv 2018;2(23): 3526–39.

74. Quesada AE, Hu Z, Routbort MJ, et al. Mixed phenotype acute leukemia contains heterogeneous genetic mutations by next-generation sequencing. Oncotarget 2018;9(9):8441–9.

75. Kern W, Grossmann V, Roller A, et al. Mixed phenotype acute leukemia, T/Myeloid, NOS (MPAL-TM) has a high DNMT3A mutation frequency and carries further genetic features of both AML and T-ALL: results of a comprehensive next-generation sequencing study analyzing 32 genes. Blood 2012;120(21):403.

76. Maude SL, Dolai S, Delgado-Martin C, et al. Efficacy of JAK/STAT pathway inhibition in murine xenograft models of early T-cell precursor (ETP) acute lymphoblastic leukemia. Blood 2015; 125(11):1759–67.

77. Van Vlierberghe P, Ambesi-Impiombato A, Perez-Garcia A, et al. ETV6 mutations in early immature human T cell leukemias. J Exp Med 2011;208(13): 2571–9.

78. Yasuda T, Tsuzuki S, Kawazu M, et al. Recurrent DUX4 fusions in B cell acute lymphoblastic leukemia of adolescents and young adults. Nat Genet 2016; 48(5):569–74.

79. Heesch S, Neumann M, Schwartz S, et al. Acute leukemias of ambiguous lineage in adults: molecular and clinical characterization. Ann Hematol 2013; 92(6):747–58.

80. Mi X, Griffin G, Lee W, et al. Genomic and clinical characterization of B/T mixed phenotype acute leukemia reveals recurrent features and T-ALL like mutations. Am J Hematol 2018;93(11):1358–67.

81. Rubnitz JE, Onciu M, Pounds S, et al. Acute mixed lineage leukemia in children: the experience of St Jude Children's Research Hospital. Blood 2009; 113(21):5083–9.

82. Cuneo A, Ferrant A, Michaux JL, et al. Cytogenetic and clinicobiological features of acute leukemia with stem cell phenotype: study of nine cases. Cancer Genet Cytogenet 1996;92(1):31–6.

83. Munker R, Brazauskas R, Wang HL, et al. Allogeneic hematopoietic cell transplantation for patients with mixed phenotype acute leukemia. Biol Blood Marrow Transplant 2016;22(6):1024–9.

84. Shimizu H, Saitoh T, Machida S, et al. Allogeneic hematopoietic stem cell transplantation for adult patients with mixed phenotype acute leukemia: results of a matched-pair analysis. Eur J Haematol 2015;95(5):455–60.

85. Lee J-H, Min YH, Chung CW, et al. Prognostic implications of the immunophenotype in biphenotypic acute leukemia. Leuk Lymphoma 2008;49(4):700–9.

86. Weir EG, Ali Ansari-Lari M, Batista DA, et al. Acute bilineal leukemia: a rare disease with poor outcome. Leukemia 2007;21(11):2264–70.

87. Tian H, Xu Y, Liu L, et al. Comparison of outcomes in mixed phenotype acute leukemia patients treated with chemotherapy and stem cell transplantation versus chemotherapy alone. Leuk Res 2016;45:40–6.

Prognostic and Predictive Biomarkers in Diffuse Large B-cell Lymphoma

Alex Chan, MD*, Ahmet Dogan, MD, PhD*

KEYWORDS

- DLBCL prognosis • Immunophenotype • Mutational profile

OVERVIEW

Diffuse large B-cell lymphoma (DLBCL) is the most common lymphoid malignancy in the Western world, accounting for 25% to 40% of adult non-Hodgkin lymphomas (NHLs), with at least 25,000 new cases in the United States estimated in 2016.[1,2] The disease is remarkably heterogeneous, with a variety of pathogenetic mechanisms, presentations, and outcomes. Since the introduction of cyclophosphamide, doxorubicin, vincristine, and prednisone plus rituximab (R-CHOP) as the standard therapy for DLBCL, approximately 60% of patients are now curable. For those who are not cured, the disease is often progressive and fatal.[1] Because of DLBCL's heterogeneity, extensive research has been performed with an aim to stratify patients based on prognosis, identify patients who would be cured by R-CHOP, and identify others who would benefit from novel therapies. This article synthesizes this research.

CLINICAL PROGNOSTIC FACTORS

The International Prognostic Index (IPI) was developed in 1993 and used clinical characteristics including age, presence of B symptoms, performance status, lactate dehydrogenase, number of sites involved, and clinical stage to stratify patients with aggressive non-Hodgkin lymphoma into distinct groups.[3] The IPI remains one of the most robust methods for predicting outcomes in DLBCL, and its value has persisted into the current era of R-CHOP therapy.[4] An enhanced IPI score was developed recently to better stratify patients in the era of R-CHOP therapy, and similarly stratifies patients into 4 distinct prognostic groups.[5] Although the IPI has persisted as a useful clinical tool, it predominantly measures extent and aggressiveness of disease but does not address underlying biological heterogeneity.

Bone marrow staging affects IPI in the stage scoring calculations, but bone marrow involvement by DLBCL is also a prognostic factor independent of IPI. Bone marrow involvement in DLBCL may be concordant, meaning involved by DLBCL, or discordant, with involvement by a small B-cell lymphoma, which may or may not be clonally related to the diagnostic DLBCL. Discordant bone marrow involvement may predict progression-free survival (PFS) but not overall survival (OS) in DLBCL.[6] Multiple studies corroborate concordant bone marrow involvement as a negative prognostic marker of both PFS and OS, and these findings are independent of IPI scoring by multivariate analyses. Extent of bone marrow involvement does not provide any valuable prognostic information.[6–8]

PHENOTYPIC PROGNOSTIC FACTORS

It has been almost 20 years from the landmark comprehensive gene expression profiling (GEP)

Disclosures: A. Dogan receives personal consultancy fees from Roche, Corvus Pharmaceuticals, Physicians' Education Resource, Seattle Genetics, Peerview Institute, Oncology Specialty Group, Pharmacyclics, Celgene, and Novartis, and research grants from National Cancer Institute, Roche. A. Chan has nothing to disclose.
Funded by: NIHHYB. Grant numbers: P30 CA008748; P50 CA192937.
Hematopathology Diagnostic Service, Department of Pathology, Memorial Sloan Kettering Cancer Center, 1275 York Avenue, New York, NY 10065, USA
* Corresponding authors.
E-mail addresses: chana7@mskcc.org (A.C.); dogana@mskcc.org (A.D.)

surgpath.theclinics.com

study by Alizadeh and colleagues,[9] which revealed that DLBCL comprised at least 2 distinct biological subtypes. This study identified 1 subgroup with gene expression like germinal center B cells (GCBs), another like activated B cells (ABCs), and a third unclassifiable group. The GCB and ABC subtypes showed distinctly different outcomes, with ABC DLBCLs having worse survival. Because GEP is impractical as a routine clinical test, several surrogate methods have been developed. The most commonly used method is immunohistochemistry (IHC), and the most common algorithm is the algorithm described by Hans and colleagues[10] (Fig. 1A). In addition, there are several other IHC-based cell-of-origin algorithms, some better correlated with GEP[11–14] (Fig. 1B, C for examples). An abbreviated GEP method applicable in formalin-fixed, paraffin-embedded specimens was developed recently but is not yet widely available outside of research applications.[15,16] Cell-of-origin subtyping was acknowledged in the 2008 World Health Organization (WHO) classification of lymphoid neoplasms, but the 2016 revision explicitly requires it, although it does not specify the methods required.[17]

The use of IHC cell-of-origin subtyping in DLBCL prognosis has been controversial. The Hans algorithm showed only 76% concordance with GEP in the original publication.[10] In addition, although GEP testing's prognostic value has been validated in several studies, the value of IHC algorithms is controversial.[16,18,19] Particularly in the R-CHOP era, IHC algorithms have had varying abilities to predict outcomes; some studies find differences in GCB and non-GCB subtypes,[20] but most show no significant differences between the two groups.[13,19,21–23] Despite the lack of prognostic significance, IHC algorithms are still used routinely in clinical practice. The subgroups have

different pathogenetic mechanisms, and the distinction aids in therapeutic decision making in the context of clinical trials.[17,24]

Several other phenotypic prognostic markers reflecting important oncogenic mechanisms in DLBCL have been established in recent years. MYC (a proto-oncogene transcription factor) overexpression is detected by IHC staining in 29% to 47% of DLBCLs, sometimes secondary to MYC gene rearrangements, but more often independent of MYC gene alterations.[25–27] Whether MYC expression by IHC alone predicts outcome is controversial; several studies show a correlation with inferior survival,[26,27] but this finding may be confounded by concurrent BCL2 expression, and has not always remained significant under multivariate analyses.[28] Furthermore, studies evaluating MYC expression by IHC have used widely variable cutoffs, making comparison between studies difficult.[26–28]

BCL2 overexpression by IHC is generally seen as a marker of DLBCL biology, without any definite effect on prognosis.[1] Some studies show correlation between expression and prognosis,[29] but their results disagree on the subtypes of DLBCL susceptible to these effects, and use widely variable cutoff percentages to establish BCL2 positivity.[28,30–32]

Evaluated individually, MYC and BCL2 IHC do not definitively provide useful prognostic information but are useful when coexpressed. Approximately 20% to 35% of cases with MYC expression show concurrent BCL2 expression, the so-called double-expresser phenotype.[25] Several studies show that expression of both MYC and BCL2 by IHC is associated with inferior outcome.[28,29,33,34] Expression of MYC and BCL2 by IHC does not necessarily reflect gene rearrangements and is frequently caused by gains or amplifications. The WHO classification system currently suggests that double-

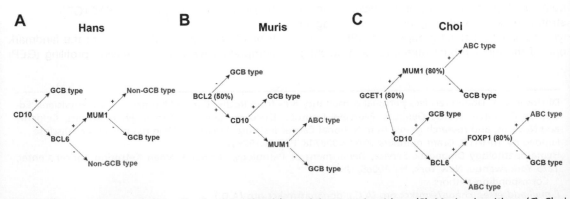

Fig. 1. Three examples of IHC cell of origin algorithms. (A) Hans algorithm. (B) Muris algorithm. (C) Choi algorithm.

expresser phenotype is a prognostic indicator but not a separate classification.[17]

CD5 is a pan–T-cell antigen that is occasionally positive in DLBCL and is associated with poor outcome. Although some CD5-positive DLBCLs represent progression of an underlying CD5+ small B-cell lymphoma such as chronic lymphocytic leukemia/small lymphocytic lymphoma (CLL/SLL) or mantle cell lymphoma, most are considered de novo DLBCL.[1] DLBCL expresses CD5 in 5% to 10% of cases, and these cases have an inferior outcome compared with CD5– DLBCL.[35–40] This finding has held over different treatment regimens.[35,36,39] In addition, although CD5 expression is often associated with older patient age, extranodal involvement, advanced clinical stage, and increased serum lactate dehydrogenase level, some studies show that CD5 also provides prognostic value independent of the IPI on multivariate analysis,[36,38,40] although others do not find an independent effect.[39]

TP53 is a tumor suppressor gene involved in several functions, including apoptosis, DNA repair, and cell cycle arrest; this function preserves genomic stability and eliminates cells that acquire pathogenic mutations.[41] Expression of p53 by IHC is a surrogate for *TP53* mutation with a cutoff of greater than 50% expression.[42] In addition, increased expression of p53 by IHC is an independent prognostic factor in DLBCL, and seems to worsen the prognostic impact of *MYC* gene rearrangement.[42,43]

CD30 IHC expression may also provide prognostic value, although study of its effect on prognosis is limited. CD30 may predict a better prognosis, except in cases associated with EBV.[44] Although studies regarding CD30 and its effects on outcome are limited, CD30 may be more useful in predicting response to therapy with the drug-antibody conjugate brentuximab vedotin, particularly in cases of relapsed or refractory DLBCL.[45] However, because brentuximab vedotin is not yet approved for treatment of DLBCL, evaluation of CD30 IHC expression is not usually required in DLBCL outside of clinical trial contexts.

Other IHC antibodies such as FOXP1 may provide useful information in DLBCL. *FOXP1* is a transcription factor involved in cell signaling and early B-cell development, and is used as a factor in several cell-of-origin algorithms, being expressed primarily in ABC-type DLBCLs.[13,14,46,47] Some studies show correlation between strong FOXP1 expression and inferior survival.[46,47] However, this finding may be related to a correlation between FOXP1 expression and other factors, such as

MYC expression, because one study did not show a significant association in multivariate analysis.[29]

There are numerous IHC biomarkers useful for predictive and prognostic purposes in DLBCL. In small biopsies, this leads to issues of prioritization of markers and tissue preservation. In addition to cell-of-origin subtyping, the authors recommend routine testing for BCL2 and MYC on all cases of DLBCL, and using cell-of-origin subtyping, BCL2, and MYC expression to guide ancillary cytogenetic testing for *BCL2*, *BCL6*, and *MYC* gene rearrangements. This initial work-up is useful for any DLBCL; any additional markers can be left to the pathologist's discretion or at the request of a clinician. To preserve tissue, cutting 3 to 5 extra unstained slides at the time of initial processing is recommended.

GENETIC PROGNOSTIC FACTORS

In the past decade, comprehensive genomic analysis has become more widely available, faster, and cheaper. Improved availability has led to numerous studies establishing genomic profiles in DLBCL, which found major differences between GCB and ABC DLBCLs in terms of mutational profile. GCB DLBCLs frequently show alterations of epigenetic modifiers such as *EZH2*, *CREBBP/EB300*, and *KMT2D/MLL2*, as well as *BCL2* alterations.[48–50] *CREBBP* and *KMT2D* mutations can also be seen in ABC DLBCL but are more frequent in GCB.[51] ABC-type DLBCLs show alterations that result in aberrant chronic B-cell receptor and Toll-like receptor signaling, ultimately leading to constitutive activation of various signaling pathways, particularly the nuclear factor kappa-B (NF-kB) pathway.[52–56]

With the possible exception of *TP53*,[57,58] single mutations show no significant prognostic value. However, combinations of mutational profiles and genetic structural analysis provide prognostic value. Two major recent studies using whole-exome sequencing identified subgroups with distinct outcomes. One study identified 5 major subgroups, including 2 major molecular subgroups of ABC DLBCLs, 2 of GCB DLBCLs, and 1 with a mixture of both. Of the 2 ABC subgroups, 1 showed concurrent *BCL6* structural variants and *NOTCH2* pathway mutations, and another had *BCL2* amplifications with concurrent *MYD88* and *CD79B* mutations, with the latter subgroup showing inferior outcome. Of the 2 predominantly GCB subgroups, 1 showed frequent mutations in histone modification proteins, and the other a combination of *EZH2* mutations, *BCL2* mutations, and translocations, with the second group having worse outcome. A fifth group showed copy number losses of chromosome 17p and *TP53* mutations, and also had a poor prognosis.[59]

Another major study published at the same time showed similar findings, with 4 major subgroups. One subgroup showed concurrent *MYD88* and *CD79B* mutations, another had concurrent *BCL6* structural variants and *NOTCH2* pathway mutations, a third harbored *NOTCH1* mutations, and the final group showed mutations in *EZH2* with concurrent *BCL2* translocations. Similarly to the previously mentioned study, this study showed inferior outcomes in the group with concurrent *MYD88* and *CD79B* mutations, although it did not find a significant survival difference between the group with *EZH2* mutations and concurrent *BCL2* translocations and other GCB-type DLBCLs.[60]

In general, *BCL2* rearrangements alone in DLBCL have no effect on prognosis in DLBCL.[29,61] However, *BCL2* combined with mutational profile may provide prognostic value.[59,60] In contrast, the finding of *MYC* rearrangements, seen in 5% to 15% of DLBCLs, has been consistently validated as a predictor of inferior survival.[25,27,61–63] In cases with *MYC* translocations, the translocation partner is also predictive of outcome; cases with *MYC-IG* translocations generally have inferior survival compared with those with non-*IG* translocations.[64,65] *MYC* copy number alterations may also be of prognostic significance.[66] However, many lymphomas with aggressive-appearing morphology and *MYC* rearrangements also show rearrangements of *BCL2* or *BCL6*,[62] and these cases should be diagnosed as high-grade B-cell lymphoma according to new classification guidelines.[17] A subset of GCB DLBCLs also show GEP signatures similar to high-grade B-cell lymphomas with rearrangements of *MYC* and *BCL2* and/or *BCL6*, and recent evidence suggests they have a poor prognosis compared with other GCB DLBCLs.[67]

Although comprehensive molecular profiling studies show the prognostic value of extensive molecular testing, it is worth noting that, even with extensive whole-exome sequencing, there is enough genetic heterogeneity in DLBCLs that many cases do not fit into any molecular subgroup. For example, in the study by Schmitz and colleagues,[60] only 44.8% of the examined cases fit into one of the 4 subgroups.[60] However, molecular profiling research also provides additional value in identifying therapeutic targets for DLBCL.[68] A simplified table of mutations associated with different subtypes of DLBCL is shown in **Table 1**. For those interested, there are several comprehensive review articles regarding DLBCL molecular pathogenesis.[51,68,69]

NEW THERAPIES AND PREDICTIVE MARKERS

Historically, the search for biomarkers revolved around identifying prognostic markers for standard of care, R-CHOP chemotherapy. These searches are now increasingly focused on identifying markers that predict response to a specific therapy. Approximately 40% of patients are not cured by R-CHOP chemotherapy, and, with current salvage chemotherapy regimens, 50% of these patients achieve either a partial response or complete response (CR).[1,70–72] Thus, new therapies for DLBCL are still needed. Based on molecular studies of pathogenesis, a variety of new therapies are currently in clinical trials, and methods for predicting efficacy are also under review.

Ibrutinib, a Bruton tyrosine kinase inhibitor, was recently approved by the US Food and Drug Administration as a first-line therapy for CLL/SLL and is in clinical trials for DLBCL. As a monotherapy for relapsed/refractory disease, ibrutinib showed a 25% overall response rate (ORR), but this finding improved to 37% in non–GCB-type

---

Table 1
Mutational profiles associated with cell of origin subtypes of diffuse large B-cell lymphoma

GCB-type DLBCL	Both GCB-type and ABC-type DLBCL	ABC-type DLBCL
• BCL2 and MYC translocations	• Other histone/chromatin modifiers: KMT2D/MLL2, CREBBP/EP300	• BCL2 and MYC amplifications
• Histone/chromatin modifiers: EZH2	• Immune surveillance: CD58, B2M/HLA-I, CIITA, PD-L1	• B-cell receptor (BCR) signaling: CD79B, CARD11
• B-cell migration: S1PR2, GNA13	• BCL6 deregulation	• Toll-like receptor signaling: MYD88 L265P mutation
• Tumor necrosis factor receptors: TNFRS14	• FOXO1 mutations	• B-cell differentiation: PRDM1/BLIMP1
		• Ubiquitination modification: TNFAIP3/A20

DLBCLs. Furthermore, 16% of patients achieved a CR, with 4 of these patients maintaining this response for more than a year.[73] Of note, patients with concurrent *CD79B* and *MYD88* mutations, which recent molecular studies identified as particularly high risk, responded the best to ibrutinib, with an 80% ORR.[59,60,73] In concert with other salvage chemotherapy regimens, ibrutinib shows better responses; a recent phase 1 study of ibrutinib in combination with rituximab, ifosfamide, carboplatin, and etoposide in relapsed/refractory DLBCL showed a 90% ORR, particularly in non–GCB-type DLBCL, which showed 100% CR.[71] Ibrutinib might find use in first-line therapies as well, because recent data showed improved survival when added to R-CHOP regimens, but only in patients less than 65 years of age.[74]

Cell-of-origin classification may also predict response to lenalidomide in DLBCL. Lenalidomide is an immunomodulatory drug that may affect NF-kB signaling. In trials of single-agent lenalidomide in relapsed/refractory DLBCL, lenalidomide showed a 53% ORR in non–GCB-type DLBCLs compared with a 9% ORR in GCB-type DLBCL.[24] Although cell-of-origin algorithms such as the Hans algorithm do not predict outcome in R-CHOP treated DLBCLs, these algorithms may retain their usefulness in predicting therapeutic responses.

Another newer agent under investigation in DLBCL is venetoclax, a BCL2 inhibitor. Because BCL2 is an antiapoptotic protein frequently overexpressed in both GCB and ABC DLBCLs, it makes an attractive target for therapy.[75] Recently approved for therapy for CLL/SLL, several trials are underway to evaluate its efficacy in DLBCL.[76,77] Expression of BCL2 by IHC seems to have no predictive value for venetoclax efficacy.[78]

Brentuximab vedotin, a CD30 targeted antibody-drug conjugate, is another drug under investigation in DLBCL. As mentioned previously, CD30 positivity may identify a subset of DLBCLs with favorable outcome.[44] In a phase 2 study of relapsed/refractory NHLs with CD30 expression including 49 DLBCL patients, monotherapy with brentuximab vedotin showed a 44% ORR. There was no correlation with CD30 expression levels and response. Samples in this study were considered positive for CD30 for any expression greater than or equal to 1% of tumor cells, suggesting that any CD30 expression predicts susceptibility to this agent.[45]

Immunotherapy agents such as checkpoint inhibitors and chimeric antigen receptor T (CAR-T) cells are a promising new class of drugs that have already shown success in treatment of melanoma, lung cancer, and acute lymphoblastic leukemias. Several trials are underway evaluating immunotherapy for treatment of NHLs, including DLBCL.[79–81] Checkpoint inhibitors have emerged as a promising treatment in classic Hodgkin lymphoma (CHL), and specific subsets of DLBCL show upregulation of PD-L1/L2 similar to CHL.[82] Although the use of checkpoint blockade in NHLs has lagged compared with in CHL, recent studies have showed objective responses in NHLs, including DLBCL.[83]

Although immunotherapy shows promise as a treatment of DLBCLs, predictive biomarkers are not yet firmly established. For example, in a phase 2 multicenter trial, CAR-T cells against CD19 showed an 82% ORR in refractory large B-cell lymphomas regardless of CD19 expression, implying that CD19 expression is not necessarily a prerequisite for efficacy at the start of therapy.[81] However, there is evidence in B lymphoblastic leukemia that loss of CD19 expression is associated with development of resistance to anti-CD19 CAR-T therapy, so the role of CD19 expression in this therapy is not entirely clear.[84] Several studies examine predictive factors in therapy with CAR-T cells, but definitive predictive biomarkers have yet to be established.[85] A summary of important emerging therapies and markers for their use is shown in **Table 2**.

Table 2	
Brief summary of emerging therapies in diffuse large B-cell lymphoma	
Medication	**Predictive Biomarkers**
Ibrutinib (Bruton tyrosine kinase inhibitor)	Cell-of-origin algorithms (non–GCB-type DLBCLs)
Lenalidomide (immunomodulatory agent)	Cell-of-origin algorithms (non–GCB-type DLBCLs)
Venetoclax (BCL2 inhibitor)	None (response not associated with BCL2 expression)
Brentuximab (CD30 targeted antibody-drug conjugate)	CD30 (cutoffs unknown, response not associated with level of CD30 expression)
Checkpoint blockade	Unknown (possibly PD-L1 amplification)
Anti-CD19 CAR-T therapy	Unknown (possibly CD19 expression)

SUMMARY

DLBCLs are a group of aggressive NHLs with remarkable heterogeneity in pathogenesis and clinical outcomes. Although most patients are cured with standard R-CHOP chemotherapy, those who are not have an unfavorable prognosis. Previous methods of prognostic stratification, including cell-of-origin subtyping and evaluation of biomarkers such as MYC, separated patients by their tumor biology. These methods are less effective at stratifying patients in the current era of R-CHOP chemotherapy. Although molecular classification may provide prognostic value in the modern era, these methods cannot stratify all patients. In the current era, the search for prognostic biomarkers increasingly revolves around identifying markers that predict responses to new therapies. In the future, combinations of molecular testing and new therapies might allow oncologists to better select patients for ideal treatment, leading to higher cure rates in this aggressive disease.

REFERENCES

1. Swerdlow SH, Campo E, Harris NL, et al. WHO classification of tumours of haematopoietic and lymphoid tissues. 4th edition. Lyon (France): International Agency for Research on Cancer; 2017.

2. Teras LR, DeSantis CE, Cerhan JR, et al. 2016 US lymphoid malignancy statistics by World Health Organization subtypes. CA Cancer J Clin 2016;66(6): 443–59.

3. The International Non-Hodgkin Lymphoma Prognostic Factors Project. A predictive model for aggressive non-Hodgkin's lymphomas. N Engl J Med 1993;329(14):987–94.

4. Vaidya R, Witzig TE. Prognostic factors for diffuse large B-cell lymphoma in the R(X)CHOP era. Ann Oncol 2014;25(11):2124–33.

5. Zhou Z, Sehn LH, Rademaker AW, et al. An enhanced International Prognostic Index (NCCN-IPI) for patients with diffuse large B-cell lymphoma treated in the rituximab era. Blood 2014;123(6): 837–42.

6. Sehn LH, Scott DW, Chhanabhai M, et al. Impact of concordant and discordant bone marrow involvement on outcome in diffuse large B-cell lymphoma treated with R-CHOP. J Clin Oncol 2011;29(11): 1452–7.

7. Yao Z, Deng L, Xu-Monette ZY, et al. Concordant bone marrow involvement of diffuse large B-cell lymphoma represents a distinct clinical and biological entity in the era of immunotherapy. Leukemia 2018; 32(2):353–63.

8. Chung R, Lai R, Wei P, et al. Concordant but not discordant bone marrow involvement in diffuse large

B-cell lymphoma predicts a poor clinical outcome independent of the International Prognostic Index. Blood 2007;110(4):1278–82.

9. Alizadeh AA, Eisen MB, Davis RE, et al. Distinct types of diffuse large B-cell lymphoma identified by gene expression profiling. Nature 2000;403: 503–11.

10. Hans CP, Weisenburger DD, Greiner TC, et al. Confirmation of the molecular classification of diffuse large B-cell lymphoma by immunohisto-chemistry using a tissue microarray. Blood 2004; 103(1):275–82.

11. Muris JJ, Meijer CJ, Vos W, et al. Immunohistochemical profiling based on Bcl-2, CD10 and MUM1 expression improves risk stratification in patients with primary nodal diffuse large B cell lymphoma. J Pathol 2006;208(5):714–23.

12. Natkunam Y, Farinha P, Hsi ED, et al. LMO2 protein expression predicts survival in patients with diffuse large B-cell lymphoma treated with anthracycline-based chemotherapy with and without rituximab. J Clin Oncol 2008;26(3):447–54.

13. Nyman H, Jerkeman M, Karjalainen-Lindsberg ML, et al. Prognostic impact of activated B-cell focused classification in diffuse large B-cell lymphoma patients treated with R-CHOP. Mod Pathol 2009;22(8): 1094–101.

14. Choi WW, Weisenburger DD, Greiner TC, et al. A new immunostain algorithm classifies diffuse large B-cell lymphoma into molecular subtypes with high accuracy. Clin Cancer Res 2009;15(17):5494–502.

15. Scott DW, Wright GW, Williams PM, et al. Determining cell-of-origin subtypes of diffuse large B-cell lymphoma using gene expression in formalin-fixed paraffin-embedded tissue. Blood 2014; 123(8):1214–7.

16. Scott DW, Mottok A, Ennishi D, et al. Prognostic significance of diffuse large B-cell lymphoma cell of origin determined by digital gene expression in formalin-fixed paraffin-embedded tissue biopsies. J Clin Oncol 2015;33(26):2848–56.

17. Swerdlow SH, Campo E, Pileri SA, et al. The 2016 revision of the World Health Organization classification of lymphoid neoplasms. Blood 2016;127(20): 2375–90.

18. Rosenwald A, Wright G, Chan WC, et al. The use of molecular profiling to predict survival after chemotherapy for diffuse large B-cell lymphoma. N Engl J Med 2002;346(25):1937–47.

19. Gutierrez-Garcia G, Cardesa-Salzmann T, Climent F, et al. Gene-expression profiling and not immunophenotypic algorithms predicts prognosis in patients with diffuse large B-cell lymphoma treated with immunochemotherapy. Blood 2011;117(18): 4836–43.

20. Chavez J, Walsh M, Hernandez-Ilizaliturri FJ, et al. Classification of newly diagnosed diffuse large B-

cell lymphoma (DLBCL) according to Han's criteria defines two groups of patients with different clinical outcomes following systemic rituximab-multi agent anthracycline-based therapy. Blood 2009; 114:623.

21. Gu K, Weisenburger DD, Fu K, et al. Cell of origin fails to predict survival in patients with diffuse large B-cell lymphoma treated with autologous hematopoietic stem cell transplantation. Hematol Oncol 2012;30(3):143–9.

22. Kumar A, Lunning MA, Zhang Z, et al. Excellent outcomes and lack of prognostic impact of cell of origin for localized diffuse large B-cell lymphoma in the rituximab era. Br J Haematol 2015;171(5):776–83.

23. Schmidt-Hansen M, Berendse S, Marafioti T, et al. Does cell-of-origin or MYC, BCL2 or BCL6 translocation status provide prognostic information beyond the International Prognostic Index score in patients with diffuse large B-cell lymphoma treated with rituximab and chemotherapy? A systematic review. Leuk Lymphoma 2017;58(10):2403–18.

24. Hernandez-Ilizaliturri FJ, Deeb G, Zinzani PL, et al. Higher response to lenalidomide in relapsed/refractory diffuse large B-cell lymphoma in nongerminal center B-cell-like than in germinal center B-cell-like phenotype. Cancer 2011;117(22):5058–66.

25. Karube K, Campo E. MYC alterations in diffuse large B-cell lymphomas. Semin Hematol 2015;52(2):97–106.

26. Kluk MJ, Chapuy B, Sinha P, et al. Immunohistochemical detection of MYC-driven diffuse large B-cell lymphomas. PLoS One 2012;7(4):e33813.

27. Horn H, Ziepert M, Becher C, et al. MYC status in concert with BCL2 and BCL6 expression predicts outcome in diffuse large B-cell lymphoma. Blood 2013;121(12):2253–63.

28. Hu S, Xu-Monette ZY, Tzankov A, et al. MYC/BCL2 protein coexpression contributes to the inferior survival of activated B-cell subtype of diffuse large B-cell lymphoma and demonstrates high-risk gene expression signatures: a report from The International DLBCL Rituximab-CHOP Consortium Program. Blood 2013;121(20):4021–31, [quiz: 4250].

29. Bellas C, Garcia D, Vicente Y, et al. Immunohistochemical and molecular characteristics with prognostic significance in diffuse large B-cell lymphoma. PLoS One 2014;9(6):e98169.

30. Iqbal J, Meyer PN, Smith LM, et al. BCL2 predicts survival in germinal center B-cell-like diffuse large B-cell lymphoma treated with CHOP-like therapy and rituximab. Clin Cancer Res 2011;17(24): 7785–95.

31. Iqbal J, Neppalli VT, Wright G, et al. BCL2 expression is a prognostic marker for the activated B-cell-like type of diffuse large B-cell lymphoma. J Clin Oncol 2006;24(6):961–8.

32. Tsuyama N, Sakata S, Baba S, et al. BCL2 expression in DLBCL: reappraisal of immunohistochemistry with new criteria for therapeutic biomarker evaluation. Blood 2017;130(4):489–500.

33. Perry AM, Alvarado-Bernal Y, Laurini JA, et al. MYC and BCL2 protein expression predicts survival in patients with diffuse large B-cell lymphoma treated with rituximab. Br J Haematol 2014;165(3): 382–91.

34. Johnson NA, Slack GW, Savage KJ, et al. Concurrent expression of MYC and BCL2 in diffuse large B-cell lymphoma treated with rituximab plus cyclophosphamide, doxorubicin, vincristine, and prednisone. J Clin Oncol 2012;30(28):3452–9.

35. Alinari L, Gru A, Quinion C, et al. De novo CD5+ diffuse large B-cell lymphoma: Adverse outcomes with and without stem cell transplantation in a large, multicenter, rituximab treated cohort. Am J Hematol 2016;91(4):395–9.

36. Thakral B, Medeiros LJ, Desai P, et al. Prognostic impact of CD5 expression in diffuse large B-cell lymphoma in patients treated with rituximab-EPOCH. Eur J Haematol 2017;98(4):415–21.

37. Yamaguchi M, Nakamura N, Suzuki R, et al. De novo CD5+ diffuse large B-cell lymphoma: results of a detailed clinicopathological review in 120 patients. Haematologica 2008;93(8):1195–202.

38. Ennishi D, Takeuchi K, Yokoyama M, et al. CD5 expression is potentially predictive of poor outcome among biomarkers in patients with diffuse large B-cell lymphoma receiving rituximab plus CHOP therapy. Ann Oncol 2008;19(11):1921–6.

39. Niitsu N, Okamoto M, Tamaru JI, et al. Clinicopathologic characteristics and treatment outcome of the addition of rituximab to chemotherapy for CD5-positive in comparison with CD5-negative diffuse large B-cell lymphoma. Ann Oncol 2010;21(10): 2069–74.

40. Xu-Monette ZY, Tu M, Jabbar KJ, et al. Clinical and biological significance of de novo CD5+ diffuse large B-cell lymphoma in Western countries. Oncotarget 2015;6(8):5616–33.

41. Xu-Monette ZY, Medeiros LJ, Li Y, et al. Dysfunction of the TP53 tumor suppressor gene in lymphoid malignancies. Blood 2012;119(16):3668–83.

42. Xie Y, Bulbul MA, Ji L, et al. p53 expression is a strong marker of inferior survival in de novo diffuse large B-cell lymphoma and may have enhanced negative effect with MYC coexpression: a single institutional clinicopathologic study. Am J Clin Pathol 2014;141(4):593–604.

43. Wang XJ, Medeiros LJ, Bueso-Ramos CE, et al. P53 expression correlates with poorer survival and augments the negative prognostic effect of MYC rearrangement, expression or concurrent MYC/BCL2 expression in diffuse large B-cell lymphoma. Mod Pathol 2017;30(2):194–203.

44. Hu S, Xu-Monette ZY, Balasubramanyam A, et al. CD30 expression defines a novel subgroup of

diffuse large B-cell lymphoma with favorable prognosis and distinct gene expression signature: a report from the International DLBCL Rituximab-CHOP Consortium Program Study. Blood 2013; 121(14):2715–24.

45. Jacobsen ED, Sharman JP, Oki Y, et al. Brentuximab vedotin demonstrates objective responses in a phase 2 study of relapsed/refractory DLBCL with variable CD30 expression. Blood 2015;125(9): 1394–402.

46. Barrans SL, Fenton JA, Banham A, et al. Strong expression of FOXP1 identifies a distinct subset of diffuse large B-cell lymphoma (DLBCL) patients with poor outcome. Blood 2004;104(9): 2933–5.

47. Yu B, Zhou X, Li B, et al. FOXP1 expression and its clinicopathologic significance in nodal and extranodal diffuse large B-cell lymphoma. Ann Hematol 2011;90(6):701–8.

48. Carbone A, Gloghini A, Kwong YL, et al. Diffuse large B cell lymphoma: using pathologic and molecular biomarkers to define subgroups for novel therapy. Ann Hematol 2014;93(8):1263–77.

49. Morin RD, Mendez-Lago M, Mungall AJ, et al. Frequent mutation of histone-modifying genes in non-Hodgkin lymphoma. Nature 2011;476(7360): 298–303.

50. Pasqualucci L, Dominguez-Sola D, Chiarenza A, et al. Inactivating mutations of acetyltransferase genes in B-cell lymphoma. Nature 2011;471(7337): 189–95.

51. Pasqualucci L, Dalla-Favera R. Genetics of diffuse large B-cell lymphoma. Blood 2018;131(21): 2307–19.

52. Nagel D, Vincendeau M, Eitelhuber AC, et al. Mechanisms and consequences of constitutive NF-kappaB activation in B-cell lymphoid malignancies. Oncogene 2014;33(50):5655–65.

53. Ngo VN, Young RM, Schmitz R, et al. Oncogenically active MYD88 mutations in human lymphoma. Nature 2011;470(7332):115–9.

54. Pfeifer M, Grau M, Lenze D, et al. PTEN loss defines a PI3K/AKT pathway-dependent germinal center subtype of diffuse large B-cell lymphoma. Proc Natl Acad Sci U S A 2013;110(30):12420–5.

55. Young RM, Shaffer AL 3rd, Phelan JD, et al. B-cell receptor signaling in diffuse large B-cell lymphoma. Semin Hematol 2015;52(2):77–85.

56. Davis RE, Ngo VN, Lenz G, et al. Chronic active B-cell-receptor signalling in diffuse large B-cell lymphoma. Nature 2010;463(7277):88–92.

57. Xu-Monette ZY, Wu L, Visco C, et al. Mutational profile and prognostic significance of TP53 in diffuse large B-cell lymphoma patients treated with R-CHOP: report from an International DLBCL Rituximab-CHOP Consortium Program Study. Blood 2012;120(19):3986–96.

58. Karube K, Enjuanes A, Dlouhy I, et al. Integrating genomic alterations in diffuse large B-cell lymphoma identifies new relevant pathways and potential therapeutic targets. Leukemia 2018;32(3):675–84.

59. Chapuy B, Stewart C, Dunford AJ, et al. Molecular subtypes of diffuse large B cell lymphoma are associated with distinct pathogenic mechanisms and outcomes. Nat Med 2018;24(5):679–90.

60. Schmitz R, Wright GW, Huang DW, et al. Genetics and pathogenesis of diffuse large B-cell lymphoma. N Engl J Med 2018;378(15):1396–407.

61. Akyurek N, Uner A, Benekli M, et al. Prognostic significance of MYC, BCL2, and BCL6 rearrangements in patients with diffuse large B-cell lymphoma treated with cyclophosphamide, doxorubicin, vincristine, and prednisone plus rituximab. Cancer 2012;118(17):4173–83.

62. Barrans S, Crouch S, Smith A, et al. Rearrangement of MYC is associated with poor prognosis in patients with diffuse large B-cell lymphoma treated in the era of rituximab. J Clin Oncol 2010;28(20):3360–5.

63. Savage KJ, Johnson NA, Ben-Neriah S, et al. MYC gene rearrangements are associated with a poor prognosis in diffuse large B-cell lymphoma patients treated with R-CHOP chemotherapy. Blood 2009; 114(17):3533–7.

64. Copie-Bergman C, Cuilliere-Dartigues P, Baia M, et al. MYC-IG rearrangements are negative predictors of survival in DLBCL patients treated with immunochemotherapy: a GELA/LYSA study. Blood 2015; 126(22):2466–74.

65. Rosenwald A, Sehn LH, Maucort-Boulch D. Prognostic significance of MYC single, double, triple hit and MYC-translocation partner status in diffuse large B-cell lymphoma - a study by the Lunenberg Lymphoma Biomarker Consortium (LLBC). Oral presentation presented at: American Society of Hematology Annual Meeting; December 1-4, 2018; San Diego, CA.

66. Quesada AE, Medeiros LJ, Desai PA, et al. Increased MYC copy number is an independent prognostic factor in patients with diffuse large B-cell lymphoma. Mod Pathol 2017;30(12): 1688–97.

67. Ennishi D, Jiang A, Boyle M, et al. The double-hit gene expression signature defines a clinically and biologically distinct subgroup within GCB-DLBCL. Oral presentation presented at: American Society of Hematology Annual Meeting; December 1-4, 2018; San Diego, CA.

68. Knittel G, Liedgens P, Korovkina D, et al. Rewired NFkappaB signaling as a potentially actionable feature of activated B-cell-like diffuse large B-cell lymphoma. Eur J Haematol 2016;97(6):499–510.

69. Pasqualucci L, Dalla-Favera R. The genetic landscape of diffuse large B-cell lymphoma. Semin Hematol 2015;52(2):67–76.

70. Crump M, Kuruvilla J, Couban S, et al. Randomized comparison of gemcitabine, dexamethasone, and cisplatin versus dexamethasone, cytarabine, and cisplatin chemotherapy before autologous stem-cell transplantation for relapsed and refractory aggressive lymphomas: NCIC-CTG LY.12. J Clin Oncol 2014;32(31):3490–6.

71. Sauter CS, Matasar MJ, Schoder H, et al. A phase 1 study of ibrutinib in combination with R-ICE in patients with relapsed or primary refractory DLBCL. Blood 2018;131(16):1805–8.

72. Gisselbrecht C, Glass B, Mounier N, et al. Salvage regimens with autologous transplantation for relapsed large B-cell lymphoma in the rituximab era. J Clin Oncol 2010;28(27):4184–90.

73. Wilson WH, Young RM, Schmitz R, et al. Targeting B cell receptor signaling with ibrutinib in diffuse large B cell lymphoma. Nat Med 2015;21(8):922–6.

74. Younes A, Sehn LH, Johnson P, et al. A Global, Randomized, Placebo-Controlled, Phase 3 Study of Ibrutinib Plus Rituximab, Cyclophosphamide, Doxorubicin, Vincristine, and Prednisone (RCHOP) in Patients with Previously Untreated Non-Germinal Center B-Cell-like (GCB) Diffuse Large B-Cell Lymphoma (DLBCL). Oral presentation presented at: American Society of Hematology Annual Meeting; December 1-4, 2018; San Diego, CA.

75. Khan N, Kahl B. Targeting BCL-2 in hematologic malignancies. Target Oncol 2018;13(3):257–67.

76. Zelenetz A, Salles G, Mason KD, et al. Results of a phase Ib study of venetoclax plus R- or G-CHOP in patients with B-cell non-Hodgkin lymphoma. Blood 2016;128(22):3032.

77. Gerecitano JF, Roberts AW, Seymour JF, et al. A phase 1 study of venetoclax (ABT-199/GDC-0199) monotherapy in patients with relapsed/refractory non-Hodgkin lymphoma. Blood 2015;126(23):254.

78. Davids MS, Roberts AW, Seymour JF, et al. Phase I first-in-human study of venetoclax in patients with relapsed or refractory non-Hodgkin lymphoma. J Clin Oncol 2017;35(8):826–33.

79. Kochenderfer JN, Dudley ME, Kassim SH, et al. Chemotherapy-refractory diffuse large B-cell lymphoma and indolent B-cell malignancies can be effectively treated with autologous T cells expressing an anti-CD19 chimeric antigen receptor. J Clin Oncol 2015;33(6):540–9.

80. Matsuki E, Younes A. Checkpoint inhibitors and other immune therapies for Hodgkin and non-Hodgkin lymphoma. Curr Treat Options Oncol 2016;17(6):31.

81. Neelapu SS, Locke FL, Bartlett NL, et al. Axicabtagene ciloleucel CAR T-cell therapy in refractory large B-cell lymphoma. N Engl J Med 2017;377(26):2531–44.

82. Hude I, Sasse S, Engert A, et al. The emerging role of immune checkpoint inhibition in malignant lymphoma. Haematologica 2017;102(1):30–42.

83. Lesokhin AM, Ansell SM, Armand P, et al. Nivolumab in patients with relapsed or refractory hematologic malignancy: preliminary results of a phase Ib study. J Clin Oncol 2016;34(23):2698–704.

84. Fry TJ, Shah NN, Orentas RJ, et al. CD22-targeted CAR T cells induce remission in B-ALL that is naive or resistant to CD19-targeted CAR immunotherapy. Nat Med 2018;24(1):20–8.

85. Rossi J, Paczkowski P, Shen YW, et al. Preinfusion polyfunctional anti-CD19 chimeric antigen receptor T cells are associated with clinical outcomes in NHL. Blood 2018;132(8):804–14.

Challenges in the Diagnosis of Gray Zone Lymphomas

Kyle Parker, MD[a], Girish Venkataraman, MD[b],*

KEYWORDS

• Gray-zone lymphoma • Approach • Classification • Hodgkin lymphoma • BCLU

Key points

- A large number of neoplastic cells need to be present to entertain GZL diagnosis. cHL or PMBL may relapse as GZL and relapse immunophenotyping is also important.
- cHL-like (more common) and PMBL-like (less common) are the two major gray zone histologic types.
- B-cell lineage markers (CD20, PAX5, CD79a, and OCT2) with CD30/CD15, MUM1, and EBER allow accurate designation in most cases.
- EBV + DLBCL, not otherwise specific (NOS) and nodular sclerosis cHL, grade 2 both need to be considered before entertaining GZL as a possibility.
- EBV is rare in cases of GZL and rare instances of EBV + GZL all exhibit features of EBV + nodular sclerosis cHL, grade 2.

ABSTRACT

The diagnosis of B-cell lymphoma unclassifiable with features intermediate between diffuse large B-cell lymphoma and classical Hodgkin lymphoma, also called gray zone lymphoma (GZL), is frequently challenging. Incorrect diagnosis as either classic Hodgkin lymphoma or diffuse large B-cell lymphoma has significant implications for choice of upfront therapy based on recent large multi-institutional series from the United States and Europe. These studies have clarified some diagnostic challenges and provided guidance on the spectrum of morphologic features in this entity. This article clarifies some of the diagnostic conundrum surrounding GZL and provides an evidence-based approach to GZL diagnosis using morphology and immunohistochemistry.

OVERVIEW

B-cell lymphoma, unclassifiable, with features intermediate between diffuse large B-cell lymphoma (DLBCL) and classic Hodgkin lymphoma (cHL), more commonly known as "gray zone lymphoma" (GZL), has recently been accepted as a distinct entity in the World Health Organization 2008 and 2016 classifications.[1,2] The term GZL was first coined in 1998 at a workshop for Hodgkin disease and related disease to help classify a subset of mediastinal B-cell lymphomas with features of overlapping Hodgkin lymphoma.[3] These lymphomas are more commonly associated with primary mediastinal occurrence and are therefore also termed as mediastinal GZL (MGZL), whereas cases occurring in the peripheral lymph nodes as the primary site are referred to as non-MGZLs.

Disclosure: Neither Dr K. Parker, nor Dr G. Venkataraman have any significant commercial of financial conflict of interest to disclose.
[a] Department of Pathology, Section of Hematopathology, University of Chicago Medical Center, Chicago, IL, USA; [b] Clinical Immunohistochemistry Lab, Department of Pathology, Section of Hematopathology, The University of Chicago Medical Center, 5841 South Maryland Avenue, TW055B, MC0008, Chicago, IL 60637, USA
* Corresponding author.
E-mail address: girish.venkataraman@uchospitals.edu

Surgical Pathology 12 (2019) 709–718
https://doi.org/10.1016/j.path.2019.03.014
1875-9181/19/© 2019 Elsevier Inc. All rights reserved.

With the growing understanding of primary mediastinal (thymic) large B-cell lymphoma (PMBL) in early 2000, a series of lymphoma cases overlapping cHL and DLBCL were described in 2005 as a link between cHL and PMBL.[4] Molecular genetic studies indicate close biologic relationship among cHL, PMBL, and GZL with evidence for biologic features overlapping cHL and PMBL demonstrated in GZL.[5,6] Observation of cases with initial presentation as cHL relapsing as PMBL or vice versa suggest origins from a common precursor B-cell with plasticity in differentiation influenced by DNA methylation states, a fact borne out by large-scale DNA methylation studies demonstrating the existence of intermediate epigenetic signature in GZL at the molecular level.[5,6]

More recently, a large 2015 retrospective study in the North American population describing clinical features, outcomes, and prognostic factors of 112 cases of GZL concluded that patients with MGZL and non-MGZL had similar outcomes.[7] Another recent study from the National Institutes of Health on GZL noted that patients treated with conventional cHL therapy (doxorubicin-bleomycin-cyclophosphamide-vinblastine-dacarbazine ± rituximab [ABVD ± R]) showed significantly worse 2-year progression-free survival than patients treated with DLBCL therapy (cyclophosphamide-doxorubicin-vincristine-prednisone ± rituximab [CHOP ± R] or dose-adjusted etoposide-doxorubicin-cyclophosphamide-vincristine-prednisone-rituximab [DA-EPOCH-R]).[8] Hence, misclassification of GZL as cHL or vice versa significantly impacts choice of appropriate frontline chemotherapy. Furthermore, a recent retrospective study of 68 cases originally diagnosed as GZL underwent expert pathologist review by consensus and only 26/68 (38%) cases were consistent with the original diagnosis of GZL, whereas most others were reclassified into non-GZL diagnostic categories, highlighting that GZL diagnosis remains (even among experienced lymphoma pathologists) an extremely challenging diagnosis.[9] This article dispels some of the confusion surrounding GZL diagnosis and discusses a simplified algorithmic approach to arriving at a diagnosis of GZL while excluding close differential diagnostic considerations in this process and also focusing on the utility of Epstein-Barr virus (EBV) in situ hybridization. Cases of sequential and composite GZL (which are uncommon forms of GZL) are not discussed here for the sake of clarity.

GROSS FEATURES

In larger series, GZL most commonly presents in young men with a median age at diagnosis within the third decade.[4,6–8] A large anterior mediastinal lesion with or without extramediastinal involvement is the most common physical presentation. If present, extramediastinal involvement most commonly includes supraclavicular and cervical lymphadenopathy with peripheral and intra-abdominal lymphadenopathy being less common. Patients who present with bulky (≥10 cm) anterior mediastinal disease may have accompanying compressive symptomatology including dyspnea and superior vena cava syndrome.[1,2] Additionally, other organ systems may be involved, such as lung by direct extension, spread to liver, spleen, and rarely bone marrow have also been described.[2,4] Patients presenting without evidence of mediastinal disease have a tendency to be older with a median age at diagnosis within the fifth decade and less likely male.[6,10]

MICROSCOPIC FEATURES AND DIAGNOSIS

There is a wide variation in the morphologic spectrum of GZL with some cases exhibiting tumor cells cytologically compatible with Hodgkin/Reed-Sternberg (HRS) cells of cHL (about two-thirds of all GZL cases; **Fig. 1**), whereas others demonstrate sheets of large cells closely resembling DLBCL or PMBL with compartmentalizing sclerosis (less common form of GZL, comprising one-third of GZL cases; **Fig. 2**). Cases with composite histology in different portions of the biopsy may also be observed. The most important feature necessary for entertaining the diagnosis of GZL is the high tumor cell content in most areas.[2] The morphologic appearance of GZL cases more closely representing PMBL/DLBCL is composed of sheets of large centroblastic lymphoid cells with clear cytoplasm, whereas other cases may demonstrate marked pleomorphism.[9] Lacunar cells may be seen. However, HRS cells are typically absent in cases with monomorphic PMBL cytomorphology unless composite histology is present.[4] Cases more closely resembling cHL show characteristic readily identifiable lacunar and HRS cells in the background of a mixed inflammatory infiltrate.[4] An important diagnostic clue is the abundance of tumor cells, often seen in confluent sheets, unlike most cHLs. Additionally, these tumor cells show nuclei with varying degrees of size and shape and less eosinophilic nucleoli compared with traditional and variants of HRS cells.[9] Another important feature of GZLs is the lack of a nodular growth pattern and fibrous bands, although focal fibrosis as seen in nodular sclerosis cHL may be present.[9] Areas of necrosis may be present; however, in contrast to cHL these areas are often scarce and lacking neutrophilic infiltrate typically seen in cHL.[1]

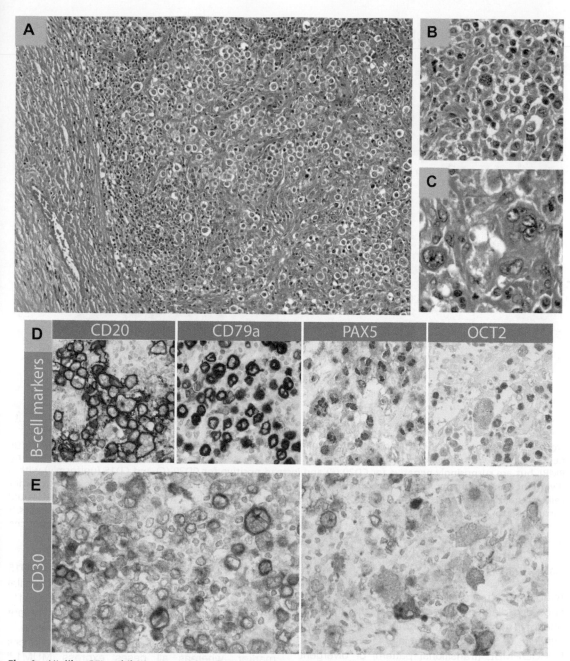

Fig. 1. cHL-like GZL exhibiting transitional immunophenotype in a 57/F with large mediastinal mass and bulky axillary adenopathy. (*A*) Low-power view depicting nodular clusters of neoplastic cells. (*B, C*) Areas with sheet-like proliferation are also noted with inflamed background milieu. Note that the neoplastic cells are fairly pleomorphic with histologic features somewhat transitional between cHL and DLBCL but still closer to cHL, nodular sclerosis grade 2 in many areas. (*D*) B-lineage markers. Most neoplastic cells express uniform CD20 and CD79a with PAX5 and OCT2 (variable with subset of Hodgkin-like cells negative for OCT2 and CD20). (*E*) CD30 expression is variable ranging from negative-weak to strong expression. Additionally, CD45 is focally positive but CD15 and EBER are both negative. Strong B-cell marker positivity in conjunction with CD45 expression is unusual for cHL, nodular sclerosis grade 2, whereas nodular architecture and minority of neoplastic cells lacking CD20 and OCT2 is not typical for DLBCL expressing CD30 and hence the morphology and staining profile is transitional between cHL and DLBCL, allowing designation as GZL in this case.

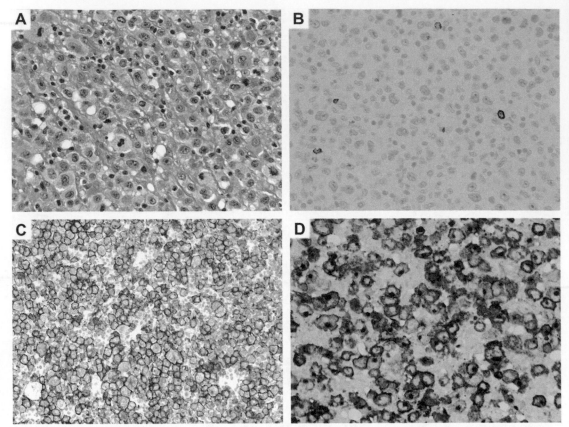

Fig. 2. PMBL-like case exhibiting cHL-like (divergent) immunophenotype. Typical case with sheets of large neoplastic cells with compartmentalizing sclerosis. The neoplastic cells have abundant cytoplasm (*A*) resembling PMBL but are surprisingly negative for CD20 (*B*) and instead positive for CD30 (*C*) and CD15 (uniformly) with a divergent immunophenotype in keeping with cHL and hence classified as GZL. Note that this is again a tumor cell–rich neoplasm as are most GZL cases. (*D*) This type of GZL comprises about a third of all GZL cases and would correspond to "group 2" cases that are the large B-cell lymphoma-like GZL described by Sarkozy and coworkers.[10] Certain PMBL-like cases expressing CD20 that also express uniform CD30 and CD15 uniformly are also categorized as GZL because uniform CD15 is not consistent with a PMBL diagnosis.

IMMUNOPHENOTYPE

Although the morphologic appearance may influence one diagnosis over the other, the immunophenotype often suggests otherwise making it difficult to classify into either pure cHL or DLBCL/PMBL (transitional pattern) or divergent in other cases (discordant cHL histology but with immunohistochemical profile of DLBCL/PMBL). As an example, cases that otherwise exhibit morphology compatible with cHL (the more common form of GZL) may show well-preserved germinal center and B-cell program with strong and uniform expression of CD20, CD79a, PAX5, OCT2, and BOB.1, whereas CD30 and sometimes CD15 are variably expressed (see **Fig. 1**).[2] Likewise, cases that are morphologically compatible with PMBL with sheets of centroblastic cells and compartmentalizing sclerosis (the less common form of GZL) may demonstrate variable loss of

B-cell program with strong CD30 and/or CD15 by immunostaining (divergent cHL immunoprofile) or demonstrate strong CD20, CD30, and CD15, so-called "group 3" cases described by the recent publication of the Lymphoma Study Association.[10] In general, most GZL express at least one B-cell marker, whereas all cases express MUM1.[9] Positivity for EBV by (EBV-encoded small RNA [EBER]) in situ hybridization is useful in that most cases of GZL are typically negative for EBER or harbor only rare EBV-positive cells.[11] However, data from other larger series in Europe and the far east indicate nearly 24% EBV positivity rate in cases classified as GZL.[7,10,12,13] Thus, it remains controversial whether EBV-positive cases should be called GZL or other EBV-related entities (discussed later).

Certain other markers, such as MAL (present in PMBLs) and CD23, are positive in a subset of

MGZL but such markers are not used widely in routine practice limiting any generalization about their utility.[10,14] Scoring systems incorporating CD45, B-lineage markers, MUM1, and EBER have also been proposed to resolve difficult cases.[15]

A recommended immunohistochemical panel for the adequate diagnosis of GZL proposed by Pilichowska and colleagues[9] includes, CD20, CD79a, PAX5, CD3, CD30, CD15, MUM1, and EBER. In cases that represent relapses, testing for PD-L1 may be informative for therapeutic purposes because most cases reportedly express PD-L1 (46%–100%).[16,17] Because of the wide variation in histomorphology, caution is advised when assessing tissue from a core needle biopsy. Thus, if possible, an excisional biopsy is favored for proper histologic evaluation.

DIFFERENTIAL DIAGNOSIS

There are few differential diagnoses for this entity once cases with low tumor cell content are excluded from being called GZL. Nevertheless, accurate distinction of the various entities is critical from a therapeutic standpoint. One should be skeptical about GZL diagnosis in cases with low tumor cell content wherein several other entities including but not limited to cHL, T-cell/histiocyte-rich large B-cell lymphoma and EBV + DLBCL, not otherwise specific (NOS) need to be considered first. The major differential diagnoses for GZL are discussed further later.

HODGKIN LYMPHOMA

Classical Hodgkin lymphoma occurs in younger patients in a mediastinal location similar to GZLs and hence, there is some clinical overlap between both entities in terms of presentation. Indeed, in the study by Pilichowska and coworkers,[9] most GZL cases that were reclassified after central review were nodular sclerosis cHL and specifically grade 2, recognized in earlier studies by the British National Lymphoma Investigation to exhibit more aggressive clinical course.[18,19] From a diagnostic standpoint, nodular sclerosis cHL (the most common subtype) is expected to show typical nodular pattern with prominent sclerosis with variable downregulation of B-cell program (CD20, PAX5, OCT2, and BOB.1) with strong CD30 and CD15 expression. However, because in routine practice, besides CD20 and PAX5, other B-lineage markers are not routinely performed, cases expressing strong and uniform CD20 pose confusion with GZL. Mere strong CD20 expression in cases otherwise typical for cHL should not warrant

designation as GZL and in such cases, GZL diagnosis may only be warranted where there is near uniform expression of several additional B-cell markers (besides CD20) in addition to CD30 (**Fig. 3**). Sometimes, grade 2 nodular sclerosis cHL cases with high content of Hodgkin cells demonstrate stronger CD20 expression at relapse and careful attention must be paid to correlate with the treatment-naive biopsy to avoid misclassification as GZL at relapse. In rare instances, cases with typical nodular sclerosis grade 2 histology but with strong and uniform EBV by In-situ hybridization may be designated as EBV + GZL if they exhibit strong CD20 and CD30.

T-CELL/HISTIOCYTE RICH LARGE B-CELL LYMPHOMA AND EPSTEIN-BARR VIRUS + DIFFUSE LARGE B-CELL LYMPHOMA, NOT OTHERWISE SPECIFIC

T/HRLBCL may sometimes express variable CD30[20] but the coexpression of CD30 and CD20 in such lymphomas with scarce tumor cells should not warrant designation as GZL. Likewise, CD20+/CD30+ cases with scarce tumor cells should also be routinely tested for EBER and if these cells express EBER, the differential between EBV + cHL versus EBV + DLBCL, NOS should be entertained more readily than GZL. EBV + cHL shows EBV expression restricted to the large Hodgkin cells, whereas in EBV + DLBCL, which may show a spectrum of pleomorphic neoplastic cells, EBV + lymphoid cells are often varied in size ranging from small to medium including larger forms consistent with EBV coinfection in the bystander small B-cells and neoplastic medium-large B-cells (**Fig. 4**).[21] Most pediatric cases of EBV + DLBCL, NOS exhibit T/HRLBCL morphology with a small subset exhibiting (15%) features compatible with nodular sclerosis grade 2 but with strong CD30 and CD20 that were classified as EBV + GZL in one study from the United States.[11] Lastly, EBV + large B-cell lymphoproliferations may arise either concurrently or subsequent to angioimmunoblastic T-cell lymphoma and hence, careful attention must be paid to background vascularity and T-cell component whenever an EBV-positive lymphoproliferation is observed because missing underlying T-cell lymphoma has significant implications for upfront therapy choices and relapse management.[22]

PRIMARY MEDIASTINAL (THYMIC) LARGE B-CELL LYMPHOMA

PMBL presents in the mediastinum but occurs more commonly in females (compared with GZL,

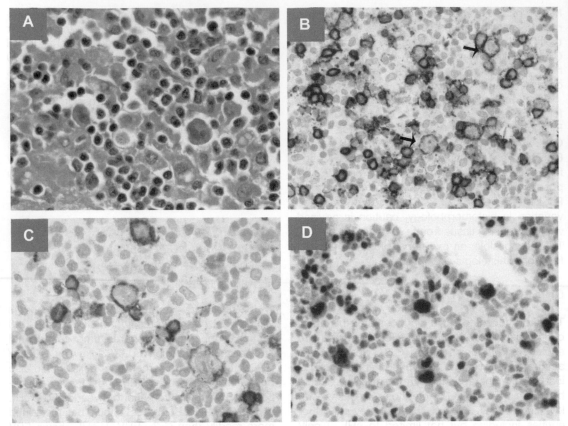

Fig. 3. Tumor cell–poor cHL with strong B-cell marker expression that is not gray zone lymphoma. (*A*) Scattered mononuclear variants of Hodgkin cells are noted in a histiocyte-rich background. The neoplastic cells expressed uniform CD20 (*B, C*) with strong OCT2 (*D*). Additionally, PAX5 and BOB.1 (not shown) were also strongly positive in addition to CD30, CD15, and MUM1. This case was initially called gray zone lymphoma and reclassified as cHL expressing strong B-cell antigens. Such tumor cell–poor neoplasms should not be considered as gray zone lymphomas despite the transitional immunophenotype.

which is more common in males) with typical compartmentalizing sclerosis on histology and can pose diagnostic confusion when there are scattered Hodgkin-like cells amid the tumor cells. These tumors also express frequent weak-moderate CD30, adding further to the confusion with GZL. The initial series by Traverse-Glehen and coworkers[4] described cases of MGZL with features of PMBL and cHL. Since then, further studies have shown cases presenting in extrame-diastinal locations and/or systemically.[6,7] Histologic examination of an otherwise typical PMBL with occasional HRS-like cells does not warrant the diagnosis of GZL.[23] Unless there is a clear morphologically distinct area of cHL within a typical PMBL biopsy, a diagnosis of GZL should not be considered. However, a small subset of GZLs with monomorphic cytology resembling PMBL may show loss of CD20.[9] In a prospective study at the National Cancer Institute, GZL

expressed CD15 more often compared with PMBL.[8]

DIFFUSE LARGE B-CELL LYMPHOMA EXPRESSING CD30

Similar confusion arises when considering a diagnosis of DLBCL with otherwise centroblastic morphology but with variable CD30. CD30 expression has been described in a minority of DLBCL cases.[24–26] However, most cases maintain expression of B-cell markers and are negative for CD15 allowing classification as DLBCL rather than GZL. Thus, in such cases, strong expression of CD30 with variable CD15 expression and loss of some B-cell markers are needed to consider a diagnosis of GZL.[27] EBV + DLBCL is another close differential because of strong CD20, CD30, with CD15 with variable downregulation of some B-cell markers along with strong EBV expression

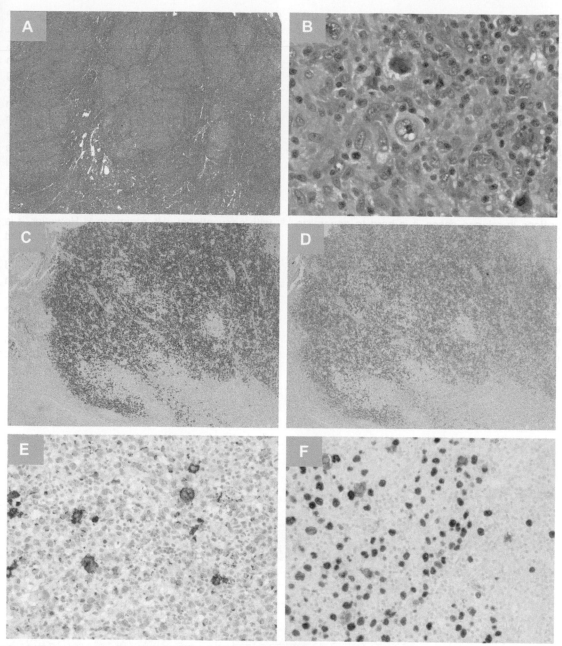

Fig. 4. EBV + large B-cell lymphoma bordering on cHL, nodular sclerosis grade 2/GZL. (*A*) This case demonstrated multifocal sheets of large neoplastic cells with a nodular architecture rich in histiocytes with focal necrosis B. Higher power depicts scattered Hodgkin-like cells and based on CD30 expression without CD20 but only strong PAX5 expression, it was thought to be consistent with cHL (*B*). Additional staining for CD20 (*C*) shows diffuse positivity, whereas CD30 (*D*) is also strongly positive. (*E*) CD15 was focally positive in some of the large Hodgkin-like cells. (*F*) EBER showed diffuse positivity in all large B-cells and some smaller background lymphoid cells allowing designation as EBV + LBCL rather than EBV + GZL.

observed in the neoplastic cells (see **Fig. 4**).[21] However, it remains unclear whether such cases should be termed as EBV + GZLs or EBV + LBCL, although data from US literature support classification as the latter.[9] Because most studies related to GZL are from retrospective

cohorts, the true impact of GZL misclassification is hard to ascertain when there is coexisting EBV infection. In my practice, nearly all EBV-positive cases (cases with significant EBV in lymphoma cells and not rare small bystander cells) are classified into one of several previously discussed entities (cHL, EBV + DLBCL, NOS, AITL with large B-cell proliferation) and I do not make a diagnosis of GZL in these instances.

Fig. 5 depicts a useful algorithm for distinguishing between a variety of differential diagnoses straddling the interface of Hodgkin and large B-cell lymphomas based on histology and commonly used immunohistochemistry stains.

PROGNOSIS

Because of heterogeneity in treatment regimens (stemming from poor recognition of GZLs) coupled with more recent availability of targeted treatment options in relapse cases, it is hard to generalize the prognostic impact of well-characterized GZL cases prospectively. However, based on large scale retrospective studies, looking at consensus-confirmed versus reclassified GZL cases, consensus-confirmed GZL cases demonstrated similar outcomes as reclassified cases in a mostly CHOP-R-treated group of patients.[9] Within confirmed GZL patients in this series, increased CD30 expression had borderline

association with inferior progression-free survival,[9] whereas receipt of front-line CHOP-R was associated with superior PFS (hazard ratio, 0.017; 95% confidence interval, 0.001–0.319) compared with patients who did not receive CHOP-R, indicating that misclassification of GZL as cHL has prognostic implications in the frontline setting. In another large series of 99 cases of GZL from Europe, GZL patients treated with standard regimens (including ABVD/R-CHOP) had worse event-free survival and overall survival compared with patients receiving intense regimens.[28]

However, cases of cHL expressing strong CD20 have been reported to exhibit poorer prognosis with conventional cHL regimens.[29] However, it is unclear if some of these cases would be called GZL by current day terminology, and whether such cases warrant addition of rituximab or would benefit from anthracycline-based regimens, such as a CHOP-R or EPOCH-R, remains to be seen. Recent studies have demonstrated the superior outcome of PMBLs with intensive chemotherapy regimens, such as EPOCH-R.[30] Misclassification of these cases as GZL may have prognostic

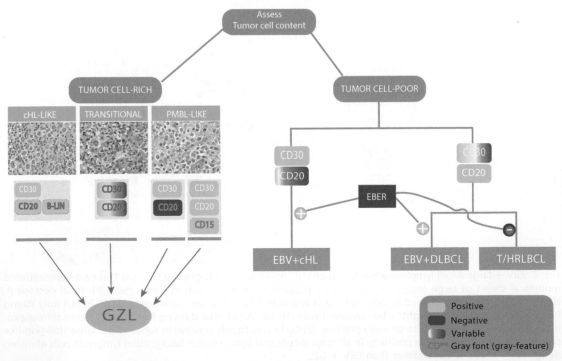

Fig. 5. Algorithm for morphologic assessment in the diagnosis of GZL using four major markers including CD20, CD30, CD15, and EBER. Gradient of colors with boxes indicate extent of positivity (*green*) or negative (*red*) in neoplastic cells for that marker. Transitional cases include cases with areas of cHL and PMBL/DLBCL within the same biopsy in different areas. Depicted image of transitional case shows composite Hodgkin-like cells in a background of large B cells with compartmentalizing sclerosis reminiscent of PMBL. Before entertaining GZL in cases with isolated strong CD20, other B-lineage markers must be performed to exclude possibility of nodular sclerosis, grade 2, which often shows variable loss of other B-lineage (B-LIN) markers including CD79a, OCT2, PAX5, and BOB.1.

implications in older patients in whom less intensive/toxic regimens, such as CHOP-R, would be beneficial. A prospective randomized trial comparing CHOP-R with EPOCH-R will clarify the most appropriate regimen for GZL in the frontline setting.

REFERENCES

1. Swerdlow SH, Campo E, Harris NL. WHO classification of tumours of haematopoietic and lymphoid tissues. 4th edition. Lyons (France): IARC press; 2008.

2. Swerdlow SH, Campo E, Harris NL, et al, editors. WHO classification of tumours of haematopoietic and lymphoid tissues (Revised 4th edition). Revised 4th edition. Lyons (France): IARC; 2017.

3. Rudiger T, Jaffe ES, Delsol G, et al. Workshop report on Hodgkin's disease and related diseases ('grey zone' lymphoma). Ann Oncol 1998;9(Suppl 5): S31–8.

4. Traverse-Glehen A, Pittaluga S, Gaulard P, et al. Mediastinal gray zone lymphoma: the missing link between classic Hodgkin's lymphoma and mediastinal large B-cell lymphoma. Am J Surg Pathol 2005;29(11):1411–21.

5. Eberle FC, Rodriguez-Canales J, Wei L, et al. Methylation profiling of mediastinal gray zone lymphoma reveals a distinctive signature with elements shared by classical Hodgkin's lymphoma and primary mediastinal large B-cell lymphoma. Haematologica 2011;96(4):558–66.

6. Eberle FC, Salaverria I, Steidl C, et al. Gray zone lymphoma: chromosomal aberrations with immunophenotypic and clinical correlations. Mod Pathol 2011;24(12):1586–97.

7. Evens AM, Kanakry JA, Sehn LH, et al. Gray zone lymphoma with features intermediate between classical Hodgkin lymphoma and diffuse large B-cell lymphoma: characteristics, outcomes, and prognostication among a large multicenter cohort. Am J Hematol 2015;90(9):778–83.

8. Wilson WH, Pittaluga S, Nicolae A, et al. A prospective study of mediastinal gray-zone lymphoma. Blood 2014;124(10):1563–9.

9. Pilichowska M, Pittaluga S, Ferry JA, et al. Clinicopathologic consensus study of gray zone lymphoma with features intermediate between DLBCL and classical HL. Blood Adv 2017;1(26):2600–9.

10. Sarkozy C, Copie-Bergmand C, Damotte D, et al. Gray-zone lymphoma between cHL and large B-cell lymphoma: a histopathologic series from the LYSA. Am J Surg Pathol 2019;43(3):341–51.

11. Nicolae A, Pittaluga S, Abdullah S, et al. EBV-positive large B-cell lymphomas in young patients: a nodal lymphoma with evidence for a tolerogenic immune environment. Blood 2015;126(7):863–72.

12. Elsayed AA, Satou A, Eladl AE, et al. Grey zone lymphoma with features intermediate between diffuse large B-cell lymphoma and classical Hodgkin lymphoma: a clinicopathological study of 14 Epstein-Barr virus-positive cases. Histopathology 2017; 70(4):579–94.

13. Quintanilla-Martinez L, de Jong D, de Mascarel A, et al. Gray zones around diffuse large B cell lymphoma. Conclusions based on the workshop of the XIV meeting of the European Association for Hematopathology and the Society of Hematopathology in Bordeaux, France. J Hematop 2009;2(4):211–36.

14. Copie-Bergman C, Gaulard P, Maouche-Chretien L, et al. The MAL gene is expressed in primary mediastinal large B-cell lymphoma. Blood 1999;94(10): 3567–75.

15. O'Malley DP, Fedoriw Y, Weiss LM. Distinguishing classical Hodgkin lymphoma, gray zone lymphoma, and large B-cell lymphoma: a proposed scoring system. Appl Immunohistochem Mol Morphol 2016; 24(8):535–40.

16. Tanaka Y, Maeshima AM, Nomoto J, et al. Expression pattern of PD-L1 and PD-L2 in classical Hodgkin lymphoma, primary mediastinal large B-cell lymphoma, and gray zone lymphoma. Eur J Haematol 2018;100(5):511–7.

17. Pelland K, Mathews S, Kamath A, et al. Dendritic cell markers and PD-L1 are expressed in mediastinal gray zone lymphoma. Appl Immunohistochem Mol Morphol 2018;26(10):e101–6.

18. von Wasielewski S, Franklin J, Fischer R, et al. Nodular sclerosing Hodgkin disease: new grading predicts prognosis in intermediate and advanced stages. Blood 2003;101(10):4063–9.

19. Haybittle JL, Hayhoe FG, Easterling MJ, et al. Review of British National Lymphoma Investigation studies of Hodgkin's disease and development of prognostic index. Lancet 1985;1(8435):967–72.

20. Lim MS, Beaty M, Sorbara L, et al. T-cell/histiocyte-rich large B-cell lymphoma: a heterogeneous entity with derivation from germinal center B cells. Am J Surg Pathol 2002;26(11):1458–66.

21. Dojcinov SD, Venkataraman G, Pittaluga S, et al. Age-related EBV-associated lymphoproliferative disorders in the Western population: a spectrum of reactive lymphoid hyperplasia and lymphoma. Blood 2011;117(18):4726–35.

22. Xu Y, McKenna RW, Hoang MP, et al. Composite angioimmunoblastic T-cell lymphoma and diffuse large B-cell lymphoma: a case report and review of the literature. Am J Clin Pathol 2002;118(6): 848–54.

23. Higgins JP, Warnke RA. CD30 expression is common in mediastinal large B-cell lymphoma. Am J Clin Pathol 1999;112(2):241–7.

24. Hao X, Wei X, Huang F, et al. The expression of CD30 based on immunohistochemistry predicts

inferior outcome in patients with diffuse large B-cell lymphoma. PLoS One 2015;10(5):e0126615.

25. Slack GW, Steidl C, Sehn LH, et al. CD30 expression in de novo diffuse large B-cell lymphoma: a population-based study from British Columbia. Br J Haematol 2014;167(5):608–17.

26. Hu S, Xu-Monette ZY, Balasubramanyam A, et al. CD30 expression defines a novel subgroup of diffuse large B-cell lymphoma with favorable prognosis and distinct gene expression signature: a report from the International DLBCL Rituximab-CHOP Consortium Program Study. Blood 2013; 121(14):2715–24.

27. Dunleavy K, Wilson WH. Primary mediastinal B-cell lymphoma and mediastinal gray zone lymphoma:

do they require a unique therapeutic approach? Blood 2015;125(1):33–9.

28. Sarkozy C, Molina T, Ghesquieres H, et al. Mediastinal gray zone lymphoma: clinico-pathological characteristics and outcomes of 99 patients from the Lymphoma Study Association. Haematologica 2017;102(1):150–9.

29. Portlock CS, Donnelly GB, Qin J, et al. Adverse prognostic significance of CD20 positive Reed–Sternberg cells in classical Hodgkin's disease. Br J Haematol 2004;125(6):701–8.

30. Dunleavy K, Pittaluga S, Maeda LS, et al. Dose-adjusted EPOCH-rituximab therapy in primary mediastinal B-cell lymphoma. N Engl J Med 2013; 368(15):1408–16.

Early Events in Lymphoid Neoplasms and Indolent Follicular Lymphomas

Sudhir Perincheri, MBBS, PhD

KEYWORDS

- In situ lymphoma • Monoclonal B-cell lymphocytosis • Indolent follicular lymphoma
- Duodenal type follicular lymphoma • In situ mantle cell neoplasia • In situ follicular neoplasia

Key Points

- Recent technical advances have led to the characterization of early and in situ lymphoid lesions.
- These early lesions share some clinicopathologic features with well-characterized mature B-cell lymphomas.
- Most of the early lesions have an indolent clinical course and have an excellent prognosis with conservative treatment regimens.

ABSTRACT

Technical advances in diagnostic modalities have led to the characterization of indolent lymphoid disorders similar to the in situ lesions described in epithelial malignancies. These early and indolent lymphoid lesions share clinicopathologic characteristics with well-characterized lymphoid malignancies such as chronic lymphocytic leukemia and follicular lymphoma. The in situ lesions have an indolent clinical course with only a minor subset shown to progress to frank malignancies. In addition to the in situ lesions, new indolent lymphoproliferative disorders have been recently characterized. Diagnosis and characterization of these indolent lesions is necessary to prevent overtreatment with aggressive therapeutic regimens.

OVERVIEW

The multihit model of tumorigenesis best exemplified by the adenoma–carcinoma sequence in colorectal carcinoma has been well-established in epithelial tumors. Until recently, however, such multistep evolution from atypical proliferations to in situ lesions to aggressive malignancies have not been typically characterized in lymphoid neoplasms. Technical advances in imaging, multiparameter flow cytometry, immunohistochemistry, and molecular diagnostics have led to the characterization of indolent and in situ lymphoproliferative disorders that may represent early events or lesions in lymphoid malignancies. These neoplasms include both definite and provisional entities in the most recent update to the World Health Organization classification of tumors of hematopoietic and lymphoid tissues.[1] They include B-cell lesions such as monoclonal B-cell lymphocytosis (MBL) and T-cell disorders such as indolent T-cell lymphoproliferative disorder of the gastrointestinal tract.

MONOCLONAL B-CELL LYMPHOCYTOSIS

Monoclonal B-cell lymphocytosis is defined by

- Monoclonal B cells less than 5×10^9/L in the peripheral blood, and
- Absence of associated lymphadenopathy, organomegaly, other extramedullary disorder, or any other feature of a B-cell lymphoproliferative disorder.[1]

Based on immunophenotype it is further subdivided into (1) chronic lymphocytic leukemia type

Disclosure Statement: The author has nothing to disclose.
Department of Pathology, Yale School of Medicine, 310 Cedar Street, Suite LB20, New Haven, CT 06510, USA
E-mail address: sudhir.perincheri@yale.edu

Surgical Pathology 12 (2019) 719–731
https://doi.org/10.1016/j.path.2019.03.004

surgpath.theclinics.com

(CLL-type; comprising approximately 75% of all MBLs), (2) atypical CLL-type, and (3) non–CLL-type.[1] Although some MBLs may be precursor lesions for CLL, monoclonal B-lymphocyte populations can be observed in the setting chronic infections and disorders of the immune system.[2]

MBL is asymptomatic and often detected incidentally by peripheral blood flow cytometry. CLL-type MBL is associated with advancing age, being virtually absent in those less than 40 years of age but affecting more than 50% of those 95 years or older.[3,4] Depending on the size of the monoclonal B-cell population, CLL-type MBL is subdivided into low-count MBL ($<0.5 \times 10^9$/L) or high-count MBL ($\geq 0.5 \times 10^9$/L).

MICROSCOPIC FEATURES

Morphologically, MBL is similar to CLL in the peripheral blood and is characterized by mature lymphocytes with round nuclei, condensed chromatin, and scant cytoplasm. Lymph node involvement by MBL shows nodal infiltration in an interfollicular or intersinusoidal pattern without proliferation centers in individuals without evidence of lymphadenopathy greater than 1.5 cm on a computed tomography scan.[5]

DIAGNOSIS

The diagnosis is often made incidentally during flow cytometry of peripheral blood and based on characteristic immunophenotype and molecular features. A subset of cases, especially high-count MBL, is detected during hematologic workup of lymphocytosis.[6]

CLL-type MBL has a similar immunophenotype to CLL

- The neoplastic cells are positive for CD19, CD20(DIM), CD5, and CD23; and
- Show dim light chain restriction or absent surface immunoglobulin.

Atypical CLL-type MBL differs from CLL-type MBL by often bright CD20 expression, being CD23 negative, and moderate to bright surface immunoglobulin positivity. Non–CLL-type MBL is often CD5 dim and shows moderate to bright surface immunoglobulin expression.[7]

Molecular Features

MBL shares many cytogenetic abnormalities with CLL such as 13q deletion and del17p. Additionally, similar to CLL, they show similar mutations in genes such as *NOTCH1*, *SF3B1*, and *TP53*. IGHV is often mutated.[8,9] A subset of non–CLL-type MBL show cytogenetic abnormalities involving chromosome 7q, a finding that has been used to invoke a relationship to splenic marginal zone lymphoma.[10]

DIFFERENTIAL DIAGNOSIS

It is important to exclude peripheral blood involvement by a systemic B-cell lymphoma-like mantle cell lymphoma, especially in cases with the atypical immunophenotype.

PROGNOSIS

Prognosis in MBL correlates with the monoclonal B-cell count. Low count MBLs usually do not progress, whereas high-count MBL can progress to CLL and is reported to require therapy at an annual rate of 1% to 2%. Most CLL cases arise from MBLs; however, not all MBLs progress to CLL.[11,12]

> ### Pathologic Key Features
> #### MONOCLONAL B-CELL LYMPHOCYTOSIS
>
> 1. MBL less than 5×10^9/L.
> 2. There are 3 types of MBLs: MBLs with a CLL phenotype (most common), MBL with an atypical CLL phenotype, and MBL with a non-CLL phenotype.
> 3. High-count MBL ($>0.5 \times 10^9$/L) is more likely to progress to CLL.

> ### Differential Diagnosis
> #### MONOCLONAL B-CELL LYMPHOCYTOSIS
>
> Peripheral blood involvement by mantle cell lymphoma or other B-cell lymphomas

> ### Pitfall
> #### DIAGNOSIS OF MONOCLONAL B-CELL LYMPHOCYTOSIS
>
> ! Cases thought to be MBL with atypical CLL or non-CLL type may represent peripheral blood involvement by a B-cell lymphoma

IN SITU MANTLE CELL NEOPLASIA

In situ mantle cell neoplasia (ISMCN) is a rare lesion characterized by presence of cyclin D1–positive lymphoid cells carrying *CCND1* rearrangements restricted to mantle cells of follicles in a background of lymphoid hyperplasia. Simultaneous peripheral blood or extranodal involvement may be present.[13]

MICROSCOPIC FEATURES

The lymph node architecture is usually preserved with intact sinuses and hyperplastic follicles. Often an incidental immunohistochemical workup to rule out a small B-cell lymphoma ends up highlighting cyclin D1–positive cells in the mantle cells.

DIAGNOSIS

The diagnosis is based on characteristic microscopic features outlined elsewhere in this article and characteristic distribution of cyclin D1–positive cells in the mantle zones, typically in the inner mantle zone (Fig. 1). In some instances, the cyclin D1–positive cells may be scattered throughout the mantle zone. The immunophenotype can sometimes be CD5 negative. Sox11 expression is often seen; however, a subset is Sox11 negative. The cyclin D1–positive cells carry the t(11;14) translocation.[13]

DIFFERENTIAL DIAGNOSIS

Involvement by early or overt mantle cell lymphoma should be excluded. In lymph node follicles where the entire mantle zone is expanded and shows a dense distribution cyclin D1–positive cells, a diagnosis of mantle cell lymphoma should be rendered. Often these cases also show interfollicular cyclin D1 positive cells.

PROGNOSIS

Most cases of ISMCN have been reported to have an indolent course. Rare cases are reported to have progressed to mantle cell lymphoma. A retrospective analysis of biopsies of patients with mantle cell lymphoma have identified ISMCN in the prior specimens. These studies imply a long latency period before ISMCN transforms to mantle cell lymphoma.[14]

Pathologic Key Features
IN SITU MANTLE CELL NEOPLASIA

1. ISMCN is rare lesion characterized by presence of cyclin D1–positive B cells in the mantle zones of lymphoid follicles.

2. They are diagnosed incidentally during immunohistochemical workup to rule out a small B-cell lymphoma in a reactive appearing lymph node.

3. Usually has an indolent course with only a minor subset reportedly progressing to mantle cell lymphoma.

Differential Diagnosis
IN SITU MANTLE CELL NEOPLASIA

Early mantle cell lymphoma: differs from ISMCN in having expanded mantle zones almost entirely replaced by cyclin D1–positive cells.

Pitfall
DIAGNOSIS OF IN SITU MANTLE CELL NEOPLASIA

! Important to differentiate from nodal involvement by early or overt nodal mantle cell lymphoma, which carries a worse prognosis.

LEUKEMIC NONNODAL MANTLE CELL LYMPHOMA

Leukemic nonnodal mantle cell lymphoma is characterized by peripheral blood, bone marrow, or splenic involvement with mantle cell lymphoma without significant adenopathy.[15]

DIAGNOSIS

The leukemic cells show mature small cell morphology. A subset is CD5 negative and, unlike classic mantle cell lymphomas, they may be CD200 positive. They are more likely to be SOX11 negative and IGHV mutated. They show the *CCDN1* translocation, but have many fewer chromosomal abnormalities than classic mantle cell lymphoma.[15–17]

PROGNOSIS

Leukemic nonnodal mantle cell lymphoma often has an indolent course. Rare cases with an aggressive course have been described, often associated with TP53 mutations.[18]

IN SITU FOLLICULAR NEOPLASIA

In situ follicular neoplasia (ISFN) is characterized by partial or total colonization of germinal centers by clonal BCL2-positive cells in an otherwise reactive lymph node.[19] The incidence of ISFN increases with age and has been associated with environmental exposure to herbicides and pesticides.[20] ISFN lesions can be seen simultaneously seen with other B-cell lymphomas and should be

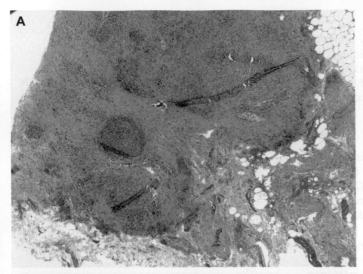

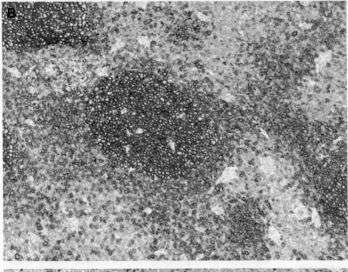

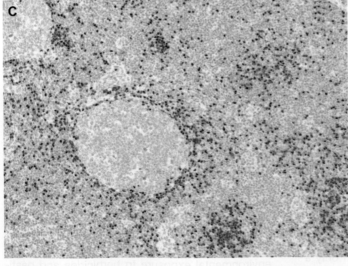

Fig. 1. ISMCN in excision of neck lymph node for localized lymphadenopathy. Hematoxylin and eosin sections show scattered small follicles in a reactive fibrotic background (*A*). CD20 highlights B cells in follicles (*B*) with cyclin D1–positive cells in the inner mantle zone (*C*). Concurrent flow cytometry showed a monoclonal CD5-positive B-cell population.

distinguished from partial involvement by follicular lymphoma (FL).[21]

MICROSCOPIC FEATURES

The lymph node architecture is preserved. As in the case of ISMCN, the diagnosis is made by immunohistochemical workup of a lymph node that looks reactive on hematoxylin and eosin evaluation (**Fig. 2**).

DIAGNOSIS

Immunostains show that the neoplastic follicles, composed almost entirely of centrocytes, are strongly BCL2 and CD10 positive (see **Fig. 2**). Adjacent noninvolved or partially involved follicles may be seen. Flow cytometry often detects a low population of CD10-positive clonal B cells in a background of polyclonal B cells.[21] Clonal IgH and BCL2 rearrangements are present; however, owing to the low level of involvement, microdissection of tissue may be necessary to increase sensitivity of detection by fluorescence in situ hybridization.[19] Very few other chromosomal abnormalities are detected by array comparative genome hybridization. Similar to nodal FLs, *EZH2* mutations and deletions of 1p36 involving the *TNFRSF14* gene have also been characterized in ISFN.[22,23]

DIFFERENTIAL DIAGNOSIS

The main differential diagnosis of ISFN is partial nodal involvement by FL that carries a worse prognosis. Unlike ISFN, partial nodal involvement by FL shows at least partial effacement of nodal architecture.[24] In addition, the follicles are usually enlarged with neoplastic follicles often seen back to back, have attenuated mantle zones, variable CD10, and BCL2 expression in contrast to the strong BCL2 and CD10 staining seen in ISFN. Follicles in reactive follicular hyperplasia are CD10 positive but BCL2 negative.

PROGNOSIS

The clinical associations of ISFN are varied. Some patients have a prior history of FL, some have concurrent lymphoma and some subsequently develop lymphoma.[19,21,24] Patients with no evidence of FL do quite well. However, given the possibility of concurrent lymphoma, in patients with ISFN and clinical or radiologic evidence of lymphadenopathy at a different site, biopsy of other enlarged lymph nodes should be recommended.

Pathologic Key Features
IN SITU FOLLICULAR NEOPLASIA

1. ISFN is often detected by immunohistochemical workup of reactive-appearing lymph nodes.

2. Characterized by partial or complete colonization of follicles by BCL2-positive B cells.

3. May be associated with FL or a B-cell lymphoma at a different site.

Differential Diagnosis
IN SITU FOLLICULAR NEOPLASIA

FL: lymph node architectural effacement, attenuated mantle zones, variable BCL2 and CD10 expression.

Reactive follicular hyperplasia: follicles are CD10 positive BCL2 negative.

Pitfall
DIAGNOSIS OF IN SITU FOLLICULAR NEOPLASIA

! Partial nodal involvement by FL may mimic ISFN but carries a worse prognosis.

DUODENAL-TYPE FOLLICULAR LYMPHOMA

Duodenal-type FL is a FL affecting the small intestine, predominantly involving the second portion of the duodenum. These indolent lymphomas are usually seen as incidental duodenal polyps during endoscopies performed for other reasons. There is often concurrent involvement of the more distal small intestine in a majority of the cases.[25] Molecular similarities to mucosa-associated lymphoid tissue (MALT) lymphoma raise the possibility of a mucosal antigen driven process.[26]

MICROSCOPIC FEATURES

The neoplastic follicles are seen submucosally and are characterized by low-grade lesions composed predominantly of centrocytes (**Fig. 3**). The cytologic grade of the follicles corresponds with grades 1 to 2 nodal FLs.

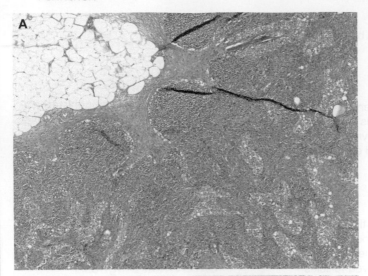

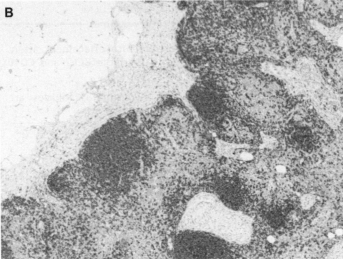

Fig. 2. ISFN in inguinal lymph node of a 59-year-old man. Note the widely spaced follicles and open sinuses (*A*). CD20 highlights the B cells in the follicles (*B*). A subset of the follicles shows colonization by ISFN with strong positivity for CD10

DIAGNOSIS

Similar to nodal FL, the neoplastic follicles are CD20, CD10, and BCL2 positive. A characteristic feature is that the follicular dendritic cell network is seen limited to the periphery with CD21 staining.[27] Although not routinely tested for, the neoplastic cells express the IgA heavy chain and the intestinal homing receptor alpha4beta7.[28] The neoplastic cells carry the t(14:18) (q32;q21) translocation. Biased IGHV use similar to MALT lymphomas has been seen raising the possibility of antigen induced pathogenesis.[26]

DIFFERENTIAL DIAGNOSIS

The main differential diagnosis is intestinal involvement by nodal FL. The lesions in FL are often more extensive and show more infiltrative pattern.[29] However, in the absence of adequate clinical and radiologic staging information, it is advisable to be cautious in rendering a definitive diagnosis. In such situations a diagnosis of involvement by FL with a discussion of the differential diagnosis is more appropriate. MALT lymphomas usually show a null immunophenotype being typically CD10 and BCL6 negative. Reactive follicular hyperplasia involving the intestinal mucosa also has a distinct immunophenotype: CD20 and CD10 positive but BCL2 negative.

PROGNOSIS

Duodenal-type FL has a favorable prognosis with only a small proportion of cases showing disease progression. There is no single defined optimal therapy given the rarity of the disease. Watch-

Fig. 2. (*continued*). (*C*) and BCL2 (*D*). Note the stronger BCL2 staining of the neoplastic cells. Flow cytometry showed a clonal CD10-positive B-cell population. The patient had concurrent retroperitoneal lymphadenopathy, biopsies of which revealed a nodal FL, WHO grades 1-2.2.

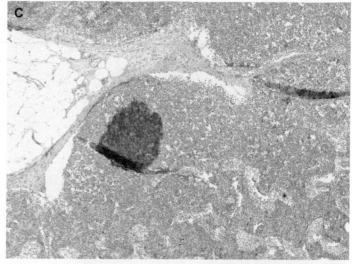

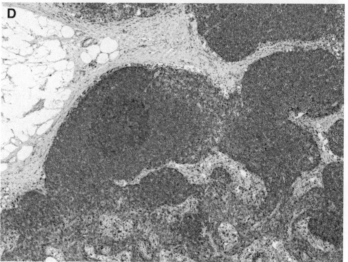

and-wait approaches, radiation, and single agent treatment with rituximab, as well as chemotherapy have been used for treatment with good outcomes.[30,31]

Pathologic Key Features
DUODENAL-TYPE FOLLICULAR LYMPHOMA

1. Submucosal involvement of duodenal mucosa with lymphoma of follicle center phenotype.

2. The neoplastic follicles are composed almost entirely of centrocytes.

3. Often associated with simultaneous involvement of distal small intestine.

4. Follicular dendritic cells are located at the periphery of the neoplastic follicles.

Differential Diagnosis
DUODENAL-TYPE FOLLICULAR LYMPHOMA

Intestinal involvement by FL

MALT lymphoma

Reactive follicular hyperplasia

Pitfall
DIAGNOSIS OF DUODENAL-TYPE FOLLICULAR LYMPHOMA

! Intestinal involvement by FL, which carries a worse prognosis.

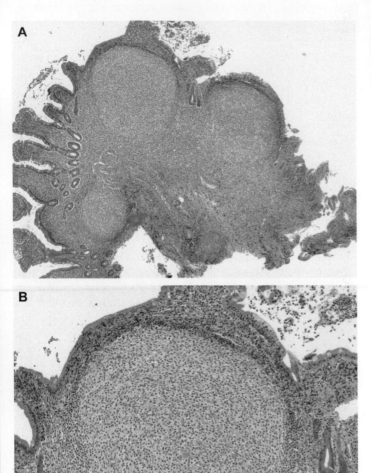

A

B

Fig. 3. Duodenal-type FL. Duodenal biopsies in a 64-year-old man showing submucosal lymphoid nodules (*A*). The nodules are almost entirely composed of centrocytes (*B*).

PEDIATRIC-TYPE FOLLICULAR LYMPHOMA

Pediatric-type FL is a lymphoma of follicular center phenotype that usually affects children and young adults (median age, 15–18 years). There is a marked male predominance with a male:female ratio of greater than 10:1. Patients usually present with peripheral lymphadenopathy, most often in the head and neck region.[32,33]

MICROSCOPIC FEATURES

The lymph node architecture is effaced by pure follicular proliferation comprised numerous expanded or serpiginous follicles. The neoplastic cells are often intermediate in size with blastoid

morphology (**Fig. 4**). Abundant admixed histiocytes can be seen, imparting a starry sky pattern.

DIAGNOSIS

The neoplastic cells are CD20 positive B cells that coexpress CD10 and BCL6 but are often negative for BCL2 (see **Fig. 4**). Unlike low-grade FLs, the Ki67 proliferation index is often high (>30%). CD21 highlights the expanded/serpiginous follicular dendritic cell networks. Flow cytometry often shows the presence of clonal CD10-positive B cells. Clonal immunoglobulin gene rearrangements are present; however, unlike nodal FL rearrangements involving *BCL2*, the *BCL6* and *IRF4* genes are absent.[33] Loss of heterozygosity at

Fig. 4. Pediatric-type FL. Neck lymph node in a 16-year old boy. Low-power view shows architectural effacement by expanded follicles with admixed histiocytes (*A*). On higher power, the neoplastic follicles show intermediate-sized cells with open chromatin and variably prominent nucleoli (*B*). CD21 highlights expanded, serpiginous FDC networks (*C*). The neoplastic B cells are CD20 positive

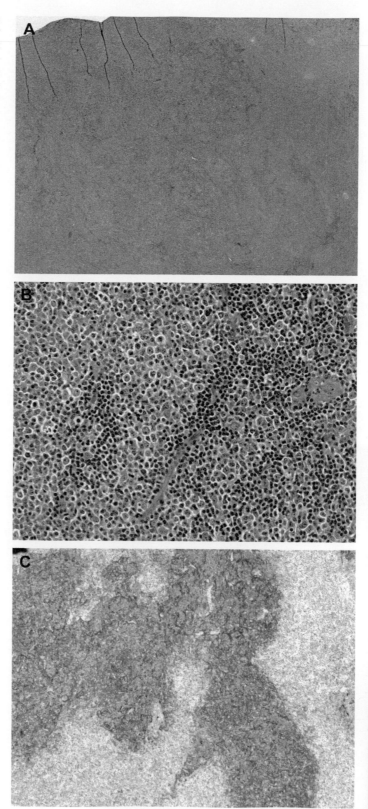

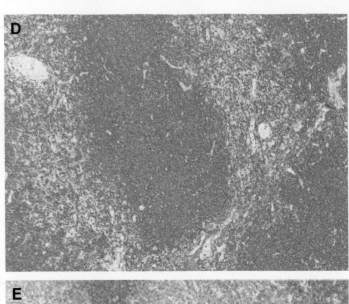

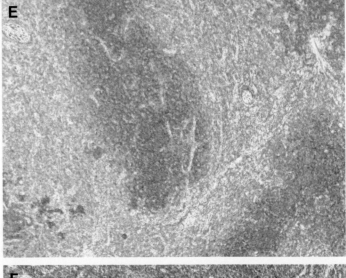

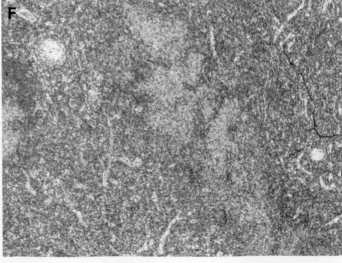

Fig. 4. *(continued)*. (*D*) and coexpress CD10 (*E*), but are negative for BCL2 (*F*).

1p36 and deletions or mutations affecting *TNFRSF14* are seen in a subset of cases. A significant number of cases have *MAP2K1* mutations.[34,35] In addition to the morphologic, immunophenotypic, and molecular characteristics, nodal and early stage (stages I–II) disease are required clinical criteria for diagnosis of pediatric type FL. The presence of areas that meet morphologic criteria for a diagnosis of diffuse large B-cell lymphoma precludes a diagnosis of pediatric-type FL.

DIFFERENTIAL DIAGNOSIS

The differential diagnosis includes neoplastic entities such as nodal involvement by grade 3 FL, large B-cell lymphoma with IRF4 rearrangement, and benign reactive follicular hyperplasia with associated clonal CD10-positive B-cell populations. The distinction from grade 3 FL is especially important in older adults, and the diagnosis of PTFL should be made with caution in those greater than 25 years. Unlike FL and large B-cell lymphoma with IRF4 rearrangement, pediatric-type FL is negative for rearrangements involving the *BCL2*, *BCL6*, *IRF4* loci and does not show aberrant rearrangements of IG. LBCL with *IRF4* rearrangement is seen primarily in the lymph nodes of the Waldeyer's ring and shows strong expression of IRF4/MUM1. Reactive follicular hyperplasia is young adults may show low levels of monoclonal CD10-positive B cells; however, monoclonal IG rearrangements are not seen in these conditions.

PROGNOSIS

The prognosis of pediatric-type FL is excellent, with most cases in children being cured by surgical excision alone. Adults treated with chemotherapeutic regimens have also been reported to show excellent survival.[35,36]

Pathologic Key Features
PEDIATRIC-TYPE FOLLICULAR LYMPHOMA

1. Pediatric-type FL is seen in young adults, shows a strong male predominance, and usually presents with isolated peripheral lymphadenopathy.

2. Pediatric-type FL is characterized by architectural effacement by large expansile follicles containing intermediate size cells with blastoid morphology.

3. They are BCL6 positive, show high Ki67 proliferation index ,and are often BCL2 negative or weakly positive.

4. Pediatric-type FL lacks *BCL2*, *BCL6*, *IRF4*, or aberrant Ig rearrangement and *BCL2* amplification.

Differential Diagnosis
OF **PEDIATRIC-TYPE FOLLICULAR LYMPHOMA**

Grade 3 FL: usually has *BCL2* or *BCL6* translocations.

Large B-cell lymphoma with *IRF4* rearrangement: high IRF4/MUM1 expression and *IRF4* rearrangement by fluorescence in situ hybridization.

Reactive follicular hyperplasia with clonal CD10 B-cells: lack clonal IG rearrangements

Pitfalls
DIAGNOSIS OF PEDIATRIC-TYPE FOLLICULAR LYMPHOMA

! Distinction from a grade 3 FL is critical, especially in older adults, but may be difficult.

REFERENCES

1. Swerlow SH, Campo E, Harris NL, et al, editors. WHO classification of tumors of hematopoietic and lymphoid tissues. 4th edition. Lyon (France): IARC; 2017.
2. Fazi C, Dagklis A, Cottini F, et al. Monoclonal B cell lymphocytosis in hepatitis C virus infected individuals. Cytometry B Clin Cytom 2010;78(Suppl 1): S61–8.
3. Ghia P, Prato G, Scielzo C, et al. Monoclonal CD5+ and CD5- B-lymphocyte expansions are frequent in the peripheral blood of the elderly. Blood 2004; 103(6):2337–42.
4. Nieto WG, Almeida J, Romero A, et al. Increased frequency (12%) of circulating chronic lymphocytic leukemia-like B-cell clones in healthy subjects using a highly sensitive multicolor flow cytometry approach. Blood 2009;114(1):33–7.
5. Gibson SE, Swerdlow SH, Ferry JA, et al. Reassessment of small lymphocytic lymphoma in the era of monoclonal B-cell lymphocytosis. Haematologica 2011;96(8):1144–52.
6. Rawstron AC, Shanafelt T, Lanasa MC, et al. Different biology and clinical outcome according to

the absolute numbers of clonal B-cells in monoclonal B-cell lymphocytosis (MBL). Cytometry B Clin Cytom 2010;78(Suppl 1):S19–23.

7. Shanafelt TD, Ghia P, Lanasa MC, et al. Monoclonal B-cell lymphocytosis (MBL): biology, natural history and clinical management. Leukemia 2010;24(3): 512–20.

8. Puente XS, Bea S, Valdes-Mas R, et al. Non-coding recurrent mutations in chronic lymphocytic leukaemia. Nature 2015;526(7574):519–24.

9. Kern W, Bacher U, Haferlach C, et al. Monoclonal B-cell lymphocytosis is closely related to chronic lymphocytic leukaemia and may be better classified as early-stage CLL. Br J Haematol 2012;157(1): 86–96.

10. Xochelli A, Kalpadakis C, Gardiner A, et al. Clonal B-cell lymphocytosis exhibiting immunophenotypic features consistent with a marginal-zone origin: is this a distinct entity? Blood 2014;123(8):1199–206.

11. Fazi C, Scarfo L, Pecciarini L, et al. General population low-count CLL-like MBL persists over time without clinical progression, although carrying the same cytogenetic abnormalities of CLL. Blood 2011;118(25):6618–25.

12. Rawstron AC, Bennett FL, O'Connor SJ, et al. Monoclonal B-cell lymphocytosis and chronic lymphocytic leukemia. N Engl J Med 2008;359(6):575–83.

13. Carvajal-Cuenca A, Sua LF, Silva NM, et al. In situ mantle cell lymphoma: clinical implications of an incidental finding with indolent clinical behavior. Haematologica 2012;97(2):270–8.

14. Adam P, Schiefer AI, Prill S, et al. Incidence of pre-clinical manifestations of mantle cell lymphoma and mantle cell lymphoma in situ in reactive lymphoid tissues. Mod Pathol 2012;25(12):1629–36.

15. Orchard J, Garand R, Davis Z, et al. A subset of t(11;14) lymphoma with mantle cell features displays mutated IgVH genes and includes patients with good prognosis, nonnodal disease. Blood 2003; 101(12):4975–81.

16. Espinet B, Ferrer A, Bellosillo B, et al. Distinction between asymptomatic monoclonal B-cell lymphocytosis with cyclin D1 overexpression and mantle cell lymphoma: from molecular profiling to flow cytometry. Clin Cancer Res 2014;20(4):1007–19.

17. Fernandez V, Salamero O, Espinet B, et al. Genomic and gene expression profiling defines indolent forms of mantle cell lymphoma. Cancer Res 2010;70(4): 1408–18.

18. Royo C, Navarro A, Clot G, et al. Non-nodal type of mantle cell lymphoma is a specific biological and clinical subgroup of the disease. Leukemia 2012; 26(8):1895–8.

19. Cong P, Raffeld M, Teruya-Feldstein J, et al. In situ localization of follicular lymphoma: description and analysis by laser capture microdissection. Blood 2002;99(9):3376–82.

20. Agopian J, Navarro JM, Gac AC, et al. Agricultural pesticide exposure and the molecular connection to lymphomagenesis. J Exp Med 2009;206(7): 1473–83.

21. Pillai RK, Surti U, Swerdlow SH. Follicular lymphoma-like B cells of uncertain significance (in situ follicular lymphoma) may infrequently progress, but precedes follicular lymphoma, is associated with other overt lymphomas and mimics follicular lymphoma in flow cytometric studies. Haematologica 2013;98(10):1571–80.

22. Schmidt J, Salaverria I, Haake A, et al. Increasing genomic and epigenomic complexity in the clonal evolution from in situ to manifest t(14;18)-positive follicular lymphoma. Leukemia 2014;28(5):1103–12.

23. Mamessier E, Song JY, Eberle FC, et al. Early lesions of follicular lymphoma: a genetic perspective. Haematologica 2014;99(3):481–8.

24. Jogalian AG, Eberle FC, Pack SD, et al. Follicular lymphoma in situ: clinical implications and comparisons with partial involvement by follicular lymphoma. Blood 2011;118(11):2976–84.

25. Misdraji J, Harris NL, Hasserjian RP, et al. Primary follicular lymphoma of the gastrointestinal tract. Am J Surg Pathol 2011;35(9):1255–63.

26. Sato Y, Ichimura K, Tanaka T, et al. Duodenal follicular lymphomas share common characteristics with mucosa-associated lymphoid tissue lymphomas. J Clin Pathol 2008;61(3):377–81.

27. Takata K, Sato Y, Nakamura N, et al. Duodenal and nodal follicular lymphomas are distinct: the former lacks activation-induced cytidine deaminase and follicular dendritic cells despite ongoing somatic hypermutations. Mod Pathol 2009;22(7):940–9.

28. Bende RJ, Smit LA, Bossenbroek JG, et al. Primary follicular lymphoma of the small intestine: alpha4-beta7 expression and immunoglobulin configuration suggest an origin from local antigen-experienced B cells. Am J Pathol 2003;162(1):105–13.

29. Shia J, Teruya-Feldstein J, Pan D, et al. Primary follicular lymphoma of the gastrointestinal tract: a clinical and pathologic study of 26 cases. Am J Surg Pathol 2002;26(2):216–24.

30. Schmatz AI, Streubel B, Kretschmer-Chott E, et al. Primary follicular lymphoma of the duodenum is a distinct mucosal/submucosal variant of follicular lymphoma: a retrospective study of 63 cases. J Clin Oncol 2011;29(11):1445–51.

31. Mori M, Kobayashi Y, Maeshima AM, et al. The indolent course and high incidence of t(14;18) in primary duodenal follicular lymphoma. Ann Oncol 2010; 21(7):1500–5.

32. Liu Q, Salaverria I, Pittaluga S, et al. Follicular lymphomas in children and young adults: a comparison of the pediatric variant with usual follicular lymphoma. Am J Surg Pathol 2013;37(3): 333–43.

33. Louissaint A Jr, Ackerman AM, Dias-Santagata D, et al. Pediatric-type nodal follicular lymphoma: an indolent clonal proliferation in children and adults with high proliferation index and no BCL2 rearrangement. Blood 2012;120(12): 2395–404.

34. Louissaint A Jr, Schafernak KT, Geyer JT, et al. Pediatric-type nodal follicular lymphoma: a biologically distinct lymphoma with frequent MAPK pathway mutations. Blood 2016;128(8): 1093–100.

35. Martin-Guerrero I, Salaverria I, Burkhardt B, et al. Recurrent loss of heterozygosity in 1p36 associated with TNFRSF14 mutations in IRF4 translocation negative pediatric follicular lymphomas. Haematologica 2013;98(8):1237–41.

36. Attarbaschi A, Beishuizen A, Mann G, et al. Children and adolescents with follicular lymphoma have an excellent prognosis with either limited chemotherapy or with a "Watch and wait" strategy after complete resection. Ann Hematol 2013;92(11): 1537–41.

New/Revised Entities in Gastrointestinal Lymphoproliferative Disorders

Sarmad H. Jassim, MD, Lauren B. Smith, MD*

KEYWORDS

• Lymphoma • Non-Hodgkin • Enteropathy-associated • EATL • MEITL

Key Points

- Enteropathy-associated T-cell lymphoma (EATL) is now a distinct and rare entity that has only one type, is associated with celiac disease, and has increased incidence in Western countries.

- Monomorphic epitheliotropic intestinal T-cell lymphoma, previously known as EATL type II, is not associated with celiac disease.

- Indolent T-cell lymphoproliferative disorder of the gastrointestinal tract is a new provisional entity and can affect multiple sites in the gastrointestinal tract.

- Intestinal T-cell lymphoma, not otherwise specified (NOS), although not considered a specific disease entity, is used when a diagnosis of intestinal T-cell lymphoma does not fit the criteria of other intestinal lymphomas, especially in small biopsies.

ABSTRACT

The gastrointestinal tract is a common extranodal site of involvement by lymphomas. These may be diagnostically challenging because they can mimic a variety of benign conditions and may be difficult to subclassify when malignant. The classification of gastrointestinal lymphomas is an evolving area with some recent changes. Although some of these entities are rare, they are important to recognize because of the variable clinical presentations, comorbidities, and treatment implications. This article explores new and revised entities in gastrointestinal lymphoproliferative disorders.

ENTEROPATHY-ASSOCIATED T-CELL LYMPHOMA

OVERVIEW

Enteropathy-associated T-cell lymphoma (EATL) is now a distinct and rare entity that has only one type. This condition tends to occur in patients of northern European descent[1–4] and is the most common subtype of primary intestinal T-cell lymphoma in Western countries.[4,5] It is a clinically aggressive intestinal lymphoma that tends to affect patients in their sixth to seventh decade with a slight male predominance (**Tables 1 and 2**).[4–9]

Disclosure Statement: The authors have nothing to disclose.
Pathology Department, University of Michigan, 2800 Plymouth Road, North Campus Research Complex, Building 36, Ann Arbor, MI, USA
* Corresponding author.
E-mail address: lbsmith@med.umich.edu

Surgical Pathology 12 (2019) 733–743
https://doi.org/10.1016/j.path.2019.03.011

Table 1
Comparison of enteropathy-associated T-cell lymphoma and monomorphic epitheliotropic intestinal T-cell lymphoma

Features	Enteropathy-Associated T-Cell Lymphoma	Monomorphic Epitheliotropic Intestinal T-Cell Lymphoma
Ethnicity	Northern European	Asian and Hispanic
Risk factors	Celiac disease (refractory type 2) HLA-DQ2/DQ8	None
Age at presentation	Adults in sixth to seventh decades	Adults
Morphology	Pleomorphic	Monomorphic
Cytology	Intermediate to large cells	Small to intermediate cells with round contours
Background pathology	Prominent eosinophils	Rare scattered eosinophils
Necrosis	Prominent necrosis	Rare necrosis
Adjacent mucosa	Villous blunting, intraepithelial lymphocytes	Intraepithelial lymphocytes near tumor
Immunophenotype	Usually CD4 and CD8 negative	Usually CD8 and CD56 positive

KEY POINTS

- Clinically aggressive and rare entity
- Northern European origin
- Associated with celiac disease (refractory type 2)
- Associated with HLA-DQ2 and HLA-DQ8
- Small intestine, most commonly the jejunum and ileum
- Grossly presents as ulcerating nodules, plaques, strictures, or less commonly large exophytic mass[4]
- Pleomorphic cells with frequent eosinophils and necrosis
- CD3$^+$, CD7$^+$, CD5$^-$, CD4$^-$, CD8$^-$, CD56$^-$, CD103$^+$, CD30$^{+/-}$, cytotoxic-positive (TIA1 > granzyme B > perforin)

Table 2
New entities in gastrointestinal lymphoproliferative disorders

Diagnosis	Site	Histology	Immunophenotype	Clinical Behavior
EATL	Small intestine	Polymorphic cellular composition Intraepithelial T lymphocytes with αβ TCR expression more than γδ	CD3$^+$, CD5$^-$, CD4$^-$, CD7$^+$, CD8$^-$, CD56$^-$, CD103$^+$, CD30$^{+/-}$, cytotoxic-positive	Aggressive
MEITL	Small intestine	Monomorphic cellular composition Intraepithelial T lymphocytes with γδ TCR expression more than αβ	CD3$^+$, CD5$^-$, CD4$^-$, CD7$^+$, CD8$^+$, CD56$^+$, CD103$^{+/-}$, CD30$^-$, cytotoxic-positive	Aggressive
Indolent T-cell lymphoproliferative disorder of the gastrointestinal tract	Multiple sites small bowel and colon	Small monotonous lamina propria infiltration of peripheral clonal mature small T lymphocytes with αβ TCR expression	CD2$^+$, CD3$^+$, CD5$^+$, CD7$^{+/-}$, CD8$^{+/-}$, CD56$^-$, CD4$^{-/+}$	Indolent
Intestinal T-cell lymphoma, NOS	Primarily Colon	Variable	Variable	Aggressive

- Usually αβ T-cell receptor expression
- Demonstrate frequent gains of 1q and 5q, amplification of 9q34 (*ABL1* and *NOTCH1* genes), and P53 overexpression

PATHOGENESIS

The pathogenesis of EATL is strongly associated with celiac disease/gluten sensitive enteropathy and is a feared complication of this condition.[10–14] Patients demonstrate higher levels of antiendomysial (or antitissue transglutaminase 2) antibodies, HLA-DQ2 or HLA-DQ8 alleles, and dermatitis herpetiformis,[15] and demonstrate gluten sensitivity with a protective effect of gluten-free diet.[4,12,16–26] Risk factors linked to EATL are duration and dose of gluten exposure, advanced age,[7,23–25] and HLA-DQ2 allele homozygosity.[4,23,26]

CLINICAL PRESENTATION

The diagnosis of celiac disease can precede EATL or be concomitant at presentation.[4] Therefore, a diagnosis of preexisting celiac disease is not a prerequisite for diagnosis. Some individuals have life-long silent gluten sensitivity and may be diagnosed with EATL after death and autopsy.[4,6–8,27,28] Although the small intestine including the jejunum and ileum[5–8] are most commonly involved, either focally or multifocally,[5,6] other parts of the gastrointestinal have also been involved including the large intestine and stomach.[4,5] Occasionally, extraintestinal manifestation is the primary presentation including skin,[29] lymph nodes, spleen, or central nervous system.[4,5,7,30,31] Symptoms at presentation are variable.[32,33] The duration of symptoms before diagnosis is also variable,[6] but usually less than 3 months.[8] High-stage disease is detected in 43% to 90%.[5–8]

CLINICAL FEATURES AND LABORATORY FINDINGS

- Abdominal pain (65%–100%)
- Diarrhea (40%–70%)
- Gluten-insensitive malabsorption (40%–70%)
- Recurrence of symptoms in patients with history of celiac disease and prior response to gluten-free diet
- Weight loss (50%–80%)
- Nausea or vomiting caused by intestinal obstruction
- Intestinal perforation (25%–50%)
- Hemorrhage
- B-symptoms (less than one-third of cases)
- Anorexia
- Fatigue

- Early satiety
- Hemophagocytic syndrome (16%–40%)
- Low serum albumin (76%–88%)
- Increased lactate dehydrogenase (LDH) (25%–62%)

REFRACTORY CELIAC DISEASE AND ITS ROLE IN ENTEROPATHY-ASSOCIATED T-CELL LYMPHOMA PATHOGENESIS

Although EATL most frequently arises from refractory celiac disease type 2, *de novo* EATL in individuals without celiac disease has also been described.[10] Based on immunophenotypic and molecular criteria,[29] refractory celiac disease is a biologically heterogeneous disorder[23,34–36] and is divided into type 1 and type 2.[4] Refractory celiac disease is defined as persistent gastrointestinal symptoms and abnormal small intestinal mucosal architecture with increased intraepithelial lymphocytes despite a strict gluten-free diet for greater than 6 to 12 months.[37] This requires exclusion of celiac disease–related conditions including bacterial overgrowth, microscopic colitis, and other small intestinal disorders, such as common variable immunodeficiency and autoimmune enteropathy.[38,39] Primary refractory celiac disease is lack of response to a gluten-free diet at diagnosis and secondary refractory celiac disease is onset of symptoms after response to a gluten-free diet.

In type 1 refractory celiac disease, the histology is similar to celiac disease and reveals intraepithelial lymphocytes with normal immunophenotype (CD8+ and CD3+) with no evidence of T-cell receptor gene rearrangement and no genetic or molecular alterations.[4] It accounts for 68% to 90% of all refractory cases,[4,23,24,34–36,40] has milder symptoms,[23] and higher survival rate (80%–96%) with low risk of developing EATL (3%–15% in 4–6 years).[23,24,34,36] In type 1 refractory celiac disease, there is sustained inflammation caused by surreptitious gluten ingestion in most cases[41] or by an autoimmune phenomenon in a minority of cases.[39,42]

In type 2 refractory celiac disease the small intestine is severely atrophic and reveals widely distributed clonal intraepithelial lymphocytes with minimal cytologic atypia.[23,43,44] An aberrant immunophenotype is present demonstrating clonality on T-cell receptor gene rearrangement studies.[4] Ulcerative jejunitis can develop in some cases.[43,45–47] Type 2 refractory celiac disease[7,23,44] is now recognized as a precursor lesion of EATL. Intensive therapy for refractory celiac disease type 2 is required to improve survival and reduce progression to EATL.[48] Identical TCR gene rearrangement between type 2 refractory celiac disease and concurrent or subsequent EATL helped establish that the aberrant intraepithelial lymphocytes are precursor cells and constitute a population of neoplastic cells, which has been variably called low-grade lymphoma of intraepithelial T lymphocytes, EATL in situ, or cryptic EATL.[43,45,46,49,50]

Symptoms in refractory celiac disease are severe in most patients with profound malnourishment caused by protein-losing enteropathy,[23,24,36] large ulcers, and stenotic areas.[23] Survival rate is low at approximately 50% with one-third to one-half of patients developing EATL over 4 to 6 years.[23,24,34,36]

GROSS AND MICROSCOPIC FEATURES OF ENTEROPATHY-ASSOCIATED T-CELL LYMPHOMA

Examination of the involved gastrointestinal specimen may reveal ulcerating nodules, plaques, strictures, or exophytic masses with common involvement of the mesentery and mesenteric lymph nodes.[4] Involvement of lymph nodes without macroscopic evidence of intestinal disease is seen occasionally.[4]

Histologically, EATL consists of large, pleomorphic lymphocytes (**Fig. 1**A, B).[4,7,51] The cells demonstrate round or angulated vesicular nuclei with prominent nucleoli and moderately abundant pale cytoplasm. Forty percent of cases show a predominance of large anaplastic cells, which are positive for CD30.[7] Other frequent histopathologic features include angiocentricity and angioinvasion and areas of extensive necrosis (**Fig. 1**D). The background inflammatory cells may consist of many eosinophils (See **Fig. 1**B), including cases with eosinophilic abscesses. Intraepithelial spread of tumor cells is variable. The neighboring mucosa usually shows features of celiac disease including villous atrophy, crypt hyperplasia, intraepithelial lymphocytes, increased lamina propria lymphocytes, and plasma cells (**Fig. 1**C).[52,50] Intraepithelial lymphocytes in the adjacent uninvolved mucosa may exhibit a normal immunophenotype in *de novo* EATL or an aberrant immunophenotype similar to EATL (See **Tables 1** and **2** for complete

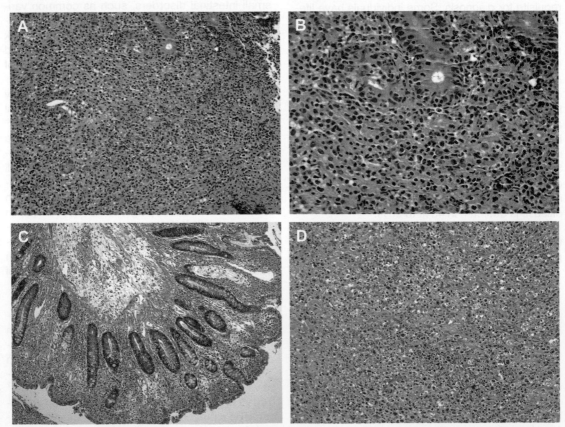

Fig. 1. EATL. (*A, B*) Pleomorphic lymphocytic infiltrate in inflammatory background prominent eosinophils (hematoxylin-eosin [H&E], original magnification ×200 [*A*] and ×400 [*B*]). (*C*) The adjacent mucosa demonstrates features of celiac disease with villous blunting and intraepithelial lymphocytes (H&E, original magnification, ×100). (*D*) Necrosis can be prominent in EATL (H&E, original magnification, ×200).

immunophenotypic signature). Studies have found that most cases reveal aberrant T lymphocytes of $\alpha\beta$ lineage.

GENETIC PROFILE

Recurrent gains of chromosome 1q22 to 44 in refractory celiac disease type 2 and EATL[23,54–57] are also suggestive of early acquisition of 1q abnormalities in the evolution of EATL. Progression to refractory celiac disease has been linked to 7p14.3 locus in one study.[58] Loss of p16 protein in absence of loss of heterozygosity at chromosome 9p21 is seen in 40% of type 2 refractory celiac disease with ulcerative jejunitis and aberrant nuclear p53 expression is detected in 57% of cases in the absence of TP53 mutations.[59]

TCRy or TCRB are clonally rearranged in all cases.[7,45,60] Most cases of EATL (80%) display gains of 9q34 region, which harbors proto-oncogenes, such as NOTCH1, ABL1, and VAV2, or alternatively show deletions of 16q12.1.[54,55,57,61] Chromosomal gains of 1q and 5q are more common in EATL when compared with monomorphic epitheliotropic intestinal T-cell lymphoma (MEITL).[55,57,62] Trisomy 1q24-q44 is noted in greater than 75% of cases.[55,62] Losses of 9p, and loss of heterozygosity at 9p21, targeting the cell cycle inhibitor CDKN2A/B, are observed in 56% of cases accompanied by loss of p16 protein expression.[57,59] Loss of 17p12 to 13.2 region containing the TP53 tumor suppressor gene is noted in 23% of EATL but aberrant nuclear p53 expression is seen in 75% of cases.[55,59] Recurrent mutations in JAK-STAT signaling in EATL,[63] and detection of JAK1 and STAT3 mutations in type 2 refractory celiac disease, indicate JAK-STAT signaling dysregulation to be an early event in pathogenesis.[64] In one study, SETD2 was described in 32% of cases of EATL as the most frequently silenced gene.[65] The same study found the JAK-STAT pathway to be the most frequently mutated pathway with frequent mutations in STAT5B, JAK1, JAK3, STAT3, and SOCS1.[65] Although the authors described overlapping gene alterations among patients with EATL type 1 and EATL type 2 (now known as MEITL), they confirmed the loss of SETD2 was associated with expansion of γδ T cells.[65]

EATL is associated with the HLA-DQA1*0501 and HLA-DQB1*0201 genotypes.[26] More than 90% of patients with EATL carry HLA-DQ2.5 heterodimers encoded by HLA-DQA1*05 and HLA-DQB1*02 alleles either in cis or trans configuration.[21]

PROGNOSIS AND THERAPY

Patients with EATL have a median survival of 7 months. Prognosis is poor because of multiple factors, including the multifocal nature of the disease,[66] high rate of intestinal recurrence,[66] low serum albumin,[7] and malnutrition.[7,34]

Disease stage and international prognostic index are not useful in predicting survival.[4] Eastern Cooperative Oncology Group score greater than 1 is noted in 88% of patients and many have poor performance status, making them poor candidates for chemotherapy.[6,8] The prognostic index for T-cell lymphoma is useful in predicting survival of EATL.[4] EATL prognostic index was developed to distinguish three risk groups and reportedly performs better than international prognostic index and the prognostic index for T cell lymphoma.[67]

Better response was reported for patients receiving intensive chemotherapy and autologous stem cell transplantation with 5-year overall survival and progression-free survival rate of 60% and 52%, respectively.[8] There is increasing evidence for the important role autologous stem cell transplant plays in management of patients with EATL.[68,69] EATL has generally a poor response to chemotherapy; however, selected patients seem to benefit from intensive chemotherapy.[70] It is now recognized that prolonged survival with chemotherapy and surgical resection is more achievable.[7] CD30+ cases may show response to monoclonal anti-CD30 therapy, such as brentuximab.[62]

MONOMORPHIC EPITHELIOTROPIC INTESTINAL T-CELL LYMPHOMA

OVERVIEW

MEITL was previously known as EATL type II, with no association with celiac disease,[3,4] and an increased incidence in Asian and Hispanic populations.[4,71–73] There is slight male predilection with a male/female ratio of 2:1.[4] All cases are clinically aggressive irrespective of cell size.[4] There is no association with HLA DQA1*0501 and DQB1*0201 genotypes (See **Tables 1** and **2**).[4]

KEY POINTS

- Clinically aggressive and rare entity
- More commonly affects those of Asian and Hispanic origin
- Not associated with celiac disease
- Monomorphic cellular composition without an inflammatory background, and less likely to be associated with necrosis

- CD3$^+$, CD7$^+$, CD5$^-$, CD4$^-$, CD8$^+$, CD56$^+$, CD103$^{+/-}$, CD30$^-$, cytotoxic-positive
- Usually $\gamma\delta$ T-cell receptor expression

CLINICAL PRESENTATION

Symptoms are variable and include abdominal pain, obstruction, or perforation with weight loss, diarrhea, and gastrointestinal bleeding.[71,74] Malabsorption is usually absent.[4]

GROSS AND MICROSCOPIC FEATURES

The disease most often affects the small intestine, most frequently the jejunum and less commonly the ileum, with tumor masses, with or without ulceration, consisting of a diffuse infiltrate of neoplastic cells.[4] Regional mesenteric lymph node involvement is common.[4] The stomach and large intestine can be involved, even if the primary site of involvement was the small intestine.[75] The stomach is involved in 5% of cases and the large intestine in 16%.[74] Dissemination of the intraepithelial lymphocytes leads to multiple sites of involvement[4,76] including extraintestinal sites.[75]

Histologically, the neoplastic cells are monomorphic and small to intermediate in size (Fig. 2A, B).[52,53] The lymphocytes are notable for a heterogeneous population of cells that typically have round nuclei with a rim of pale cytoplasm, finely dispersed chromatin, and inconspicuous nucleoli, which diffusely infiltrate the epithelium and adjacent mucosa.[4] Numerous mitoses are present. In comparison with EATL, there is little or no inflammatory background and necrosis is not prominent.[4] There is epitheliotropism with distorted and broadly expanded villi[4]; however, this does not indicate concomitant celiac disease. The immunophenotype of MEITL is distinct with usual expression of CD8 and CD56 without CD5, which suggests $\gamma\delta$ T-cell origin (Fig. 2C, D). The cytotoxic molecules TIA1 is usually positive, but granzyme B and perforin are less common.[77] Aberrant CD20 expression may be seen.[78] TCRγ is positive in most cases, but TCRβ[2,78] have been reported. In a minority of cases, the tumor

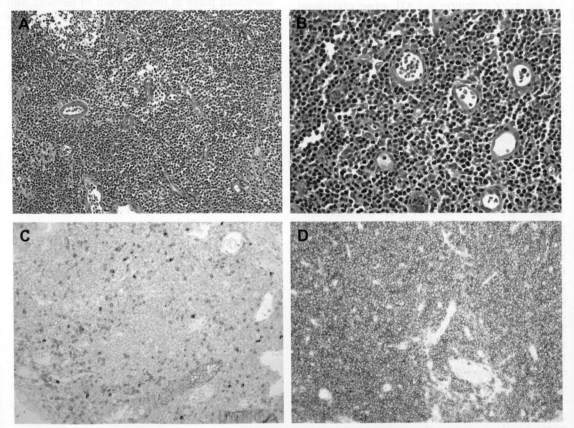

Fig. 2. MEITL. (*A, B*) Monotonous cellular composition of small-to-intermediate-sized cells without a prominent inflammatory background (H&E, original magnification, ×200 [*A*] and ×400 [*B*]). (*C*) The neoplastic cells demonstrate loss of expression of CD5, which is also seen in EATL (immunohistochemistry, original magnification ×200). (*D*) The neoplastic cells demonstrate expression of CD56, unlike EATL (immunohistochemistry, original magnification, ×200).

cells are TCR silent or rarely both $TCR\beta$ and $TCR\gamma$ are expressed.[71]

GENETIC PROFILE

Extra signals for *MYC* at 8q14 are common in MEITL.[55,62] Gains at 9q34.3 by fluorescence in situ hybridization and copy number analysis are identified and are the most common genetic change see in greater than 75% of cases.[55,57,77,79] Other aberrations include 1q32.1, 4p15.1, 5q34, 7q34, 8p11.23, 9q22.31, 9q33.2, 8q24 (*MYC* locus), and 12p13.31 and losses of 7p14.1 and 16q12.1.[4,62,77,80] EATL has other more frequent aberrations in 1q32.2 to 41 and 5q34 to 35.5.[80]

STAT5B activating mutations are found in a high proportion of cases,[81] up to 63% of cases by whole exome sequencing.[80] *STAT5B* mutations are seen in $\gamma\delta$ and $\alpha\beta$ cases.[4] *JAK3* and *GNAI2* are also mutated in some cases.[4,80] *SETD2* is the most common mutated gene in one study in more than 90% of cases.[82,83]

PROGNOSIS AND THERAPY

The prognosis of MEITL is poor with a median survival of 7 months.[4] The 5-year survival and complete response rates are poor at 46% and 48%, respectively.[4] Although limited data are available, studies show that MEITL has a worse prognosis than EATL.[74,84] Involvement of the *JAK-STAT* pathway has suggested the utility of ruxolitinib as a therapeutic option.[62]

INDOLENT T-CELL LYMPHOPROLIFERATIVE DISORDER OF THE GASTROINTESTINAL TRACT

OVERVIEW

This clonal intestinal T-cell disorder is a new provisional entity in the World Health Organization classification and can affect multiple sites in the gastrointestinal tract, most commonly the small intestine[85] and colon. It is important to differentiate them from other T-cell/natural killer cell lymphomas[86] because they behave less aggressively. There is a characteristic lymphocytic infiltrate in the lamina propria without destruction and some cases show epitheliotropism.[4,85,87] The clinical course is usually indolent, although many have been treated with chemotherapy.[4] Rare cases have more aggressive disease, progress to high-grade T-cell lymphoma, and spread beyond the gastrointestinal tract, and are probably a different entity.[4]

Patients affected are usually adults with a slight male predominance.[85] Some patients have a history of Crohn disease.[85] Although all sites in the gastrointestinal tract can be involved,[88] the small intestine or colon are the most common sites.[4,89] Clinical features are variable[85,90] and include abdominal pain, diarrhea, vomiting, dyspepsia, and weight loss. Chronic relapsing clinical course with poor response to conventional chemotherapy is seen.[4] Patients may have prolonged survival with persistent disease.[87,90]

GROSS AND MICROSCOPIC FEATURES

The mucosa is thickened with prominent folds, nodules, and polyps that may mimic lymphomatous polyposis.[91,92] The cells that infiltrate the lamina propria are monotonous small round and mature lymphocytes. Admixed inflammatory cells are rare and epithelioid granulomas may be appreciated, focally mimicking Crohn's disease.[4,87,93]

These cases are usually CD3+ and CD8+ but a significant number of cases have CD4 expression.[87,89,90] The CD8+ cases express TIA1. Other T-cell markers are also positive including CD2, and CD5 and CD7 (variable). All cases express $\alpha\beta$ T-cell receptor. CD56 is negative but expression of CD103 has been reported in some cases.[4] Ki-67 demonstrates an extremely low proliferative index (<10%) in all cases.[4] Because rare cases have been reported with disease progression to aggressive T-cell lymphoma, close follow-up is warranted.[94]

GENETIC PROFILE

All cases demonstrate clonal rearrangement of T-cell receptor genes, either *TCRγ* or *TCRβ*.[85,87] Recurrent mutations or translocations have not been identified.[4] Few cases revealed absence of activating mutations of *STAT3*.[4,85]

INTESTINAL T-CELL LYMPHOMA, NOT OTHERWISE SPECIFIED (NOS)

This terminology, although not considered a specific disease entity, is used when a diagnosis of intestinal T-cell lymphoma does not fit the criteria for classic EATL or MEITL. This may be caused by biopsy size or insufficient immunophenotypic data.[4] All cases are clinically aggressive and most affect the colon.[2] The morphology and immunophenotype are heterogenous.[4] Many of these may also fit into the category of peripheral T-cell lymphoma, not otherwise specified (NOS).

DUODENAL-TYPE FOLLICULAR LYMPHOMA

This lymphoma is discussed elsewhere in this issue (See Sudhir Perincheri's article, "Early events in Lymphoid Neoplasms and Indolent Follicular Lymphomas," in this issue.).

REFERENCES

1. Skinnider BF. Lymphoproliferative disorders of the gastrointestinal tract. Arch Pathol Lab Med 2018; 142(1):44–52.
2. Attygalle AD, Cabeçadas J, Gaulard P, et al. Peripheral T-cell and NK-cell lymphomas and their mimics; taking a step forward. Report on the lymphoma workshop of the XVIth meeting of the European Association for Haematopathology and the Society for Hematopathology. Histopathology 2014;64(2): 171–99.
3. Swerdlow SH, Jaffe ES, Brousset P, et al. Cytotoxic T-cell and NK-cell lymphomas: current questions and controversies. Am J Surg Pathol 2014;38(10): e60–71.
4. Jaffe ES, Bhagat G, Chott A, et al. Intestinal T-cell lymphoma. In: Swerdlow SH, Campo E, Harris NL, et al, editors. WHO classification of tumours of the haematopoietic and lymphoid tissues. Revised 4th edition. Lyon (France): IARC; 2017. p. 372–80.
5. Delabie J, Holte H, Vose JM, et al. Enteropathy-associated T-cell lymphoma: clinical and histological findings from the international peripheral T-cell lymphoma project. Blood 2011;118(1):148–55.
6. Gale J, Simmonds PD, Mead GM, et al. Enteropathy-type intestinal T-cell lymphoma: clinical features and treatment of 31 patients in a single center. J Clin Oncol 2000;18(4):795–803.
7. Malamut G, Chandesris O, Verkarre V, et al. Enteropathy associated T cell lymphoma in celiac disease: a large retrospective study. Dig Liver Dis 2013;45(5): 377–84.
8. Sieniawski M, Angamuthu N, Boyd K, et al. Evaluation of enteropathy-associated T-cell lymphoma comparing standard therapies with a novel regimen including autologous stem cell transplantation. Blood 2010;115(18):3664–70.
9. Verbeek WH, Van De Water JM, Al-Toma A, et al. Incidence of enteropathy–associated T-cell lymphoma: a nation-wide study of a population-based registry in The Netherlands. Scand J Gastroenterol 2008;43(11):1322–8.
10. Chander U, Leeman-Neill RJ, Bhagat G. Pathogenesis of enteropathy-associated T cell lymphoma. Curr Hematol Malig Rep 2018;13(4):308–17.
11. Green PH, Cellier C. Celiac disease. N Engl J Med 2007;357(17):1731–43.
12. O'Farrelly C, Feighery C, O'Briain DS, et al. Humoral response to wheat protein in patients with coeliac disease and enteropathy associated T cell lymphoma. Br Med J (Clin Res Ed) 1986;293(6552): 908–10.
13. Swinson CM, Slavin G, Coles EC, et al. Coeliac disease and malignancy. Lancet 1983;1(8316):111–5.
14. Zing NPC, Fischer T, Zain J, et al. Peripheral T-cell lymphomas: incorporating new developments in diagnostics, prognostication, and treatment into clinical practice-PART 2: ENNKTL, EATL, indolent T-cell lymphoproliferative disease of the GI tract, ATLL, and hepatosplenic T-cell lymphoma. Oncology (Williston Park) 2018;32(7):e74–82.
15. Collin P, Salmi TT, Hervonen K, et al. Dermatitis herpetiformis: a cutaneous manifestation of coeliac disease. Ann Med 2017;49(1):23–31.
16. Askling J, Linet M, Gridley G, et al. Cancer incidence in a population-based cohort of individuals hospitalized with celiac disease or dermatitis herpetiformis. Gastroenterology 2002;123(5):1428–35.
17. Corrao G, Corazza GR, Bagnardi V, et al. Mortality in patients with coeliac disease and their relatives: a cohort study. Lancet 2001;358(9279):356–61.
18. Green PH, Fleischauer AT, Bhagat G, et al. Risk of malignancy in patients with celiac disease. Am J Med 2003;115(3):191–5.
19. Holmes GK, Prior P, Lane MR, et al. Malignancy in coeliac disease: effect of a gluten free diet. Gut 1989;30(3):333–8.
20. Holmes GK. Coeliac disease and malignancy. Dig Liver Dis 2002;34(3):229–37.
21. Howell WM, Leung ST, Jones DB, et al. HLA-DRB, -DQA, and -DQB polymorphism in celiac disease and enteropathy-associated T-cell lymphoma. Common features and additional risk factors for malignancy. Hum Immunol 1995;43(1):29–37.
22. Silano M, Volta U, Vincenzi AD, et al. Effect of a gluten-free diet on the risk of enteropathy-associated T-cell lymphoma in celiac disease. Dig Dis Sci 2008;53(4):972–6.
23. Malamut G, Afchain P, Verkarre V, et al. Presentation and long-term follow-up of refractory celiac disease: comparison of type I with type II. Gastroenterology 2009;136(1):81–90.
24. Ilus T, Kaukinen K, Virta LJ, et al. Refractory coeliac disease in a country with a high prevalence of clinically-diagnosed coeliac disease. Aliment Pharmacol Ther 2014;39(4):418–25.
25. Malamut G, Cellier C. Refractory coeliac disease. Curr Opin Oncol 2013;25(5):445–51.
26. Al-Toma A, Goerres MS, Meijer JW, et al. Human leukocyte antigen-DQ2 homozygosity and the development of refractory celiac disease and enteropathy-associated T-cell lymphoma. Clin Gastroenterol Hepatol 2006;4(3):315–9.
27. Daum S, Ullrich R, Heise W, et al. Intestinal non-Hodgkin's lymphoma: a multicenter prospective clinical study from the German Study Group on

Intestinal non-Hodgkin's Lymphoma. J Clin Oncol 2003;21(14):2740–6.

28. Novakovic BJ, Novakovic S, Frkovic-Grazio S. A single-center report on clinical features and treatment response in patients with intestinal T cell non-Hodgkin's lymphomas. Oncol Rep 2006;16(1):191–5.

29. Webster A, Crea P, Bamford MW, et al. Enteropathy-associated T-cell lymphoma presenting as cutaneous deposits. Br J Haematol 2017;176(1):7.

30. Gobbi C, Buess M, Probst A, et al. Enteropathy-associated T-cell lymphoma with initial manifestation in the CNS. Neurology 2003;60(10):1718–9.

31. Tutt AN, Brada M, Sampson SA. Enteropathy associated T cell lymphoma presenting as an isolated CNS lymphoma three years after diagnosis of coeliac disease: T cell receptor polymerase chain reaction studies failed to show the original enteropathy to be a clonal disorder. Gut 1997;40(6):801–3.

32. Spijkerman M, Tan IL, Kolkman JJ, et al. A large variety of clinical features and concomitant disorders in celiac disease: a cohort study in the Netherlands. Dig Liver Dis 2016;48(5):499–505.

33. Daum S, Cellier C, Mulder CJ. Refractory coeliac disease. Best Pract Res Clin Gastroenterol 2005;19(3):413–24.

34. Al-Toma A, Verbeek WH, Hadithi M, et al. Survival in refractory coeliac disease and enteropathy-associated T-cell lymphoma: retrospective evaluation of single-centre experience. Gut 2007;56(10):1373–8.

35. Roshan B, Leffler DA, Jamma S, et al. The incidence and clinical spectrum of refractory celiac disease in a North American referral center. Am J Gastroenterol 2011;106(5):923–8.

36. Rubio-Tapia A, Kelly DG, Lahr BD, et al. Clinical staging and survival in refractory celiac disease: a single center experience. Gastroenterology 2009;136(1):99–107.

37. Rubio-Tapia A, Murray JA. Classification and management of refractory celiac disease. Gut 2010;59(4):547–57.

38. O'Mahony S, Howdle PD, Losowsky MS. Review article: management of patients with non-responsive coeliac disease. Aliment Pharmacol Ther 1996;10(5):671–80.

39. Ciccocioppo R, Croci GA, Biagi F, et al. Intestinal T-cell lymphoma with enteropathy-associated T-cell lymphoma-like features arising in the setting of adult autoimmune enteropathy. Hematol Oncol 2018;36(2):481–8.

40. Daum S, Ipczynski R, Schumann M, et al. High rates of complications and substantial mortality in both types of refractory sprue. Eur J Gastroenterol Hepatol 2009;21(1):66–70.

41. Hollon JR, Cureton PA, Martin ML, et al. Trace gluten contamination may play a role in mucosal and clinical recovery in a subgroup of diet-adherent non-responsive celiac disease patients. BMC Gastroenterol 2013;13:40.

42. Malamut G, Meresse B, Cellier C, et al. Refractory celiac disease: from bench to bedside. Semin Immunopathol 2012;34(4):601–13.

43. Cellier C, Delabesse E, Helmer C, et al. Refractory sprue, coeliac disease, and enteropathy-associated T-cell lymphoma. French Coeliac Disease Study Group. Lancet 2000;356(9225):203–8.

44. Verkarre V, Asnafi V, Lecomte T, et al. Refractory coeliac sprue is a diffuse gastrointestinal disease. Gut 2003;52(2):205–11.

45. Ashton-Key M, Diss TC, Pan L, et al. Molecular analysis of T-cell clonality in ulcerative jejunitis and enteropathy-associated T-cell lymphoma. Am J Pathol 1997;151(2):493–8.

46. Bagdi E, Diss TC, Munson P, et al. Mucosal intraepithelial lymphocytes in enteropathy-associated T-cell lymphoma, ulcerative jejunitis, and refractory celiac disease constitute a neoplastic population. Blood 1999;94(1):260–4.

47. Fernandes A, Ferreira AM, Ferreira R, et al. Refractory celiac disease type II: a case report that demonstrates the diagnostic and therapeutic challenges. GE Port J Gastroenterol 2015;23(2):106–12.

48. Nijeboer P, van Wanrooij R, van Gils T, et al. Lymphoma development and survival in refractory coeliac disease type II: histological response as prognostic factor. United Eur Gastroenterol J 2017;5(2):208–17.

49. Carbonnel F, Grollet-Bioul L, Brouet JC, et al. Are complicated forms of celiac disease cryptic T-cell lymphomas? Blood 1998;92(10):3879–86.

50. Wright DH, Jones DB, Clark H, et al. Is adult-onset coeliac disease due to a low-grade lymphoma of intraepithelial T lymphocytes? Lancet 1991;337(8754):1373–4.

51. Wright DH. Enteropathy associated T cell lymphoma. Cancer Surv 1997;30:249–61.

52. Chott A, Haedicke W, Mosberger I, et al. Most CD56+ intestinal lymphomas are CD8+CD5-T-cell lymphomas of monomorphic small to medium size histology. Am J Pathol 1998;153(5):1483–90.

53. Chott A, Vesely M, Simonitsch I, et al. Classification of intestinal T-cell neoplasms and their differential diagnosis. Am J Clin Pathol 1999;111:S68–74.

54. Baumgärtner AK, Zettl A, Chott A, et al. High frequency of genetic aberrations in enteropathy-type T-cell lymphoma. Lab Invest 2003;83(10):1509–16.

55. Deleeuw RJ, Zettl A, Klinker E, et al. Whole-genome analysis and HLA genotyping of enteropathy-type T-cell lymphoma reveals 2 distinct lymphoma subtypes. Gastroenterology 2007;132(5):1902–11.

56. Verkarre V, Romana SP, Cellier C, et al. Recurrent partial trisomy 1q22-q44 in clonal intraepithelial

lymphocytes in refractory celiac sprue. Gastroenterology 2003;125(1):40–6.

57. Zettl A, Ott G, Makulik A, et al. Chromosomal gains at 9q characterize enteropathy-type T-cell lymphoma. Am J Pathol 2002;161(5):1635–45.

58. Hrdlickova B, Mulder CJ, Malamut G, et al. A locus at 7p14.3 predisposes to refractory celiac disease progression from celiac disease. Eur J Gastroenterol Hepatol 2018;30(8):828–37.

59. Obermann EC, Diss TC, Hamoudi RA, et al. Loss of heterozygosity at chromosome 9p21 is a frequent finding in enteropathy-type T-cell lymphoma. J Pathol 2004;202(2):252–62.

60. Murray A, Cuevas EC, Jones DB, et al. Study of the immunohistochemistry and T cell clonality of enteropathy-associated T cell lymphoma. Am J Pathol 1995;146(2):509–19.

61. Cejkova P, Zettl A, Baumgärtner AK, et al. Amplification of NOTCH1 and ABL1 gene loci is a frequent aberration in enteropathy-type T-cell lymphoma. Virchows Arch 2005;446(4):416–20.

62. Couronné L, Bastard C, Gaulard P, et al. Molecular pathogenesis of peripheral T cell lymphoma (2): extranodal NK/T cell lymphoma, nasal type, adult T cell leukemia/lymphoma and enteropathy associated T cell lymphoma. Med Sci (Paris) 2015;31(11):1023–33.

63. Nicolae A, Xi L, Pham TH, et al. Mutations in the JAK/STAT and RAS signaling pathways are common in intestinal T-cell lymphomas. Leukemia 2016;30(11):2245–7.

64. Ettersperger J, Montcuquet N, Malamut G, et al. Interleukin-15-dependent T-cell-like innate intraepithelial lymphocytes develop in the intestine and transform into lymphomas in celiac disease. Immunity 2016;45(3):610–25.

65. Moffitt AB, Ondrejka SL, McKinney M, et al. Enteropathy-associated T cell lymphoma subtypes are characterized by loss of function of SETD2. J Exp Med 2017;214(5):1371–86.

66. Chott A, Dragosics B, Radaszkiewicz T. Peripheral T-cell lymphomas of the intestine. Am J Pathol 1992; 141(6):1361–71.

67. De Baaij LR, Berkhof J, van de Water JM, et al. A new and validated clinical prognostic model (EPI) for enteropathy-associated T-cell lymphoma. Clin Cancer Res 2015;21(13):3013–9.

68. Kharfan-Dabaja MA, Kumar A, Ayala E, et al. Clinical practice recommendations on indication and timing of hematopoietic cell transplantation in mature T cell and NK/T cell lymphomas: an international collaborative effort on behalf of the guidelines committee of the American Society for Blood and Marrow Transplantation. Biol Blood Marrow Transplant 2017; 23(11):1826–38.

69. Ondrejka S, Jagadeesh D. Enteropathy-associated T-cell lymphoma. Curr Hematol Malig Rep 2016; 11(6):504–13.

70. Armitage JO. The aggressive peripheral T-cell lymphomas: 2017. Am J Hematol 2017;92(7):706–15.

71. Chan JK, Chan AC, Cheuk W, et al. Type II enteropathy-associated T-cell lymphoma: a distinct aggressive lymphoma with frequent γδ T-cell receptor expression. Am J Surg Pathol 2011;35(10): 1557–69.

72. Garcia-Herrera A, Song JY, Chuang SS, et al. Non-hepatosplenic γδ T-cell lymphomas represent a spectrum of aggressive cytotoxic T-cell lymphomas with a mainly extranodal presentation. Am J Surg Pathol 2011;35(8):1214–25.

73. Sun J, Lu Z, Yang D, et al. Primary intestinal T-cell and NK-cell lymphomas: a clinicopathological and molecular study from China focused on type II enteropathy-associated T-cell lymphoma and primary intestinal NK-cell lymphoma. Mod Pathol 2011;24(7):983–92.

74. Tse E, Gill H, Loong F, et al. Type II enteropathy-associated T-cell lymphoma: a multicenter analysis from the Asia Lymphoma Study Group. Am J Hematol 2012;87(7):663–8.

75. Chan TSY, Lee E, Khong PL, et al. Positron emission tomography computed tomography features of monomorphic epitheliotropic intestinal T-cell lymphoma. Hematology 2018;23(1):10–6.

76. Ishibashi H, Nimura S, Kayashima Y, et al. Multiple lesions of gastrointestinal tract invasion by monomorphic epitheliotropic intestinal T-cell lymphoma, accompanied by duodenal and intestinal enteropathy-like lesions and microscopic lymphocytic proctocolitis: a case series. Diagn Pathol 2016;11(1):66.

77. Tomita S, Kikuti YY, Carreras J, et al. Genomic and immunohistochemical profiles of enteropathy-associated T-cell lymphoma in Japan. Mod Pathol 2015;28(10):1286–96.

78. Tan SY, Chuang SS, Tang T, et al. Type II EATL (epitheliotropic intestinal T-cell lymphoma): a neoplasm of intra-epithelial T-cells with predominant CD8αα phenotype. Leukemia 2013;27(8):1688–96.

79. Ko YH, Karnan S, Kim KM, et al. Enteropathy-associated T-cell lymphoma: a clinicopathologic and array comparative genomic hybridization study. Hum Pathol 2010;41(9):1231–7.

80. Nairismägi ML, Tan J, Lim JQ, et al. JAK-STAT and G-protein-coupled receptor signaling pathways are frequently altered in epitheliotropic intestinal T-cell lymphoma. Leukemia 2016;30(6): 1311–9.

81. Küçük C, Jiang B, Hu X, et al. Activating mutations of STAT5B and STAT3 in lymphomas derived from γδ-T or NK cells. Nat Commun 2015;6:6025.

82. Roberti A, Dobay MP, Bisig B, et al. Type II enteropathy-associated T-cell lymphoma features a unique genomic profile with highly recurrent SETD2 alterations. Nat Commun 2016;7:12602.

83. Vallois D, Roberti A, Bisig B, et al. Molecular onco-genesis of lymphomas: role of the *SETD2* gene in intestinal T-cell lymphomas. Med Sci (Paris) 2017; 33(5):469–73, [in French].
84. Mehta-Shah N, Horwitz S. Zebras and hen's teeth: recognition and management of rare T and NK lymphomas. Hematology Am Soc Hematol Educ Program 2015;2015:545–9.
85. Perry AM, Warnke RA, Hu Q, et al. Indolent T-cell lymphoproliferative disease of the gastrointestinal tract. Blood 2013;122(22):3599–606.
86. Matnani R, Ganapathi KA, Lewis SK, et al. Indolent T- and NK-cell lymphoproliferative disorder of the gastrointestinal tract: a review and update. Hematol Oncol 2017;35(1):3–16.
87. Margolskee E, Jobanputra V, Lewis SK, et al. Indolent small intestinal CD4+ T-cell lymphoma is a distinct entity with unique biologic and clinical features. PLoS One 2013;8(7):e68343.
88. Egawa N, Fukayama M, Kawaguchi K, et al. Relapsing oral and colonic ulcers with monoclonal T-cell infiltration. A low grade mucosal T-lymphoproliferative disease of the digestive tract. Cancer 1995; 75(7):1728–33.
89. Ranheim EA, Jones C, Zehnder JL, et al. Spontaneously relapsing clonal, mucosal cytotoxic T-cell lymphoproliferative disorder: case report and review of the literature. Am J Surg Pathol 2000; 24(2):296–301.
90. Carbonnel F, d'Almagne H, Lavergne A, et al. The clinicopathological features of extensive small intestinal CD4 T cell infiltration. Gut 1999;45(5):662–7.
91. Hirakawa K, Fuchigami T, Nakamura S, et al. Primary gastrointestinal T-cell lymphoma resembling multiple lymphomatous polyposis. Gastroenterology 1996; 111(3):778–82.
92. Isomoto H, Maeda T, Akashi T, et al. Multiple lymphomatous polyposis of the colon originating from T-cells: a case report. Dig Liver Dis 2004; 36(3):218–21.
93. Carbonnel F, Lavergne A, Messing B, et al. Extensive small intestinal T-cell lymphoma of low-grade malignancy associated with a new chromosomal translocation. Cancer 1994;73(4):1286–91.
94. Perry AM, Bailey NG, Bonnett M, et al. Disease progression in a patient with indolent T-cell lymphoproliferative disease of the gastrointestinal tract. Int J Surg Pathol 2019;27(1):102–7.

EBV–Associated Lymphoproliferative Disorders: Update in Classification

Sherif A. Rezk, MD[a], Lawrence M. Weiss, MD[a,b,*]

KEYWORDS

- EBV • B-cell lymphoproliferative disorders • T-cell lymphoproliferative disorders
- Immunodeficiency-related lymphoproliferative disorders

Key Points

- Although about 90% of the world's population is infected by Epstein-Barr virus (EBV), only a small subset of the related infections result in neoplastic transformation.
- The number of EBV-related neoplasms discovered has been increasing over the years and it is anticipated that more EBV-related neoplastic associations will be reported.
- EBV has proved to be a versatile oncogenic agent involved in a multitude of various hematopoietic, epithelial, and mesenchymal neoplasms, but the precise role of EBV in the pathogenesis of many of the associated lymphoid/histiocytic proliferations discussed in this article remains hypothetical or not completely understood.
- Additional studies and use of evolving technologies such as high-throughput next-generation sequencing may help address this knowledge gap and may lead to enhanced diagnostic assessment and the development of potential therapeutic interventions.

ABSTRACT

Although about 90% of the world's population is infected by EBV only a small subset of the related infections result in neoplastic transformation. EBV is a versatile oncogenic agent involved in a multitude of hematopoietic, epithelial, and mesenchymal neoplasms, but the precise role of EBV in the pathogenesis of many of the associated lymphoid/histiocytic proliferations remains hypothetical or not completely understood. Additional studies and use of evolving technologies such as high-throughput next-generation sequencing may help address this knowledge gap and may lead to enhanced diagnostic

assessment and the development of potential therapeutic interventions.

OVERVIEW

EBV was the first known oncogenic virus and more than 90% of the adult population worldwide are estimated to be infected by the virus.[1] EBV has lytic (productive) stage that is asymptomatic in most individuals and a latent (nonproductive) stage, in which the viral DNA persists as an episome in the nucleus of circulating B cells, thus making it capable of evading immune clearance and persisting for the life of the host.[1,2] Three distinct latency programs have been described that correlate with the differentiation state of B

Conflict of interests: The authors declare that there is no conflict of interests regarding the publication of this article and there have been no significant financial contributions for this work that could have influenced its outcome.

[a] Department of Pathology and Laboratory Medicine, University of California Irvine (UCI) Medical Center, 101 The City Drive, Orange, CA 92868, USA; [b] NeoGenomics Laboratories, 31 Columbia, Aliso Viejo, CA 92656, USA
* Corresponding author. NeoGenomics Laboratories, 31 Columbia, Aliso Viejo, CA 92656.
E-mail address: weiss11111@gmail.com

cells and are thought to have enabled EBV-infected cells to survive an adaptive immune response and surveillance.[3] EBV has been linked to many human neoplasms, including hematopoietic, epithelial, and mesenchymal tumors. This article only discusses the EBV-associated lymphoproliferative disorders, which can be classified into reactive proliferations (including reactive lesions with no malignant potential and reactive lesions with varied malignant potential), B-cell proliferations (including Hodgkin lymphoma and plasma cell neoplasms), T/natural killer (NK) cell proliferations, and immunodeficiency-related lymphoid proliferations (**Fig. 1**).

EBV–ASSOCIATED REACTIVE LYMPHOID PROLIFERATIONS

Reactive lymphoid proliferations are divided into reactive proliferations with no or minimal malignant potential that are usually benign and self-limited and reactive

proliferations with varied malignant potential. The EBV-infected cells represent B cells as well as NK/T cells.

REACTIVE PROLIFERATIONS WITH NO OR MINIMAL MALIGNANT POTENTIAL

EBV–Positive Reactive Lymphoid Hyperplasia

Definition and clinical picture
No specific definition or disease-associated symptoms exist and it is usually dependent on the condition causing stimulation of the lymph node.

Morphologic picture
Scattered small EBV-positive cells can be detected by in situ hybridization in normal lymph nodes or in lymph nodes with minimal hyperplasia. They are usually located in the interfollicular areas, although they can be seen, rarely, in the follicles. Stimulated/activated lymph nodes with follicular hyperplasia, paracortical hyperplasia, plasma cell hyperplasia, or Castleman-like changes may

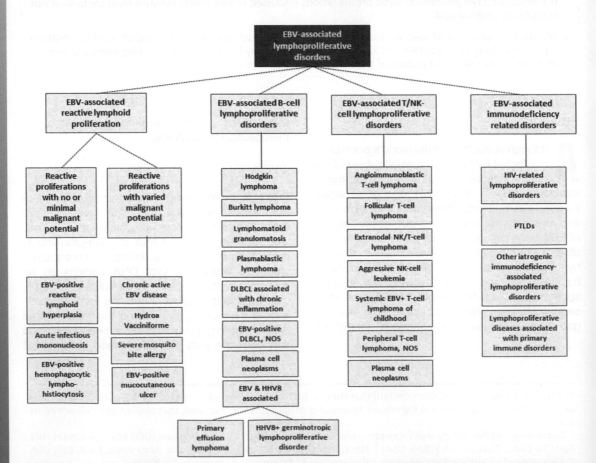

Fig. 1. The classification scheme for EBV-associated lymphoproliferative disorders. DLBCL, diffuse large B-cell lymphoma; HHV8, human virus herpes 8; HIV, human immunodeficiency virus; NOS, not otherwise specified; PTLDs, posttransplant lymphoproliferative disorders.

contain increased numbers of EBV-positive cells, mainly in older individuals and in certain immunodeficiency conditions.[4] The nodal architecture is usually preserved and no atypical cells are present. Cases in which the nodal architecture is effaced and atypical cells are identified are referred to as polymorphic lymphoproliferative disorders, reminiscent of posttransplant lymphoproliferative disorder (PTLD) but in immunocompetent patients.[4]

Pathogenesis
The EBV-positive cells presumably represent circulating latently infected EBV-positive cells that increase in number in tandem with the overall number of lymphocytes in activated state.[5]

Clinical course and prognosis
EBV expression does not alter the clinical course and a high rate of spontaneous resolution has been reported in these patients.[4]

EBV staining pattern by in situ hybridization (EBER)
EBV-positive cells are mostly small and are localized within the paracortical areas, although they can be rarely seen in the germinal centers.

Acute Infectious Mononucleosis

Definition and clinical picture
This infectious disorder is characterized by sore throat, fever, markedly enlarged tonsils, and lymphadenopathy, particularly cervical lymph nodes.[6] Most initial infections occur asymptomatically in children less than 5 years of age but symptomatic infectious mononucleosis occurs in all age groups except childhood.[7] The disorder is usually suspected clinically and lymphocytosis with 10% to 20% atypical lymphocytes is usually noted on examination of the peripheral blood smear. The diagnosis is confirmed serologically by the Monospot test or by the more specific EBV antibody titer studies. In addition to the peripheral blood findings, the bone marrow is often involved, although not frequently sampled.

Morphologic picture
An immunoblastic proliferation is the characteristic feature, accompanied by reactive follicular hyperplasia. Foci of monocytoid B-cell hyperplasia may be present or may precede the immunoblastic proliferation. Abundant plasma cells are usually seen and foci of necrosis may be present. Most of the proliferating immunoblasts are CD30 positive. The exuberant immunoblastic proliferation and architectural distortion seen in some cases can lead to misdiagnosis of infectious mononucleosis as a lymphoma, especially diffuse large B-cell

lymphoma (DLBCL). The localization of the lesion to the tonsils or cervical lymph nodes in a young patient, the heterogeneity of the cellular infiltrate, and the presence of few residual hyperplastic germinal centers and distended sinuses are factors that support a diagnosis of infectious mononucleosis, but the main distinction can be achieved by in situ hybridization.

Pathogenesis
The lytic cycle of EBV infection and the profound cellular immune response leads to destruction of virus-infected cells and the eventual release of inflammatory cytokines, which are the main cause of symptoms.[8]

Clinical course and prognosis
This condition is self-limiting in immunocompetent patients, although persistence into chronic active EBV disease can occur and progression to fatal sporadic infectious mononucleosis may occur, which is now classified under the systemic EBV-positive T-cell lymphoma of childhood category in the 2016 World Health Organization (WHO) classification.[9,10]

EBV staining pattern by in situ hybridization (EBER)
This expression pattern is characteristic of EBV, with many EBV-positive small and large cells present, mainly in the paracortical area, but scattered cells are usually present in the germinal centers and the monocytoid B-cell areas. Many negative cells are also present. This pattern contrasts with EBV-positive lymphomas, which usually have a much higher proportion and uniformity of EBV-positive cells, mainly large .[7] Most of the EBV-positive cells represent B cells with a low proportion of the cells (<10%) representing T and NK cells.[11-13]

EBV–Positive Hemophagocytic Lymphohistiocytosis

Definition and clinical picture
In the absence of primary genetic aberrations, EBV-positive hemophagocytic lymphohistiocytosis (HLH) usually occurs in young children, mainly Asian, with a median age of 4 years.[14] These patients usually have a high EBV viral load in the blood. The diagnosis of HLH can be established on a molecular basis or by the presence of 5 of the 8 clinical criteria: fever, splenomegaly, cytopenias affecting at least 2 lineages, hypertriglyceridemia or hypofibrinogenemia, morphologic evidence of hemophagocytosis, low or absent NK-cell activity, increased ferritin level, and increased soluble CD25 level.[14]

Morphologic picture

The affected organs show an infiltration of benign-appearing histiocytes with hemophagocytosis, predominantly of red blood cells and neutrophils. Bone marrow is the tissue most widely used for diagnostic examination, and bone marrow aspirate smears may best show hemophagocytosis. T-cell receptor gene clonality may be detected in EBV-positive HLH but it does not necessarily indicate an underlying T-cell lymphoma.[15]

Pathogenesis

This condition represents an exaggerated immune response secondary to acute EBV infection in most cases. EBV can infect B cells but mainly infects T and NK cells in this disorder, and infection of CD8+ T cells results in a cytokine storm with increased levels of tumor necrosis factor and interferon leading to secondary and systemic activation of histiocytes and macrophages.[16]

Clinical course and prognosis

The HLH 2004 treatment is effective in most cases, with remissions achieved in many cases.

EBV staining pattern by in situ hybridization (EBER)

EBV is detected mainly in T cells, usually in an interstitial pattern with scattered positive bystander B cells. The EBV-positive cells are mainly small and lack any atypical features.

REACTIVE PROLIFERATIONS WITH VARIED MALIGNANT POTENTIAL

Chronic Active EBV Disease

Definition and clinical picture

This condition is a rare systemic entity related to persistent EBV infection (>3 months) that is usually preceded by an acute EBV infection in patients without known immunodeficiency. Patients usually show markedly increased EBV DNA levels or antibodies to EBV in the peripheral blood; show EBV-positive cells in tissues; and clinically present with fever, lymphadenopathy, and hepatosplenomegaly.[17,18] Occurrence of hemophagocytic syndrome as a secondary finding may occur in some patients and progressive loss of B cells leading to hypogammaglobulinemia can occur in a subset of the patients.[19] Although EBV usually resides in B cells in healthy individuals, most chronic active EBV (CAEBV) cases (mainly from Japan and other Asian countries, as well as in Native Americans) have EBV detected in T and NK cells (T/NK-cell type) but cases with EBV detected in B cells (B-cell type) are more common in the United States and occur rarely in Japan.[19,20]

Morphologic picture

For CAEBV of T/NK-cell type, a T/NK-cell infiltrate (more commonly T cells) is noted, which is usually sinusoidal in the liver and spleen, sinusoidal/interstitial in the bone marrow, and interstitial/diffuse in the paracortical areas of the lymph nodes. The architecture of the affected tissue is usually preserved and cytologic atypia is absent within the EBV-positive cells. Hemophagocytosis is commonly seen and the expanded activated histiocytes alter the histologic picture in some cases. For CAEBV of B-cell type, it morphologically shows a PTLD-like picture but with an increased number of proliferating immunoblasts, plasma cells, occasional Reed-Sternberg–like cells, and paracortical hyperplasia.

Pathogenesis

This condition likely involves a cellular immune defect that failed to control the proliferation of EBV latently infected lymphocytes with expression of viral lytic proteins and the subsequent production of antibodies to these proteins.[19]

Clinical course and prognosis

CAEBV can be polyclonal, oligoclonal, or monoclonal, and clonality can be used as a prognostic factor and for subclassification purposes.[21] Allogeneic stem cell transplant can be curative for CAEBV disease if considered early in the course of the disease. Some patients respond temporarily to immunomodulating agents, immunosuppressive therapy, or cytotoxic chemotherapy, but these treatments are not curative, and most patients succumb to their disease.[19]

EBV staining pattern by in situ hybridization (EBER)

For CAEBV of T/NK-cell type, EBV is uniformly expressed in many cytotoxic T cells in most cases.[18] For CAEBV of B-cell type, the EBV expression pattern is similar to infectious mononucleosis, in which many small and large EBV-positive cells are identified with many EBV-negative cells present.

Hydroa Vacciniforme

Definition and clinical picture

Hydroa vacciniforme (HV) is a rare idiopathic photodermatosis that is considered as a subcategory of CAEBV. It usually occurs during childhood and is characterized by vesicles and crust formation after sunlight exposure and typically heals by vacciniform scarring.[22] The classic form of the disease has a low risk of progression and usually resolves spontaneously in adolescence; however, many patients show disease progression and develop severe and extensive skin lesions with facial edema and ulceration that are not limited to sun-exposed areas along with systemic manifestations including fever, hepatosplenomegaly, and lymphadenopathy.[15] Many patients eventually develop a clonal T-cell population but, given the lack of reliable clinical or molecular criteria that can predict clinical outcomes, it is not designated as a lymphoma but as HV-like lymphoproliferative disorder in the 2016 WHO classification to encompass the broad clinical spectrum of the disease.[10]

Morphologic picture
A dermal lymphoid infiltrate with angiocentric and angiodestructive features is usually seen and is composed in most cases of CD8-positive cytotoxic T cells, but cases with CD4-positive or NK-cell phenotype have been reported.

Pathogenesis
The cause of the disorder is largely unknown. Although the EBV status was not studied in the initial Western studies on the classic HV cases, studies on Asian populations showed that HV is an EBV-associated disorder.[23,24] Genetic predisposition may play a major role given the geographic and ethnic distribution of the disorder, similar to that seen in other EBV-associated T/NK-cell lymphoproliferative disorders.[10]

Clinical course and prognosis
The clinical course is variable, with many patients experiencing recurrent skin lesions for 10 to 15 years before systemic progression. T-cell clonality, the density of the infiltrate, and the number of EBV-positive cells do not predict clinical outcome or disease progression.[10]

EBV latency pattern
Latency II.

EBV staining pattern by in situ hybridization (EBER)
The number of EBV-positive cells by in situ hybridization varies from one case to another, but many EBV-positive T cells are usually seen.[10]

Severe Mosquito Bite Allergy

Definition and clinical picture
This allergy is a rare, exaggerated reaction to mosquito bites in children that presents as intense local skin lesions, including erythema, bullae, ulcers, skin necrosis, and deep scarring. Patients have circulating EBV-positive NK cells in the peripheral blood and are at an increased risk of developing hemophagocytic syndrome and progression to an overt NK/T-cell lymphoma or aggressive NK-cell leukemia over the long-standing course of the disease.[10] Patients usually

have high serum immunoglobulin (Ig) E titers and high EBV DNA load in the peripheral blood in addition to the NK-cell lymphocytosis.

Morphologic picture
A dermal infiltrate that extends into the subcutaneous tissue with features of angiodestruction is usually seen. Most of the infiltrating cells have an NK-cell phenotype.

Pathogenesis
The pathogenesis of the disease is unknown, although it is thought that the severe mosquito bite allergy may play a role in the reactivation of EBV in NK cells inducing the expression of LMP1, which stimulates NK-cell proliferation and the eventual development of aggressive NK-cell leukemia in some patients.[10,25,26]

Clinical course and prognosis
Most patients have a prolonged clinical course with increased risk of HLH and aggressive NK-cell leukemia after a median of 12 years.[10]

EBV latency pattern
Latency II.

EBV staining pattern by in situ hybridization (EBER)
A fraction of the NK cells are usually positive for Epstein-Barr encoding region (EBER) and a much higher density of EBV-positive cells should raise suspicion of NK-cell lymphoma/leukemia.

EBV–Positive Mucocutaneous Ulcer

Definition and clinical picture
EBV-positive mucocutaneous ulcer (MCU) is an entity described in immunosuppressed patients who present with painful, well-circumscribed ulcer arising at mucosal or cutaneous sites, with the oropharyngeal mucosa as the most common site of presentation.[27] No mass lesion or lymphadenopathies are detected clinically or by imaging. The cause of immunosuppression is variable and includes elderly individuals, after therapeutic immunosuppression for immune-mediated disorders, and after solid and allogeneic stem cell transplant.[27] Methotrexate is the most commonly implicated drug, mainly in the setting of rheumatoid arthritis; by the same token, EBV plus MCU is the most common EBV-associated lymphoproliferative disorder to be reported with methotrexate as a therapy complication.[28–30]

Morphologic picture
A well-circumscribed ulcer is noted with a mixed inflammatory background and a variable number of CD30-positive, EBV-positive large immunoblasts.[27,28] Some of the immunoblasts can look

atypical or Reed-Sternberg–like. The base of the lesion is usually sharply demarcated by a rim of CD3-positive small lymphocytes.

Pathogenesis

The cause of the disorder is not fully known but it is hypothesized that the immune surveillance of T cells is diminished, either because of age-related immune senescence or iatrogenic immunosuppression, to a level that is only just enough to maintain the virus dormant systemically but additional exposure to a site-restricted immune-modulating factor leads to a localized EBV-driven proliferation.[27,28]

Clinical course and prognosis

Spontaneous regression in elderly immunocompetent individuals or following reduction in immunosuppression usually occurs.

EBV latency pattern

The EBV latency pattern has not been fully studied but the transformed cells are commonly positive for LMP1 and EBER,[31] which may be suggestive of latency II or latency III pattern.

EBV staining pattern by in situ hybridization (EBER)

EBV is variably expressed, with most cases showing scattered EBV-positive cells that range in size from small to large, tend to be concentrated near the surface of the ulcer and away from the base, and are composed predominantly of B cells.

EBV–ASSOCIATED B-CELL LYMPHOPROLIFERATIVE DISORDERS

Because of EBV's preferential infection of B cells, B-cell lymphomas predominate among the EBV-related lymphoproliferative disorders. The list of EBV-associated B-cell lymphoproliferative disorders has grown over the years and includes Hodgkin lymphoma, Burkitt lymphoma, lymphomatoid granulomatosis, plasmablastic lymphoma, primary effusion lymphoma, DLBCL associated with chronic inflammation, human herpesvirus (HHV) 8–positive germinotropic lymphoproliferative disorder, EBV-positive diffuse large cell lymphoma not otherwise specified, and a subset of plasma cell neoplasms. Hodgkin lymphoma is discussed among the B-cell disorders because it has a B-cell origin, and the role of EBV in the pathogenesis of the disease is probably mediated through infected B cells. Plasma cell neoplasms are discussed here because plasma cells are the product of terminal differentiation of B cells. T-cell lymphomas such as angioimmunoblastic T-cell lymphoma are discussed in the context of T/NK-cell disorders despite EBV acting predominantly through infecting B cells and not T cells.

HODGKIN LYMPHOMA

Definition and Clinical Picture

Hodgkin lymphoma is a distinct lymphoma that is derived from germinal center B cells as a result of crippling mutations,[32] although a T-cell origin has also been postulated in about 1% to 2% of the cases.[33] Hodgkin lymphoma is classified into 2 distinct entities based on different morphologic, phenotypic, and molecular features: nodular lymphocyte–predominant Hodgkin lymphoma (NLPHL) and classic Hodgkin lymphoma, which includes nodular sclerosis, mixed-cellularity, lymphocyte-rich, and lymphocyte-depleted subtypes.[34] EBV is detected in 30% to 50% of Hodgkin lymphoma cases and is more commonly associated with classic Hodgkin lymphoma, especially the mixed-cellularity and lymphocyte-depleted subtypes.[35] NLPHL cases are very rarely associated with EBV (<5%). Underdeveloped countries have an increased incidence of EBV-positive cases, which may be attributed to the existence of an underlying immunosuppression.[34] This possibility is supported by the near-100% EBV-positive expression in patients with human immunodeficiency virus (HIV)–positive Hodgkin lymphoma.[36] Sex and ethnicity are also factors in the epidemiology of EBV-positive Hodgkin cases; men from a Hispanic or Asian origin tend to be more commonly affected.[37] A bimodal age distribution has been recognized for patients with EBV-positive Hodgkin lymphoma; children and older age groups tend to have much higher rates than young adults, which correlates with the competency of the immune surveillance at those age groups.[37]

Morphologic Picture

The characteristic large mononucleated or multinucleated neoplastic cells, known as Hodgkin and Reed-Sternberg cells (HRS), are interspersed among an inflammatory background and only constitute about 1% to 3% of total tumor mass.

Pathogenesis

Certain transforming events in the germinal center cause HRS cells to escape and survive the programmed cell death process designed for cells lacking intraclonal diversity or carrying crippling mutations. LMP1 and LMP2A may mimic and replace survival signals induced by activated CD40 and B-cell receptor (BCR), respectively.

LMP1 resembles a constitutively active CD40 receptor,[38] whereas LMP2A has been reported to mimic the presence of BCR in transgenic mice.[39] In addition, LMP1 has also been postulated to prohibit apoptosis by upregulating the antiapoptotic protein bcl-2 and mediating the activation of the nuclear factor κB (NFκB) signaling pathway.[40,41] The activated NFκB pathway plays a crucial role in the induction of proliferation in HRS cells.[41] LMP1 is also presumed to downregulate and transcriptionally reduce the expression of CD99, which has been reported to be associated with generation of B cells with classic Hodgkin lymphoma immunophenotype.[42]

Clinical Course and Prognosis

Overall, prognosis is favorable for patients with Hodgkin lymphoma, with a cure rate of ~85% in classic Hodgkin lymphoma cases.[34] The prognostic impact of EBV in patients with Hodgkin lymphoma is controversial, although some population-based studies have reported an adverse outcome in older individuals with EBV-positive Hodgkin lymphoma, likely caused by LMP1-induced activation and secretion of cytokines (interleukin [IL]-13, macrophage inflammatory protein [MIP]–1α, MIP-1β) that contribute to the systemic symptoms and overall accelerated clinical course in these patients.[35,43]

EBV Latency Pattern

Latency II.

EBV Staining Pattern by in Situ Hybridization (EBER)

EBV is usually positive in all HRS cells, although some cases show partial expression, likely caused by RNA degradation. In many cases, small EBV-positive cells are identified but these represent latently infected cells rather than being part of the neoplastic process.

BURKITT LYMPHOMA

Definition and Clinical Picture

Burkitt lymphoma a highly proliferative B-cell lymphoma that includes 3 variants: endemic (affecting children in equatorial Africa and New Guinea), sporadic (children and young adults throughout the world), and immunodeficiency related (primarily in association with HIV infection).[44] The detection of somatic hypermutations in the variable region of the immunoglobulin genes and the phenotype of the neoplastic cells indicate a germinal center cell origin of the lymphoma.[45] EBV has been detected in virtually all cases of the endemic variant, 20% to 30% of the sporadic variant, and 30% to 40% of the immunodeficiency-related variant.[44,46]

Morphologic Picture

A diffuse monotonous proliferation of medium-sized lymphocytes is noted. Markedly increased mitotic figures, apoptotic bodies, and numerous tingible body macrophages with a starry-sky pattern are also seen.

Pathogenesis

Constitutive activation of the MYC oncogene through its translocation into one of the immunoglobulin loci is the key factor in the oncogenesis.[44,46] Mutations in TCF3 or its negative regulator ID3 activate the phosphatidylinositol 3 kinase (PI3K)/BCR signaling pathway and have been reported in 70% of sporadic and 40% of endemic cases.[47,48] The near absence of these mutations in DLBCL may suggest a critical role that these mutations may play in the oncogenesis of Burkitt lymphoma in addition to MYC.[47,48] Moreover, recent studies suggest that a cryptic deletion at 11q can be a key factor in the pathogenesis of Burkitt lymphoma in the absence of MYC translocation[49] and, as such, the provisional entity of Burkitt-like lymphoma with 11q abnormality has been included in the 2016 WHO classification.[50] The variable EBV association in the 3 variants and the restrictive latency pattern has prompted many clinicians to speculate that the virus is a passenger in the neoplastic process and not the initiating factor. EBNA1 plays a crucial role in the maintenance and replication of the viral genome but its oncogenic potential is highly controversial.[46] Because the EBERs are thought to possess antiapoptotic activities as well as the ability to induce IL-10, which may promote cell growth and survival, they may play a role in the oncogenesis of Burkitt lymphoma.[51] More recent data point to a possible polymicrobial disease pathogenesis involving EBV, Plasmodium falciparum, and herpesviruses, among others.[44,52,53]

Clinical Course and Prognosis

Burkitt lymphoma is highly aggressive but potentially curable in many patients, with long-term overall survival of 70% to 90%. EBV association does not have any reported prognostic implication.

EBV Latency Pattern

The EBV latency patterns in Burkitt lymphoma are heterogeneous but almost all cases show a highly restrictive pattern, only expressing EBNA1 and the EBERs (latency I).[46] Some cases are reported to express EBNAs 3A, 3B, 3C, and leader protein in addition to EBNA1 and the EBERs, but they still lack EBNA2 and the latent membrane proteins.[54] Another distinct latency pattern involving the expression of LMP2 along with that of lytic genes has been reported, postulating that LMP2A increases *MYC*-driven lymphoid proliferations through activation of the PI3K pathway.[44,55]

EBV Staining Pattern by in Situ Hybridization (EBER)

The EBV-positive cases show diffuse EBER staining in most of the lymphoma cells.

LYMPHOMATOID GRANULOMATOSIS

Definition and Clinical Picture

Lymphomatoid granulomatosis is a rare angiocentric and angiodestructive B-cell lymphoproliferative disorder that usually occurs in the lungs, with less frequent involvement of other extranodal sites such as the central nervous system (CNS), skin, kidney, and liver.[56] It is associated with underlying immunodeficiency in most cases, and careful clinical or laboratory analysis usually yields evidence of reduced immune status in patients presenting without an apparent underlying immunodeficiency.[57]

Morphologic Picture

This condition is an angiocentric and angiodestructive lesion that is composed predominantly of reactive T cells and fewer interspersed neoplastic EBV-positive B cells. A 3-tier grading system for lymphomatoid granulomatosis exists that has been slightly modified in the 2016 WHO classification and relates to the number of EBV-positive B cells within each patient (grade 1, <5 positive cells with minimal necrosis and without cytologic atypia; grade 2, 5–20 positive cells, but can reach up to 50 cells occasionally with necrosis and minimal atypia; and grade 3, >50 positive cells with extensive necrosis and evident atypia).[57] EBV-positive cells may, rarely, be absent in grade 1 lesions. Some clinicians argue that quantitating the number of large B cells rather than counting the number of EBV-positive cells for establishing grade is a more accurate method, given that extensive areas of necrosis can lead to poor RNA preservation for EBV detection by in situ hybridization.[56]

Pathogenesis

The near-100% EBV association with lymphomatoid granulomatosis and the presumed wide expression of EBV latent encoded proteins may indicate that EBV is not just an innocent bystander but likely plays a crucial role in the pathogenesis of the disease. The presence of lymphomatoid granulomatosis in a considerable number of immunosuppressed patients and the presumed latency III pattern suggest that EBV plays a similar transformative role to that seen in PTLD.

Clinical Course and Prognosis

The clinical course is widely variable, with some patients asymptomatic and just presenting with pulmonary nodules. Other patients may have multiorgan involvement and may even progress to EBV-positive DLBCL. The overall survival rate has improved to ~70% following the use of dose-adjusted EPOCH-R therapy (Etoposide, Prednisone, Vincristine, Cyclophosphamide, Doxorubicin, and Rituximab).[57]

EBV Latency Pattern

The latency pattern for EBV has not been extensively studied in lymphomatoid granulomatosis, but a type III latency pattern is the most commonly reported pattern given the detection of LMP1 and EBNA2 by immunohistochemistry.[57–59]

EBV Staining Pattern by in Situ Hybridization (EBER)

EBV is positive in the large neoplastic B cells and the number of EBV-positive cells determines the grade, as previously mentioned.

PLASMABLASTIC LYMPHOMA

Definition and Clinical Picture

Plasmablastic lymphoma is a highly aggressive B-cell lymphoma that was originally described in the oral cavity in association with HIV infection but can occur at other sites, mainly extranodal, and in association with other causes of immunodeficiency.[60] Disseminated involvement, including bone marrow involvement, is seen in 75% of HIV-positive individuals but in only 25% of patients with no apparent immunodeficiency.[61] EBV is detected in about 60% to 70% of the cases, more frequently in HIV-positive cases.[60,61] *MYC* translocation has been reported in almost half of the cases, more frequently in EBV-positive cases (74%) than in EBV-negative cases (43%).[60,62]

Morphologic Picture

A morphologic spectrum is noted that ranges from a diffuse proliferation of immunoblastlike large cells resembling DLBCL to cells with more notable plasmacytic differentiation. Patients with prior plasma cell myeloma should be considered as plasmablastic transformation of myeloma and should not be included in this category.[60] Plasmablastic transformation from low-grade small B-cell lymphomas, mainly chronic lymphocytic leukemia and follicular lymphoma, can also occur but no notable association with EBV infection, immunodeficiency, or *MYC* translocation has been described in these cases.[63]

Pathogenesis

The pathogenesis of plasmablastic lymphoma is not fully known but a potential role for *MYC* gene rearrangements in association with EBV has been described.[61] In contrast with most other B-cell lymphoproliferative disorders, EBV expression is usually restricted to the EBERs with rare expression of LMP1, which correlates with previous work showing a marked reduction of the expression of EBV latent proteins with terminal B-cell differentiation into plasma cells.[64,65]

Clinical Course and Prognosis

The prognosis is grave for most patients, with an overall survival rate of less than 1 year.

EBV Latency Pattern

An overall restricted EBV latency pattern is noted (latency I/latency 0).

EBV staining pattern by in situ hybridization (EBER)

Most of the lymphoma cells are diffusely positive for EBER.

DIFFUSE LARGE B-CELL LYMPHOMA ASSOCIATED WITH CHRONIC INFLAMMATION

Definition and Clinical Picture

A mass-forming lesion that is considered to be a subcategory of DLBCL mostly involving body cavities. It was primarily defined from pyothorax-associated lymphoma (PAL), which was first described in Japanese patients in 1987[66] and was later incorporated into the WHO classification of lung and pleural tumors in 2004.[67] In the 2008 WHO classification of tumors of hematopoietic and lymphoid tissues, PAL was incorporated into the DLBCL with chronic inflammation (DLBCL-CI) entity.[68] With discontinuation of artificial pneumothorax for treatment of pulmonary tuberculosis, the incidence of PAL has decreased but other causes for DLBCL-CI, including chronic osteomyelitis,

metallic implants, and chronic skin ulcers, have been described.[69,70] The interval between the inciting event and the development of lymphoma is usually greater than 10 years.[69] Its reported association with EBV has ranged from 70% to 100% of the cases.[67] Recently, a small number of cases of fibrin-associated EBV-positive large B-cell proliferations has been reported in immunocompetent patients in association with hematomas, thrombi in sites with prior vascular surgery, prosthetic cardiac valves, atrial myxomas, and pseudocysts.[71–74] It has been incorporated in the 2016 WHO classification as a subtype of DLBCL-CI, labeled fibrin-associated DLBCL.[75] Compared with DLBCL-CI, patients with this entity have non–mass-forming lesions, shorter latency, lower genetic complexity, and an indolent clinical course with significantly lower mortality.[76]

Morphologic Picture

This condition typically presents with clusters of large lymphoma cells that show immunoblastic/centroblastic morphology. An angiocentric growth pattern and massive necrosis can be seen. For the fibrin-associated subtype, these cases show discontiguous foci of large B cells in a background of abundant fibrin.[76]

Pathogenesis

The exact role of EBV in the pathogenesis has yet to be determined, although some studies have suggested that the production of IL-6 and IL-10 by EBV in addition to the ability of EBNA1-expressing and LMP1-expressing B cells to escape immunosurveillance in immunocompromised patients may provide some clues for a potential role for EBV.[77,78] For the fibrin-associated subtype, the focal nature of these proliferations is hypothesized to be related to localized immune suppression[72,79] but other investigators postulated a pathogenesis related to the lack of ability of the transformed and immortalized EBV-positive cells to proliferate outside immune-privileged spaces.[76]

Clinical Course and Prognosis

DLBCL-CI is an aggressive lymphoma with an overall 5-year survival rate of 20% to 35%.[68] However, the fibrin-associated subtype has a more favorable clinical course in most cases, even with surgical excision alone.

EBV Latency Pattern

Latency III.

EBV Staining Pattern by in Situ Hybridization (EBER)

Most of the lymphoma cells are positive for EBER.

EBV–POSITIVE DIFFUSE LARGE B-CELL LYMPHOMA, NOT OTHERWISE SPECIFIED

Definition and Clinical Picture

The 2008 WHO classification recognized a provisional entity, DLBCL of the elderly.[80,81] It was defined as an EBV-associated B-cell lymphoma in immunocompetent patients more than 50 years-old with a predilection for involvement of extranodal sites and an overall poor outcome.[80,81] However, recent studies have shown that the age cutoff of 50 years is arbitrary and that EBV-positive large cell lymphomas are not restricted to older individuals but can occur in younger immunocompetent patients, with a predilection toward a nodal distribution pattern and an overall more favorable outcome than in the elderly.[82] In the 2016 WHO classification, the term elderly was dropped and the entity was designated as EBV-positive DLBCL, not otherwise specified (NOS).[83] The NOS designation is used to emphasize the exclusion of more specific types of EBV-positive lymphomas, previously described. EBV plus DLBCL accounts for 10% to 15% of DLBCL cases in Asian and Latin patients but less than 5% of Western patients.[83]

Morphologic Picture

EBV plus DLBCL usually has a nongerminal center cell B-cell phenotype and shows a broader morphologic spectrum that ranges from monomorphic lesions to polymorphic lesions including cases described as T-cell/histiocyte-rich large B-cell lymphoma (THRLBCL)–like or Hodgkin-like.[82,84] The polymorphic pattern is commonly seen in younger patients and in some cases can be mistaken for Hodgkin lymphoma or THRLBCL.[82] Although CD30 is frequently positive, the intact B-cell phenotype, CD45 expression within the large lymphoma cells, the lack of CD15 positivity in most cases, and the strong and uniform expression of LMP-1 are factors that support a diagnosis of EBV plus DLBCL rather than Hodgkin lymphoma. THRLBCLs are EBV negative by definition and lack the focal residual B-cell areas usually seen in polymorphic EBV plus DLBCL cases. Rare cases of gray zone lymphomas with features intermediate between DLBCL and Hodgkin lymphoma have been reported to be EBV positive; however, given the difficulty in differentiating these lymphomas from EBV plus DLBCL, extreme caution is recommended before making a diagnosis of gray zone lymphoma when EBV is positive.[82,85]

Pathogenesis

EBV is detected in all cases that typically have various levels of immunosuppression. Alteration in T-cell responses with diminished functionality likely plays a role in the pathogenesis, at least in elderly patients.[83]

Clinical Course and Prognosis

The prognosis is significantly different between elderly and young patients. An aggressive course with an overall median survival rate of 2 years is noted in the elderly, whereas an excellent prognosis with a long-term complete remission is noted in ~80% of younger patients.[83] As expected, cases with polymorphic pattern have a more favorable prognosis than monomorphic cases in young patients.

EBV Latency Pattern

A latency III program was initially reported to be the most commonly encountered, although some cases lacked EBNA2 expression (latency II), especially in younger individuals.[80,86] The variable presence of EBNA2 expression may be attributed to the variable degrees of immune surveillance in aging individuals. The redefinition of the lymphoma in the 2016 WHO classification and the reports from more recent studies indicate more frequent EBV latency II occurrence, given the evident predominance of latency II in younger patients, a pattern more in keeping with immunocompetent individuals.[82,87]

EBV Staining Pattern by in Situ Hybridization (EBER)

Most of the large atypical neoplastic cells are EBV positive. Scattered bystander small reactive B cells may also be positive and should not be the sole reason for calling the lymphoma EBV positive.

HUMAN HERPESVIRUS 8–ASSOCIATED B-CELL LYMPHOPROLIFERATIVE DISORDERS

HHV8 was initially discovered in association with Kaposi sarcoma but since then it has also been linked to 4 lymphoproliferative disorders: a subset of multicentric Castleman disease (MCD), HHV8-positive DLBCL, primary effusion lymphoma (PEL), and germinotropic lymphoproliferative disorder.[88] Of these 4 disorders, concurrent EBV infection is seen in PEL and germinotropic lymphoproliferative disorder (described later). In addition, other rare cases of HHV8+/EBV+ disorders have been described and include a rare case of intravascular large cell lymphoma in an HIV-positive patient with many subcutaneous nodules, a Hodgkin-like lymphoma case with scattered large highly atypical HHV8+/EBV+ cells interspersed in a reactive background, rare cases of MCD with dual positivity for HHV8 and EBV, and 2 cases of mass-forming PEL-like lymphoma in immunocompetent patients.[88–91] These reported cases are suggestive that HHV8+/EBV+ lymphoproliferative disorders may represent a spectrum of overlapping disorders and that EBV may play a possible cofactor role in the proliferation of lymphoma cells with HHV8 latent proteins being the driving force.

PRIMARY EFFUSION LYMPHOMA

Definition and Clinical Picture

Primary effusion lymphoma is a distinct HHV8-positive B-cell lymphoma that affects body cavities, usually without detectable extracavitary tumor masses, although rare HHV8-positive tumors can present as solid tumor masses and are labeled as extracavitary PEL.[92] It usually occurs in the setting of immunodeficiency, mainly HIV infection, but can also occur in the solid organ transplant setting.[92,93] Occurrence in elderly individuals in the absence of immunodeficiency has also been reported and these cases are usually HHV8 positive but EBV negative.[94] EBV-negative PEL cases usually occur in HHV-8 endemic areas such as the Mediterranean.[92,95] A rare HHV8-negative effusion based lymphoma with PEL-like morphology has also been described; these cases are usually EBV and HIV negative, occur in elderly individuals with no apparent immunosuppression, and are likely associated with chronic inflammation that causes fluid overload in body cavities.[96]

Morphologic Picture

An immunoblastic to anaplastic plasmacytoid morphology is seen in almost all cases. Some cases contain few highly pleomorphic cells with a Reed-Sternberg–like appearance. The extracavitary cases show a similar morphologic picture to that seen in effusions and frequently involve nodal sinuses and vascular channels.

Pathogenesis

EBV is detected in most PEL cases (~70%) and a defined role in the pathogenesis is not supported given the presence of EBV-negative cases and the restricted expression patterns in the positive cases.[92] However, other investigators describe a possible cofactor role for EBV in the development and proliferation of lymphoma cells, with the latent proteins of HHV8 being the driving force.[97–100] One study reported a potential role of EBV in promoting establishment of latency in HHV8 by inhibiting its lytic replication.[101]

Clinical Course and Prognosis

An extremely aggressive clinical course is noted in most patients, with an overall survival rate of less than 1 year.

EBV Latency Pattern

The expression of EBV latent encoded proteins is restricted to EBNA1, LMP2A, and EBERs, although heterogeneous LMP1 expression has been reported in some cases, which is suggestive of a latency I/latency II pattern.[99]

EBV Staining Pattern by in Situ Hybridization (EBER)

Most of the lymphoma cells are positive for EBER in the EBV-positive cases.

HUMAN HERPESVIRUS 8–POSITIVE GERMINOTROPIC LYMPHOPROLIFERATIVE DISORDER

Definition and Clinical Picture

HHV8-positive germinotropic lymphoproliferative disorder (HHV8+GLPD) is a novel HHV8-positive entity that was described in 2002.[102] Patients are usually immunocompetent, present with localized lymphadenopathy, and have an overall favorable clinical course with good response to chemotherapy and radiation. However, more recent studies reported its occurrence in HIV-positive individuals as well as presentation with generalized lymphadenopathy.[103,104] Progression or transformation to large B-cell lymphoma has not been described yet, although one study reported progression to DLBCL in 1 of the cases, but the phenotype (EBV+, HHV8−) may have been suggestive of a separate independent clone.[103]

Morphologic Picture

The nodal architecture is generally preserved and clusters of HHV8-positive, EBV-positive plasmablasts are identified in a subset of the germinal centers. These clusters may coalesce to form aggregates reminiscent of the microlymphomas seen in MCD with HHV8-positive plasmablasts; however, the characteristic follicular changes, the interfollicular plasmacytosis, and the vascular proliferation seen in Castleman disease are generally absent. A germinal center cell origin has been postulated given the detection of somatic mutations and intraclonal diversity within the microdissected HHV8-positive, EBV-positive plasmablasts.[102]

Pathogenesis

The role of EBV in the pathogenesis of the disease is largely unknown and rare EBV-negative cases have been reported.[104] Given the small number of cases reported for HHV8+GLPD, it is likely that the outline and disease course of this disorder will be better defined in the future once more cases are studied.

Clinical Course and Prognosis

A favorable clinical course is seen in most patients, with good response to chemotherapy or radiation therapy.

EBV Latency Pattern

EBV latency I pattern was reported in one of the studies based on the negativity for LMP1, EBNA2, and BZLF-1 protein expression in 2 cases.[103]

EBV Staining Pattern by in Situ Hybridization (EBER)

Clusters of EBV-positive large cells are seen in some germinal centers that correlate with HHV8 expression.

PLASMA CELL NEOPLASMS

Definition and Clinical Picture

Plasma cell neoplasms are a group that encompasses a spectrum of plasma cell disorders that include non-IgM monoclonal gammopathy of undetermined significance (MGUS), plasmacytoma, plasma cell myeloma and variants, monoclonal immunoglobulin deposition disease, and plasma cell neoplasms associated with paraneoplastic syndrome according to the 2016 WHO classification.[105] True plasma cell neoplasms have been rarely reported to be associated with EBV expression, except in the setting of immunodeficiency. Posttransplant and severely immunocompromised patients, especially those with established HIV infection, have a slightly increased incidence of EBV-positive plasma cell neoplasms.[106,107] A recent study by our group (in press) examining EBV expression in 147 cases with plasma cell neoplasms in a diverse ethnic population detected no EBV expression in immunocompetent patients with plasma cell myeloma and MGUS but detected about 14% (3 out of 21 cases) EBV expression in immunocompetent patients with plasmacytoma, usually with focal plasmablastic features. Another recent study detected 10% (4 out of 46 cases) EBV-positive expression in an immunocompetent plasmacytoma patient cohort.[108] The study reported no association with plasmablastic features, no difference in overall survival time, but an increased likelihood of disease relapse/progression to plasma cell myeloma compared with their EBV-negative patients.[108] Other case reports describing EBV expression in immunocompetent patients with plasmacytoma exist,[109–111] but a larger meta-analysis study may be needed to confirm any potential association of EBV with plasmacytomas.

Morphologic Picture

The morphologic features of the neoplastic plasma cells in EBV-positive cases have been mainly described as plasmablastic, focally plasmablastic, or anaplastic.[112]

Pathogenesis

In healthy individuals that are seropositive for EBV, terminal differentiation of EBV-infected memory B cells into plasma cells has been reported to be associated with viral replication and initiation of the EBV lytic cycle.[113,114] This finding may explain to an extent the rarity of EBV expression in plasma cell neoplasms; the rare tumors with plasmacytic differentiation that are associated with EBV, such as PEL or plasmablastic lymphoma, usually establish a latent cycle and show a restrictive EBV latency pattern.

Clinical Course and Prognosis

The clinical course depends on the type of plasma cell neoplasm involved.

EBV Latency Pattern

No studies have extensively studied the latency patterns in EBV-positive plasma cell neoplasms in immunocompetent patients, but most cases studied are LMP1 negative, suggestive of a more restricted latency pattern.

EBV Staining Pattern by in Situ Hybridization (EBER)

In the few published EBV-positive plasmacytoma cases, EBV is usually positive focally, mainly in cells that show plasmablastic morphology, although normal-appearing plasma cells can also be positive for EBER.

EBV–ASSOCIATED T/NATURAL KILLER–CELL LYMPHOPROLIFERATIVE DISORDERS

EBV can infect CD4-positive and CD8-positive peripheral blood T cells as well as NK cells in a minority of patients with infectious mononucleosis, but most EBV-associated T-cell lymphomas have a cytotoxic phenotype, which suggests that these tumors may have resulted somehow from the proliferating cytotoxic T cells trying to kill the EBV-infected cells.[115,116] T/NK-cell lymphoproliferative disorders that have been reported to be EBV associated include angioimmunoblastic T-cell lymphoma, follicular T-cell lymphoma, extranodal nasal NK/T-cell lymphoma, aggressive NK-cell leukemia, systemic EBV-positive T-cell lymphoma of childhood, and a subset of peripheral T-cell lymphoma, NOS.

ANGIOIMMUNOBLASTIC T-CELL LYMPHOMA

Definition and Clinical Picture

Angioimmunoblastic T-cell lymphoma (AITL) is a systemic lymphoproliferative disorder that mainly affects older individuals and is characterized by constitutional symptoms including generalized lymphadenopathy, fever, skin rash, hepatosplenomegaly, and polyclonal hypergammaglobulinemia.[117] Mature T-follicular helper cells represents the cells of origin for the lymphoma, and clonal rearrangements of the T-cell receptor genes have been detected in most cases.[118] Scattered EBV-positive B cells are seen in nearly all the cases. Expansion of EBV-positive cells is seen in nearly 75% of the cases and EBV-driven B-cell lymphomas can also superimpose or complicate the course of AITL in some of these cases, in which the AITL-associated immunodeficiency followed by the immunosuppressive effects of chemotherapy may have created an ideal environment for the variable number of EBV-infected B cells to proliferate and transform.[117,119]

Morphologic Picture

Effacement of the nodal architecture by a polymorphous lymphoid infiltrate, florid vascular proliferation, and follicular dendritic cell (FDC) proliferation, usually around blood vessels. Variable numbers of B immunoblasts are seen, some of which are EBV positive.

Pathogenesis

Given the presence of EBV-positive B cells in nearly all the cases, a potential role for EBV in the pathogenesis has been postulated, likely through antigen drive. The EBV-positive B cells have been determined to have ongoing somatic mutations, a hallmark of germinal center cells; however, these mutations are nonfunctional.[120] These crippling mutations are almost restricted to the EBV-infected cells and not detected in EBV-negative cells, which assumes a potential influence of EBV on these proliferating cells.[120] The sustained somatic hypermutation status likely leading to escaping apoptosis could be caused by the stimulation by the rich FDC meshwork and the increased number of CD4-positive helper T cells.[45,121]

Clinical Course and Prognosis

The clinical course is variable but the overall prognosis is poor, with an overall survival of less than 3 years.

EBV Latency Pattern

The latency pattern for EBV is not known, although some investigators have assumed a restricted latency II program similar to that seen in other EBV-associated T-cell lymphoproliferative disorders.[120] This postulation can also be supported by the fact that most of the subsequent EBV-associated B-cell proliferations that sometimes follow AITL express LMP1 and the EBERs, which is consistent with type II latency.[119]

EBV Staining Pattern by in Situ Hybridization (EBER)

EBV is positive in a variable number of the B immunoblasts, which vary in size, although they are mainly large. Significantly increased number of EBV-positive cells can be seen in some cases, especially in cases with B-cell progression.

FOLLICULAR T-CELL LYMPHOMA

Definition and Clinical Picture

Follicular T-cell lymphoma is a rare nodal lymphoma with occasional skin and bone marrow involvement that has a predominantly follicular growth pattern and arises from mature follicular helper T cells but lacks the characteristic features of AITL, such as vascular proliferation and extrafollicular FDC proliferation.[117] It was incorporated in the 2016 WHO classification under angioimmunoblastic T-cell lymphoma and other nodal lymphomas of T-follicular helper cell origin.[117] A relatively specific translocation t(5;9) has been described in about 20% of the cases.[122,123]

Morphologic Picture

Two distinct growth patterns have been described: a follicular lymphomalike pattern, in which the neoplastic T cells form well-defined nodules, and a progressive transformation of germinal centers–like pattern, in which the neoplastic T cells form large irregular nodules, surrounded by many IgD-positive mantle cells.[122]

Pathogenesis

EBV is reported to be positive in B immunoblasts in about 50% to 60% of the cases, and its role in the pathogenesis is hypothetical, similar to that described in AITL.

Clinical Course and Prognosis

An overall aggressive course is reported, although the clinical course and prognosis are not well characterized given the rarity of the disorder and its recent definition as a distinct entity.

EBV Latency Pattern

The EBV latency is not known but it may be similar to latency II, which is postulated for AITL cases.

EBV Staining Pattern by in Situ Hybridization (EBER)

EBV is usually positive in large B immunoblasts and sometimes in large Reed-Sternberg–like cells.[117,122]

EXTRANODAL NATURAL Killer/T-CELL LYMPHOMA, NASAL TYPE

Definition and Clinical Picture

Extranodal natural killer/T-cell lymphoma, nasal type, is an angiocentric and angiodestructive neoplasm associated with prominent necrosis that predominantly involves extranodal sites, particularly the upper aerodigestive track, and has a geographic predilection for Asia and Central America.[124] Most cases seem to show a pure NK-cell phenotype but some cases have a cytotoxic T-cell phenotype and hence the NK/T-cell designation. A near-100% EBV association is described, irrespective of the ethnic origin.[124,125] Although secondary nodal involvement occurs in occasional cases of nasal NK/T-cell lymphoma, primary EBV-positive nodal NK/T-cell lymphomas should be classified as a variant of peripheral T-cell lymphoma; these cases usually lack the angiodestruction and necrosis and occur in elderly individuals or in the setting of immunodeficiency.[126]

Morphologic Picture

A diffuse lymphoid infiltrate is noted with an angiocentric and angiodestructive growth pattern. Extensive coagulative necrosis is seen in many cases.

Pathogenesis

Earlier studies described a minimal role for EBV in the pathogenesis of the lymphoma, because reduction of LMP1 levels in treated cell lines did not lead to growth inhibition or apoptosis within the neoplastic cells.[127] However, more recent studies describe a similar role for EBV in inducing transformation and promoting cell survival to that seen in Hodgkin lymphoma and B-cell lymphomas by activation of the NFκB pathway via LMP1 protein.[128,129] Another study suggested that LMP1 may increase the sensitivity of the NK cell to the growth-promoting effects of IL-2 receptor alpha.[130]

Clinical Course and Prognosis

An overall poor prognosis and low survival rate have been reported historically but survival has improved in recent years with more intensive chemotherapy. Higher levels of circulating EBV DNA in the peripheral blood and presence of EBV-positive cells in the bone marrow are usually associated with a more aggressive disease and poor survival.[126,131]

EBV Latency Pattern

Latency II.

EBV Staining Pattern by in Situ Hybridization (EBER)

The EBV expression pattern is characteristic, in which virtually all the lymphoma cells are positive for EBER.

AGGRESSIVE NATURAL KILLER CELL LEUKEMIA

Definition and Clinical Picture

Aggressive NK-cell leukemia is a rare systemic neoplastic proliferation of NK cells that is characterized by an aggressive and often fatal clinical course.[132] The most frequently involved sites are bone marrow, peripheral blood, spleen, and liver. In rare cases, the leukemia arises from chronic lymphoproliferative disorders of NK cells and, in younger patients, it may evolve from chronic active EBV infection.[124,132,133] EBV is reported to be positive in 85% to 100% of aggressive NK-cell leukemia cases.[132] The EBV-negative cases can occur de novo or as a progression of chronic lymphoproliferative disorder of NK cells.[132,134] Some investigators think that aggressive NK-cell leukemia may represent the leukemic counterpart of nasal NK/T-cell lymphoma. This hypothesis is mainly based on the similar ethnic background, morphologic picture, immunophenotype, strong EBV association, and genotype (lack of T-cell receptor gene rearrangements).[135] At present, the most accepted differentiating features between the two entities are that aggressive NK-cell leukemia often presents at a younger age (almost a decade younger, with a median age of 40 years), shows B symptoms, has more frequent hepatosplenic and bone marrow involvement, has a lower frequency of cutaneous involvement and more frequent expression of CD16 (positive in 75% of cases), and usually disseminates early in presentation.[136–138] Moreover, an array-based comparative genomic hybridization study has reported significance differences in genetic changes between the two disorders, in which 7p−, 17p−, and 1q+ are more frequent in aggressive NK-cell leukemia, whereas 6q− is more common in nasal NK-cell lymphoma.[139]

Morphologic Picture

A monotonous NK-cell infiltrate is noted that can range from a subtle infiltrate in the bone marrow to a massive diffuse infiltrate. Necrosis is common and an increased number of apoptotic bodies is usually seen.

Pathogenesis

A potential role for EBV in inducing transformation and promoting cell survival through activation of the NFκB pathway via LMP1 protein has been postulated, similar to that seen in nasal NK/T-cell lymphoma.

Clinical Course and Prognosis

A fulminant clinical course is noted in most cases, with an overall survival rate of 2 to 3 months.

EBV Latency Pattern

Latency II.

EBV Staining Pattern by in Situ Hybridization (EBER)

Almost all of the leukemia cells are positive for EBER, similar to that seen in nasal NK/T-cell lymphoma.

SYSTEMIC EBV–POSITIVE T-CELL LYMPHOMA OF CHILDHOOD

Definition and Clinical Picture

Systemic EBV-positive T-cell lymphoma of childhood is a rare, aggressive, systemic T-cell lymphoma that usually occurs in children and young adults, mainly Asian, and is derived from T cells, usually with an activated cytotoxic phenotype.[10]

Despite its name, it can occur in adolescents and young adults as well, with a reported median age at diagnosis of 20 years.[140,141] The most commonly involved sites are liver and spleen, followed by lymph nodes, bone marrow, and skin. It can occur after acute EBV infection or in the setting of CAEBV, and severe CAEBV cases with monoclonal EBV-positive T-cell proliferation are considered by many clinicians as part of the spectrum of systemic EBV-positive T-cell lymphoma of childhood.[21,142] Hemophagocytic syndrome is present in nearly all cases. EBV has been detected in all cases.

Morphologic Picture

A sinusoidal infiltration pattern with evident hemophagocytosis is usually noted. The cortical areas of the lymph node (B-cell areas) and white pulp of the spleen are usually depleted. Necrosis may be present.

Pathogenesis

The cause of the lymphoma is unknown, but its ethnic predilection and its strong association with EBV infection may be suggestive of a genetic defect of the immune system response to EBV.[10,142,143]

Clinical Course and Prognosis

A rapidly progressive and often lethal clinical course is described, similar to that seen in aggressive NK-cell leukemia.

EBV Latency Pattern

The EBV latency pattern has not been adequately studied and is unknown.

EBV Staining Pattern by in Situ Hybridization (EBER)

EBV is positive in almost all neoplastic T cells, similar to that seen in nasal NK-cell lymphoma and aggressive NK-cell leukemia cases.

PERIPHERAL T-CELL LYMPHOMA, NOT OTHERWISE SPECIFIED

Definition and Clinical Picture

Peripheral T-cell lymphoma (PTCL), NOS, is a heterogeneous group of nodal and extranodal T-cell lymphomas that do not correspond with any of the defined categories in the 2016 WHO classification.[144] It is very rare in children and usually presents in older adults. EBV expression in PTCL, NOS, has been variably reported in the literature but about 30% of all cases are EBV positive (any positivity), with 10% to 15%

showing strong EBER positivity.[11,145] More commonly, EBV is positive in background small and large B cells but it can also be positive in the neoplastic T cells.[144,145]

Morphologic Picture

A diffuse or paracortical infiltrate with broad cytologic spectrum is usually noted that causes effacement of the nodal architecture. Clusters of epithelioid histiocytes and mild vascular hyperplasia may be seen.

Pathogenesis

The exact role of EBV in the oncogenesis of peripheral T-cell lymphomas is still hypothetical; although one study reported that increased IL-9 levels induced by the EBERs possess antiapoptotic effects and promote T-cell proliferation and transformation.[146] Also, similar to Hodgkin lymphoma pathogenesis, LMP1 may mimic or act as a viral analogue for members of the family of tumor necrosis factor (TNF) receptors, thereby transmitting growth signals through cytoplasmic TNF receptor–associated factors.[147] Members of the TNF family include CD40, which was previously discussed in relation to Hodgkin lymphoma.

Clinical Course and Prognosis

A very aggressive clinical course is noted, especially in older patients. The presence of strong EBER positivity is reported to be associated with a more aggressive clinical course.[145,148] Because TNF-α levels, which may be the cause of fever and weight loss in T-cell lymphomas, are thought to reliably correlate with disease activity and with EBV infection, a few investigators suggested that TNF-α levels would be a useful prognostic marker to monitor in EBV-associated peripheral T-cell lymphoma.[149]

EBV Latency Pattern

The EBV latency pattern has not been widely studied but it is thought to represent a restricted pattern (latency II), similar to other EBV-positive T/NK-cell lymphoproliferative disorders.

EBV Staining Pattern by in Situ Hybridization (EBER)

A variable staining pattern is noted, with only a few cases showing diffuse strong EBER staining of the neoplastic T cells.

EBV AND IMMUNODEFICIENCY-RELATED LYMPHOPROLIFERATIVE DISORDERS

The EBV-associated/immunodeficiency-related lymphoproliferative disorders include HIV-related lymphoproliferative disorders, PTLD, other iatrogenic immunodeficiency-associated lymphoproliferative disorders, and lymphoproliferative diseases associated with primary immune disorders.

HUMAN IMMUNODEFICIENCY VIRUS–RELATED LYMPHOPROLIFERATIVE DISORDERS

Definition and Clinical Picture

HIV-related lymphoproliferative disorders are a heterogeneous group of disorders that can range from HIV-related polyclonal lymphoid proliferations in some patients to full-blown monoclonal proliferations in most patients, which is suggestive of a multistep lymphomagenesis.[150] HIV-related lymphomas tend to have an increased propensity to involve extranodal sites and are generally divided into 3 groups: (1) lymphomas that can occur in immunocompetent individuals (HIV negative), such as DLBCL and Burkitt lymphoma; (2) lymphomas that occur predominantly in the setting of HIV infection, such as PEL, plasmablastic lymphoma of the oral cavity, and HHV8-positive DLBCL; and (3) lymphomas occurring in other immunodeficiency states, such as polymorphic B-cell lymphomas (PTLD-like).[151] EBV has been reported to be detected in approximately 40% of all HIV-related lymphomas, including nearly 100% of primary CNS lymphomas, 80% of DLBCL with immunoblastic features (~30% of all other types of DLBCL), 30% to 50% of Burkitt lymphomas, 60% to 70% of plasmablastic lymphomas, 70% to 80% of PEL, and nearly 100% of classic Hodgkin lymphomas arising in the setting of HIV.[150–153]

Morphologic Picture

The morphologic picture depends on the type of lymphoma involved.

Pathogenesis

Several factors play a role in the pathogenesis of HIV-related lymphomas, including genetic abnormalities, chronic antigen stimulation, cytokine deregulation, and possible roles for HHV8 and EBV.[154] As with many EBV-associated lymphoproliferative disorders, the role of EBV in the pathogenesis of the HIV-related disorders is speculative at the current time. In DLBCL with immunoblastic features and classic Hodgkin lymphoma, some researchers strongly believe that the high EBV association with these tumors and the consistent expression of LMP1 indicate an EBV-driven proliferation.[151,155]

Clinical Course and Prognosis

Almost all HIV-associated lymphoproliferative disorders are highly aggressive and of a B-cell origin.[156] Primary CNS lymphoma constitutes about 20% of all HIV-related lymphomas and used to have a 1000-fold increased incidence in HIV-positive individuals before the introduction of combined antiretroviral therapy.[151] Classic Hodgkin lymphoma is also increased in the setting of HIV infection and is reported to have an 8-fold increased incidence, with mixed cellularity and lymphocyte-depleted subtypes being the most commonly reported.[157]

EBV Latency Pattern

Because of the heterogeneity of the HIV-related disorders, different patterns of latent EBV gene expression have been described. In the first group of disorders that can occur in immunocompetent individuals, the pattern of EBV expression coincides with the histologic subtype of lymphoma irrespective of the HIV status. In the second group of disorders (HIV near-specific lymphomas), EBV expression in plasmablastic lymphomas is usually restricted to the EBERs with rare expression of LMP1 and, in PEL, the expression of EBV latent encoded proteins is restricted to EBNA1, LMP2A, and EBERs, although heterogeneous LMP1 expression has been reported in some cases, which is suggestive of a latency I/latency II pattern for this group of lymphomas. In primary CNS lymphoma, all EBV latent encoded proteins are detected in most cases (latency III).[158] In the third group (HIV-related lymphoma in other immunodeficiency states), an EBV latency pattern similar to that seen in PTLD is postulated (latency III).

EBV Staining Pattern by in Situ Hybridization (EBER)

The EBV expression patterns are dependent on the type of lymphoma involved.

POSTTRANSPLANT LYMPHOPROLIFERATIVE DISORDERS

Definition and Clinical Picture

PTLDs are clinicopathologic entities encompassing a heterogeneous group of disorders that follow solid organ or stem cell transplant as a consequence of immunosuppression and range

from polyclonal proliferations to malignant monoclonal forms.[159,160] The 2016 WHO classification divides PTLD into nondestructive PTLD (plasmacytic hyperplasia, florid follicular hyperplasia, and infectious mononucleosis), polymorphic PTLD, monomorphic PTLD (B-cell or T-cell lymphoma), and classic Hodgkin lymphoma lesions.[161] The monomorphic PTLDs encompass a variety of B-cell and T-cell neoplasms that usually represent high-grade lesions. Indolent B-cell lymphomas are not considered part of PTLD, with the exception of EBV-positive mucosa-associated lymphoid tissue (MALT) lymphoma, which typically occurs in the skin/subcutaneous tissue of allograft recipients.[161,162] The EBV-positive monomorphic PTLDs are usually of a nongerminal center cell origin, whereas most EBV-negative cases are of germinal center cell origin.[161] The risk of developing PTLD varies considerably, which mainly depends on several factors such as the transplant type, age of the patient, the immunosuppressive regimen, and the EBV status, with EBV seronegativity at time of transplant considered to be the most important risk factor.[161] EBV has been linked to most PTLDs, with a near 100% association in the early-occurring cases (within a year) and in PTLD-associated Hodgkin lymphoma.[163] The EBV-negative PTLDs constitute about 20% to 40% of all cases, are more common in adults, have a tendency to late occurrence (>5 years posttransplant), tend to present as monomorphic PTLD, and have a largely unknown cause.[161]

Morphologic Picture

The morphologic picture depends on the type of PTLD identified.

Pathogenesis

The wide expression of the latent EBV encoded proteins and the high EBV viral loads measured by polymerase chain reaction are factors that suggest an important role that EBV plays in the oncogenic process. EBV is thought to contribute to the pathogenesis of PTLD in a similar manner to its presumed role in classic Hodgkin lymphoma, in which EBV rescues germinal center B cells lacking a functional BCR from an imminent programmed cell death.[164,165] LMP1 and LMP2A may replace survival signals induced by activated BCR and CD40 receptors and may also activate the NFκB signaling pathway inducing proliferation of neoplastic cells. The decreased cytotoxic T-cell surveillance caused by immunosuppression in patients with PTLD also facilitates the actions of EBV.[164,165] Recently, increasing evidence points to a potential role that the lytic program of EBV may play in the early stages of B-cell transformation of PTLD and its association with plasmacytic differentiation.[160] One study reported that EBV lytic replication has an important role in the aggressive behavior of some PTLD and was associated in their study with early onset, short survival, and tumoral XBP-1 expression.[166]

Clinical Course and Prognosis

The clinical course depends on the type of PTLD identified.

EBV Latency Pattern

PTLD is thought to have a type III EBV latency pattern, although more restricted latency patterns have also been reported.[167]

EBV Staining Pattern by in Situ Hybridization (EBER)

The EBV expression patterns depend on the subtype of PTLD identified. In nondestructive plasmacytic hyperplasia, the EBV expression is variable, with few EBV-positive cells usually identified, which are mainly composed of polyclonal B cells that range in size from small to large along with rare interspersed T cells. In most cases, the plasma cells are EBV negative.[168] In nondestructive infectious mononucleosis, many small to large EBV-positive cells are identified and are composed predominantly of polyclonal B cells along with rare admixed T cells. In nondestructive florid follicular hyperplasia, the EBV expression is variable but usually few cells are EBV positive, mainly inside the germinal centers. The EBV-positive cells usually represent polyclonal B cells along with scattered interspersed T cells. In polymorphic lesions, numerous EBV-positive cells of variable sizes are identified, and are composed mainly of polyclonal B cells admixed with scattered T cells. In monomorphic and classic Hodgkin lymphoma lesions, the EBV staining pattern is similar to their counterparts in the immunocompetent setting. In EBV-positive MALT lymphoma, which is considered part of monomorphic PTLD, numerous EBV-positive cells are detected, which consist of monoclonal B cells (mainly small) along with admixed EBV-positive plasma cells[162]

OTHER IATROGENIC IMMUNODEFICIENCY-ASSOCIATED LYMPHOPROLIFERATIVE DISORDERS

Definition and Clinical Picture

Iatrogenic immunodeficiency-associated lymphoproliferative disorders (IILDs) are lymphoid proliferations arising in patients treated with immunosuppressive drugs for conditions outside of a transplant setting. In patients receiving autologous stem cell transplants, the development of a PTLD-like lesion may be related to an additional high-dose immunosuppressive regimen, and these patients are better categorized under the umbrella term of IILD.[161] Similar to PTLD, IILD constitutes a spectrum ranging from polymorphic proliferations to full-blown lymphomas.[169] Methotrexate was the first immunosuppressive agent reported to be associated with IILD and is still the most commonly reported, mainly in patients treated for rheumatoid arthritis.[170,171] Other drugs include antithymocyte globulin, mainly used in aplastic anemia,[172,173] and TNF antagonists.[169,174] An increased risk of T-cell lymphoma, particularly hepatosplenic T-cell lymphoma, has been well documented in association with anti-TNF therapy.[175]

Morphologic Picture

The morphologic picture depends on the type involved but an increase in the frequency of Hodgkin lymphoma and lymphoproliferative disorders with Hodgkin-like features are noted compared with other immunodeficiency settings.

Pathogenesis

EBV association with IILD is variable, with more frequent association with polymorphic proliferations (near 100%), IILD-related Hodgkin lymphoma (80%), and patients with rheumatoid arthritis treated with methotrexate (40%).[169,176] EBV is not associated with the reported hepatosplenic T-cell lymphoma cases. Several factors may affect the risk of developing EBV-positive lymphoid proliferations in these patients, including the degree and duration of immunosuppression, the degree of inflammation/chronic antigenic stimulation, and the ethnic background.[169,177]

Clinical Course and Prognosis

The clinical course depends on the type involved, but patients with methotrexate-related disorders usually show partial regression following drug withdrawal.

EBV Latency Pattern

A latency type II is reported to be more common than type III latency in patients with IILD.[169,178]

EBV Staining Pattern by in Situ Hybridization (EBER)

Many large and small EBV-positive cells are noted in polymorphic lesions. In monomorphic lymphomas, the staining pattern is similar to their counterparts in the immunocompetent setting.

LYMPHOPROLIFERATIVE DISEASES ASSOCIATED WITH PRIMARY IMMUNE DISORDERS

Definition and Clinical Picture

Lymphoproliferative diseases (LPDs) associated with primary immune disorders (PIDs) are variable lymphoid proliferations that arise as a result of a primary immunodeficiency or an immunoregulatory disorder and include ataxia telangiectasia, Wiskott-Aldrich syndrome, common variable immunodeficiency, severe combined immunodeficiency (SCID), X-linked lymphoproliferative disorder (XLP), hyper-IgM syndrome, and autoimmune lymphoproliferative syndrome as the most frequent abnormalities.[179] Lymphomas occurring in association with LPD-PID are usually of B-cell lineage and are not different from those occurring in the immunocompetent setting.

Morphologic Picture

Similar to other immunodeficiency-related disorders, a spectrum of lymphoid proliferations is noted that ranges from reactive hyperplasia to polymorphic and monomorphic infiltrates.

Pathogenesis

EBV has been reported to be involved in most of these disorders and is thought to be primarily related to the diminished or absent T-cell immune surveillance in these patients.[179,180] In patients with severely diminished or absent T-cell surveillance, such as in XLP and SCID, fatal infectious mononucleosis can occur.[179,181]

Clinical Course and Prognosis

The clinical course is related to the underlying PID and the type of lymphoproliferative disorder.

EBV Latency Pattern

An EBV latency III or latency II has been described in LPD-PID.[179]

EBV Staining Pattern by in Situ Hybridization (EBER)

The EBV expression pattern by in situ hybridization is similar to that seen in PTLD.

SUMMARY

Although about 90% of the world's population is infected by EBV, only a small subset of the related infections result in neoplastic transformation. The number of EBV-related neoplasms discovered has been increasing over the years, and it is anticipated that more EBV-related neoplastic associations will be reported. EBV has proved to be a versatile oncogenic agent involved in a multitude of various hematopoietic, epithelial, and mesenchymal neoplasms, but the precise role of EBV in the pathogenesis of many of the associated lymphoid/histiocytic proliferations discussed in this article remains hypothetical or not completely understood. Additional studies and the use of evolving technologies, such as high-throughput next-generation sequencing, may help address this knowledge gap and may lead to enhanced diagnostic assessment and the development of potential therapeutic interventions.

REFERENCES

1. Williams H, Crawford DH. Epstein-Barr virus: the impact of scientific advances on clinical practice. Blood 2006;107(3):862–9.
2. Rezk SA, Weiss LM. Epstein-Barr virus-associated lymphoproliferative disorders. Hum Pathol 2007; 38(9):1293–304.
3. Thorley-Lawson DA. Epstein-Barr virus: exploiting the immune system. Nat Rev Immunol 2001;1(1): 75–82.
4. Dojcinov SD, Venkataraman G, Pittaluga S, et al. Age-related EBV-associated lymphoproliferative disorders in the Western population: a spectrum of reactive lymphoid hyperplasia and lymphoma. Blood 2011;117(18):4726–35.
5. Niedobitek G, Herbst H, Young LS, et al. Patterns of Epstein-Barr virus infection in non-neoplastic lymphoid tissue. Blood 1992;79(10):2520–6.
6. Dunmire SK, Hogquist KA, Balfour HH. Infectious mononucleosis. Curr Top Microbiol Immunol 2015; 390(Pt 1):211–40.
7. Weiss L. Acute infectious mononucleosis. In: Weiss L, editor. Lymph nodes. New York: Cambridge University Press; 2008. p. 39–42.
8. Rezk SA, Zhao X, Weiss LM. Epstein-Barr virus (EBV)-associated lymphoid proliferations, a 2018 update. Hum Pathol 2018;79:18–41.
9. Wick MJ, Woronzoff-Dashkoff KP, McGlennen RC. The molecular characterization of fatal infectious mononucleosis. Am J Clin Pathol 2002;117(4): 582–8.
10. Quintanilla-Martinez L, Ko Y, Kimura H, et al. EBV-positive T-cell and NK-cell lymphoproliferative disease of childhood. In: Swerdlow SH, Campo E, Jaffe ES, et al, editors. WHO classification of hematopoietic and lymphoid tissues. Lyon (France): IARC; 2017. p. 355–63.
11. Gru AA, Haverkos BH, Freud AG, et al. The Epstein-Barr virus (EBV) in T cell and NK cell

lymphomas: time for a reassessment. Curr Hematol Malig Rep 2015;10(4):456–67.

12. Hudnall SD, Ge Y, Wei L, et al. Distribution and phenotype of Epstein-Barr virus-infected cells in human pharyngeal tonsils. Mod Pathol 2005; 18(4):519–27.

13. Trempat P, Tabiasco J, Andre P, et al. Evidence for early infection of nonneoplastic natural killer cells by Epstein-Barr virus. J Virol 2002;76(21): 11139–42.

14. Henter JI, Horne A, Arico M, et al. HLH-2004: diagnostic and therapeutic guidelines for hemophagocytic lymphohistiocytosis. Pediatr Blood Cancer 2007;48(2):124–31.

15. Gratzinger D, de Jong D, Jaffe ES, et al. T- and NK-cell lymphomas and systemic lymphoproliferative disorders and the immunodeficiency setting: 2015 SH/EAHP workshop report-part 4. Am J Clin Pathol 2017;147(2):188–203.

16. Rezk S, Usmani N, Woda B. Non-neoplastic histiocytic proliferations of lymph nodes and bone marrow. In: Jaffe ES, Campo E, Harris NL, et al, editors. Hematopathology. 2nd edition. Philadelphia: Elsevier; 2017. p. 957–68.

17. Cohen JI, Kimura H, Nakamura S, et al. Epstein-Barr virus-associated lymphoproliferative disease in non-immunocompromised hosts: a status report and summary of an international meeting, 8-9 September 2008. Ann Oncol 2009;20(9):1472–82.

18. Pittaluga S. Viral-associated lymphoid proliferations. Semin Diagn Pathol 2013;30(2):130–6.

19. Cohen JI, Jaffe ES, Dale JK, et al. Characterization and treatment of chronic active Epstein-Barr virus disease: a 28-year experience in the United States. Blood 2011;117(22):5835–49.

20. Kimura H, Hoshino Y, Kanegane H, et al. Clinical and virologic characteristics of chronic active Epstein-Barr virus infection. Blood 2001;98(2): 280–6.

21. Ohshima K, Kimura H, Yoshino T, et al. Proposed categorization of pathological states of EBV-associated T/natural killer-cell lymphoproliferative disorder (LPD) in children and young adults: overlap with chronic active EBV infection and infantile fulminant EBV T-LPD. Pathol Int 2008;58(4):209–17.

22. Gupta G, Man I, Kemmett D. Hydroa vacciniforme: a clinical and follow-up study of 17 cases. J Am Acad Dermatol 2000;42(2 Pt 1):208–13.

23. Iwatsuki K, Satoh M, Yamamoto T, et al. Pathogenic link between hydroa vacciniforme and Epstein-Barr virus-associated hematologic disorders. Arch Dermatol 2006;142(5):587–95.

24. Iwatsuki K, Xu Z, Takata M, et al. The association of latent Epstein-Barr virus infection with hydroa vacciniforme. Br J Dermatol 1999;140(4):715–21.

25. Asada H, Miyagawa S, Sumikawa Y, et al. CD4+ T-lymphocyte-induced Epstein-Barr virus reactivation in a patient with severe hypersensitivity to mosquito bites and Epstein-Barr virus-infected NK cell lymphocytosis. Arch Dermatol 2003; 139(12):1601–7.

26. Asada H, Saito-Katsuragi M, Niizeki H, et al. Mosquito salivary gland extracts induce EBV-infected NK cell oncogenesis via CD4 T cells in patients with hypersensitivity to mosquito bites. J Invest Dermatol 2005;125(5):956–61.

27. Dojcinov SD, Venkataraman G, Raffeld M, et al. EBV positive mucocutaneous ulcer–a study of 26 cases associated with various sources of immunosuppression. Am J Surg Pathol 2010;34(3):405–17.

28. Natkunam Y, Goodlad JR, Chadburn A, et al. EBV-positive B-cell proliferations of varied malignant potential: 2015 SH/EAHP workshop report-part 1. Am J Clin Pathol 2017;147(2):129–52.

29. Sadasivam N, Johnson RJ, Owen RG. Resolution of methotrexate-induced Epstein-Barr virus-associated mucocutaneous ulcer. Br J Haematol 2014;165(5):584.

30. Yamakawa N, Fujimoto M, Kawabata D, et al. A clinical, pathological, and genetic characterization of methotrexate-associated lymphoproliferative disorders. J Rheumatol 2014;41(2):293–9.

31. Gaulard P, Harris NL, Sundstrom C, et al. EBV-positive mucocutaneous ulcer. In: Swerdlow SH, Campo E, Jaffe ES, et al, editors. WHO classification of tumors of hematopoietic and lymphoid tissues. Lyon (France): IARC; 2017. p. 307–8.

32. Kanzler H, Kuppers R, Hansmann ML, et al. Hodgkin and Reed-Sternberg cells in Hodgkin's disease represent the outgrowth of a dominant tumor clone derived from (crippled) germinal center B cells. J Exp Med 1996;184(4):1495–505.

33. Kuppers R, Schwering I, Brauninger A, et al. Biology of Hodgkin's lymphoma. Ann Oncol 2002; 13(Suppl 1):11–8.

34. Stein HPS, Weiss LM, Poppema S, et al. Hodgkin lymphoma, introduction. In: Swerdlow SH, Campo E, Jaffe ES, et al, editors. WHO classification of tumors of hematopoietic and lymphoid tissues. Revised 4th edition. Lyon (France): IARC; 2017. p. 424–30.

35. Chang KC, Chen PC, Chang Y, et al. Epstein-Barr virus latent membrane protein-1 up-regulates cytokines and correlates with older age and poorer prognosis in Hodgkin lymphoma. Histopathology 2017;70(3):442–55.

36. Uccini S, Monardo F, Stoppacciaro A, et al. High frequency of Epstein-Barr virus genome detection in Hodgkin's disease of HIV-positive patients. Int J Cancer 1990;46(4):581–5.

37. Flavell KJ, Murray PG. Hodgkin's disease and the Epstein-Barr virus. Mol Pathol 2000;53(5):262–9.

38. Kilger E, Kieser A, Baumann M, et al. Epstein-Barr virus-mediated B-cell proliferation is dependent

upon latent membrane protein 1, which simulates an activated CD40 receptor. EMBO J 1998;17(6): 1700–9.

39. Caldwell RG, Wilson JB, Anderson SJ, et al. Epstein-Barr virus LMP2A drives B cell development and survival in the absence of normal B cell receptor signals. Immunity 1998;9(3):405–11.

40. Henderson S, Rowe M, Gregory C, et al. Induction of bcl-2 expression by Epstein-Barr virus latent membrane protein 1 protects infected B cells from programmed cell death. Cell 1991;65(7): 1107–15.

41. Krappmann D, Emmerich F, Kordes U, et al. Molecular mechanisms of constitutive NF-kappaB/Rel activation in Hodgkin/Reed-Sternberg cells. Oncogene 1999;18(4):943–53.

42. Kim SH, Shin YK, Lee IS, et al. Viral latent membrane protein 1 (LMP-1)-induced CD99 downregulation in B cells leads to the generation of cells with Hodgkin's and Reed-Sternberg phenotype. Blood 2000;95(1):294–300.

43. Diepstra A, van Imhoff GW, Schaapveld M, et al. Latent Epstein-Barr virus infection of tumor cells in classical Hodgkin's lymphoma predicts adverse outcome in older adult patients. J Clin Oncol 2009;27(23):3815–21.

44. Leoncini L, Stein H, Harris NL, et al. Burkitt lymphoma. In: Swerdlow SH, Harris NL, Jaffe ES, et al, editors. WHO classification of tumors of hematopoietic and lymphoid tissues. Lyon (France): IARC; 2017. p. 262–4.

45. Kuppers R. B cells under influence: transformation of B cells by Epstein-Barr virus. Nat Rev Immunol 2003;3(10):801–12.

46. Young LS, Rickinson AB. Epstein-Barr virus: 40 years on. Nat Rev Cancer 2004;4(10):757–68.

47. Love C, Sun Z, Jima D, et al. The genetic landscape of mutations in Burkitt lymphoma. Nat Genet 2012;44(12):1321–5.

48. Schmitz R, Young RM, Ceribelli M, et al. Burkitt lymphoma pathogenesis and therapeutic targets from structural and functional genomics. Nature 2012; 490(7418):116–20.

49. Salaverria I, Martin-Guerrero I, Wagener R, et al. A recurrent 11q aberration pattern characterizes a subset of MYC-negative high-grade B-cell lymphomas resembling Burkitt lymphoma. Blood 2014;123(8):1187–98.

50. Leoncini L, Stein H, Harris NL, et al. Burkitt-like lymphoma with 11q aberration. In: Swerdlow SH, Campo E, Jaffe ES, et al, editors. WHO classification of tumors of hematopoietic and lymphoid tissues. Lyon (France): IARC; 2017. p. 334.

51. Kitagawa N, Goto M, Kurozumi K, et al. Epstein-Barr virus-encoded poly(A)(-) RNA supports Burkitt's lymphoma growth through interleukin-10 induction. EMBO J 2000;19(24):6742–50.

52. Abate F, Ambrosio MR, Mundo L, et al. Distinct viral and mutational spectrum of endemic Burkitt lymphoma. PLoS Pathog 2015;11(10):e1005158.

53. Chene A, Donati D, Orem J, et al. Endemic Burkitt's lymphoma as a polymicrobial disease: new insights on the interaction between Plasmodium falciparum and Epstein-Barr virus. Semin Cancer Biol 2009; 19(6):411–20.

54. Kelly GL, Milner AE, Baldwin GS, et al. Three restricted forms of Epstein-Barr virus latency counteracting apoptosis in c-myc-expressing Burkitt lymphoma cells. Proc Natl Acad Sci U S A 2006; 103(40):14935–40.

55. Dittmer DP. Not like a wrecking ball: EBV fine-tunes MYC lymphomagenesis. Blood 2014;123(4):460–1.

56. Katzenstein AL, Doxtader E, Narendra S. Lymphomatoid granulomatosis: insights gained over 4 decades. Am J Surg Pathol 2010;34(12):e35–48.

57. Pittaluga S, Jaffe ES. Lymphomatoid granulomatosis. In: Swerdlow SH, Campo E, Jaffe ES, et al, editors. WHO classification of tumors of hematopoietic and lymphoid tissues. Lyon (France): IARC; 2017. p. 312–4.

58. Song JY, Pittaluga S, Dunleavy K, et al. Lymphomatoid granulomatosis–a single institute experience: pathologic findings and clinical correlations. Am J Surg Pathol 2015;39(2):141–56.

59. Taniere P, Thivolet-Bejui F, Vitrey D, et al. Lymphomatoid granulomatosis–a report on four cases: evidence for B phenotype of the tumoral cells. Eur Respir J 1998;12(1):102–6.

60. Campo E, Montserrat E, Harris NL, et al. B-cell prolymphocytic leukemia. In: Swerdlow SH, Campo E, Jaffe ES, et al, editors. WHO classification of tumors of hematopoietic and lymphoid tissues. Lyon (France): IARC; 2017. p. 222–3.

61. Castillo JJ, Bibas M, Miranda RN. The biology and treatment of plasmablastic lymphoma. Blood 2015; 125(15):2323–30.

62. Valera A, Balague O, Colomo L, et al. IG/MYC rearrangements are the main cytogenetic alteration in plasmablastic lymphomas. Am J Surg Pathol 2010;34(11):1686–94.

63. Martinez D, Valera A, Perez NS, et al. Plasmablastic transformation of low-grade B-cell lymphomas: report on 6 cases. Am J Surg Pathol 2013;37(2): 272–81.

64. Dong HY, Scadden DT, de Leval L, et al. Plasmablastic lymphoma in HIV-positive patients: an aggressive Epstein-Barr virus-associated extramedullary plasmacytic neoplasm. Am J Surg Pathol 2005;29(12):1633–41.

65. Rochford R, Hobbs MV, Garnier JL, et al. Plasmacytoid differentiation of Epstein-Barr virus-transformed B cells in vivo is associated with reduced expression of viral latent genes. Proc Natl Acad Sci U S A 1993;90(1):352–6.

66. Iuchi K, Ichimiya A, Akashi A, et al. Non-Hodgkin's lymphoma of the pleural cavity developing from long-standing pyothorax. Cancer 1987;60(8): 1771–5.

67. Banks PM, Warnke RA, Gaulard PH. Lymphomas. In: Travis WD, Muller-Hermelink HK, Harris CC, editors. World Health Organization classification of tumors. Pathology and genetics of tumors of the lung, pleura, thymus, and heart. Lyon (France): IARC; 2004. p. 137–40.

68. Chan JK, Gaulard P. DLBCL associated with chronic inflammation. In: Swerdlow SHCE, Jaffe ES, Pileri SA, et al, editors. WHO classification of tumors of hematopoietic and lymphoid tissues. Lyon (France): IARC; 2008. p. 245–6.

69. Cheuk W, Chan AC, Chan JK, et al. Metallic implant-associated lymphoma: a distinct subgroup of large B-cell lymphoma related to pyothorax-associated lymphoma? Am J Surg Pathol 2005; 29(6):832–6.

70. Copie-Bergman C, Niedobitek G, Mangham DC, et al. Epstein-Barr virus in B-cell lymphomas associated with chronic suppurative inflammation. J Pathol 1997;183(3):287–92.

71. Bartoloni G, Pucci A, Giorlandino A, et al. Incidental Epstein-Barr virus associated atypical lymphoid proliferation arising in a left atrial myxoma: a case of long survival without any postsurgical treatment and review of the literature. Cardiovasc Pathol 2013;22(3):e5–10.

72. Boroumand N, Ly TL, Sonstein J, et al. Microscopic diffuse large B-cell lymphoma (DLBCL) occurring in pseudocysts: do these tumors belong to the category of DLBCL associated with chronic inflammation? Am J Surg Pathol 2012;36(7):1074–80.

73. Gruver AM, Huba MA, Dogan A, et al. Fibrin-associated large B-cell lymphoma: part of the spectrum of cardiac lymphomas. Am J Surg Pathol 2012; 36(10):1527–37.

74. Miller DV, Firchau DJ, McClure RF, et al. Epstein-Barr virus-associated diffuse large B-cell lymphoma arising on cardiac prostheses. Am J Surg Pathol 2010;34(3):377–84.

75. Chan J, Gaulard P. Diffuse large B-cell lymphoma associated with chronic inflammation. In: Swerdlow SH, Campo E, Jaffe ES, et al, editors. WHO classification of tumors of hematopoietic and lymphoid tissues. Lyon (France): IARC; 2017. p. 309–11.

76. Boyer DF, McKelvie PA, de Leval L, et al. Fibrin-associated EBV-positive large B-cell lymphoma: an indolent neoplasm with features distinct from diffuse large B-cell lymphoma associated with chronic inflammation. Am J Surg Pathol 2017; 41(3):299–312.

77. Aozasa K. Pyothorax-associated lymphoma. J Clin Exp Hematop 2006;46(1):5–10.

78. Kanno H, Naka N, Yasunaga Y, et al. Role of an immunosuppressive cytokine, interleukin-10, in the development of pyothorax-associated lymphoma. Leukemia 1997;11(Suppl 3):525–6.

79. Aguilar C, Beltran B, Quinones P, et al. Large B-cell lymphoma arising in cardiac myxoma or intracardiac fibrinous mass: a localized lymphoma usually associated with Epstein-Barr virus? Cardiovasc Pathol 2015;24(1):60–4.

80. Oyama T, Ichimura K, Suzuki R, et al. Senile EBV+ B-cell lymphoproliferative disorders: a clinicopathologic study of 22 patients. Am J Surg Pathol 2003;27(1):16–26.

81. Nakamura S, Swerdlow SH. EBV positive diffuse large B-cell lymphoma of the elderly. In: Swerdlow SH, Harris NL, Jaffe ES, et al, editors. WHO classification of tumors of hematopoietic and lymphoid tissues, vol. 243-245. Lyon (France): IARC; 2008.

82. Nicolae A, Pittaluga S, Abdullah S, et al. EBV-positive large B-cell lymphomas in young patients: a nodal lymphoma with evidence for a tolerogenic immune environment. Blood 2015;126(7):863–72.

83. Nakamura S, Swerdlow SH. EBV-positive diffuse large B-cell lymphoma, not otherwise specified (NOS). In: Swerdlow SH, Campo E, Jaffe ES, et al, editors. WHO classification of tumors of hematopoietic and lymphoid tissues. Lyon (France): IARC; 2017. p. 304–6.

84. Hsi ED. 2016 WHO classification update-what's new in lymphoid neoplasms. Int J Lab Hematol 2017;39(Suppl 1):14–22.

85. Jaffe ES, Swerdlow SH, Campo E, et al. B-cell lymphoma, unclassifiable, with features intermediate between diffuse large B-cell lymphoma and classic Hodgkin lymphoma. In: Swerdlow SH, Campo E, Jaffe ES, et al, editors. WHO classification of tumours of hematopoietic and lymphoid tissues. Lyon (France): IARC; 2016. p. 342–4.

86. Shimoyama Y, Oyama T, Asano N, et al. Senile Epstein-Barr virus-associated B-cell lymphoproliferative disorders: a mini review. J Clin Exp Hematop 2006;46(1):1–4.

87. Said J. The expanding spectrum of EBV+ lymphomas. Blood 2015;126(7):827–8.

88. Wang W, Kanagal-Shamanna R, Medeiros LJ. Lymphoproliferative disorders with concurrent HHV8 and EBV infection: beyond primary effusion lymphoma and germinotropic lymphoproliferative disorder. Histopathology 2018;72(5):855–61.

89. Crane GM, Ambinder RF, Shirley CM, et al. HHV-8-positive and EBV-positive intravascular lymphoma: an unusual presentation of extracavitary primary effusion lymphoma. Am J Surg Pathol 2014;38(3): 426–32.

90. Ferry JA, Sohani AR, Longtine JA, et al. HHV8-positive, EBV-positive Hodgkin lymphoma-like large

B-cell lymphoma and HHV8-positive intravascular large B-cell lymphoma. Mod Pathol 2009;22(5): 618–26.

91. Lee YM, Kim JM, Kim SY. Human herpes virus 8/ Epstein-Barr virus-copositive, plasmablastic microlymphoma arising in multicentric Castleman's disease of an immunocompetent patient. J Pathol Transl Med 2017;51(1):99–102.

92. Said J, Cesarman E. Primary effusion lymphoma. In: Swerdlow SH, Campo E, Jaffe ES, et al, editors. WHO classification of tumors of hematopoietic and lymphoid tissues. Lyon (France): IARC; 2017. p. 323–4.

93. Luppi M, Barozzi P, Santagostino G, et al. Molecular evidence of organ-related transmission of Kaposi sarcoma-associated herpesvirus or human herpesvirus-8 in transplant patients. Blood 2000; 96(9):3279–81.

94. Cobo F, Hernandez S, Hernandez L, et al. Expression of potentially oncogenic HHV-8 genes in an EBV-negative primary effusion lymphoma occurring in an HIV-seronegative patient. J Pathol 1999; 189(2):288–93.

95. Song JY, Jaffe ES. HHV-8-positive but EBV-negative primary effusion lymphoma. Blood 2013; 122(23):3712.

96. Wu W, Youm W, Rezk SA, et al. Human herpesvirus 8-unrelated primary effusion lymphoma-like lymphoma: report of a rare case and review of 54 cases in the literature. Am J Clin Pathol 2013; 140(2):258–73.

97. Fan W, Bubman D, Chadburn A, et al. Distinct subsets of primary effusion lymphoma can be identified based on their cellular gene expression profile and viral association. J Virol 2005;79(2):1244–51.

98. Mack AA, Sugden B. EBV is necessary for proliferation of dually infected primary effusion lymphoma cells. Cancer Res 2008;68(17):6963–8.

99. Szekely L, Chen F, Teramoto N, et al. Restricted expression of Epstein-Barr virus (EBV)-encoded, growth transformation-associated antigens in an EBV- and human herpesvirus type 8-carrying body cavity lymphoma line. J Gen Virol 1998; 79(Pt 6):1445–52.

100. Trivedi P, Takazawa K, Zompetta C, et al. Infection of HHV-8+ primary effusion lymphoma cells with a recombinant Epstein-Barr virus leads to restricted EBV latency, altered phenotype, and increased tumorigenicity without affecting TCL1 expression. Blood 2004;103(1):313–6.

101. Xu D, Coleman T, Zhang J, et al. Epstein-Barr virus inhibits Kaposi's sarcoma-associated herpesvirus lytic replication in primary effusion lymphomas. J Virol 2007;81(11):6068–78.

102. Du MQ, Diss TC, Liu H, et al. KSHV- and EBV-associated germinotropic lymphoproliferative disorder. Blood 2002;100(9):3415–8.

103. Bhavsar T, Lee JC, Perner Y, et al. KSHV-associated and EBV-associated germinotropic lymphoproliferative disorder: new findings and review of the literature. Am J Surg Pathol 2017;41(6): 795–800.

104. Gonzalez-Farre B, Martinez D, Lopez-Guerra M, et al. HHV8-related lymphoid proliferations: a broad spectrum of lesions from reactive lymphoid hyperplasia to overt lymphoma. Mod Pathol 2017; 30(5):745–60.

105. McKenna RW, Kuehl WM, Harris NL, et al. Plasma cell neoplasms. In: Swerdlow SH, Campo E, Jaffe ES, et al, editors. WHO classification of tumors of hematopoietic and lymphoid tissues. Lyon (France): IARC; 2017. p. 241–58.

106. Engels EA, Clarke CA, Pfeiffer RM, et al. Plasma cell neoplasms in US solid organ transplant recipients. Am J Transplant 2013;13(6):1523–32.

107. Ouedraogo DE, Makinson A, Vendrell JP, et al. Pivotal role of HIV and EBV replication in the long-term persistence of monoclonal gammopathy in patients on antiretroviral therapy. Blood 2013; 122(17):3030–3.

108. Yan J, Wang J, Zhang W, et al. Solitary plasmacytoma associated with Epstein-Barr virus: a clinicopathologic, cytogenetic study and literature review. Ann Diagn Pathol 2017;27:1–6.

109. Aguilera NS, Kapadia SB, Nalesnik MA, et al. Extramedullary plasmacytoma of the head and neck: use of paraffin sections to assess clonality with in situ hybridization, growth fraction, and the presence of Epstein-Barr virus. Mod Pathol 1995;8(5):503–8.

110. Scarberry K, Jegalian A, Valent J, et al. Solitary extramedullary plasmacytoma of the penis. Urol Ann 2014;6(3):242–3.

111. Tomita Y, Ohsawa M, Hashimoto M, et al. Plasmacytoma of the gastrointestinal tract in Korea: higher incidence than in Japan and Epstein-Barr virus association. Oncology 1998;55(1):27–32.

112. Chang ST, Liao YL, Lu CL, et al. Plasmablastic cytomorphologic features in plasma cell neoplasms in immunocompetent patients are significantly associated with EBV. Am J Clin Pathol 2007; 128(2):339–44.

113. Anastasiadou E, Vaeth S, Cuomo L, et al. Epstein-Barr virus infection leads to partial phenotypic reversion of terminally differentiated malignant B cells. Cancer Lett 2009;284(2):165–74.

114. Laichalk LL, Thorley-Lawson DA. Terminal differentiation into plasma cells initiates the replicative cycle of Epstein-Barr virus in vivo. J Virol 2005;79(2): 1296–307.

115. Mitarnun W, Suwiwat S, Pradutkanchana J, et al. Epstein-Barr virus-associated peripheral T-cell and NK-cell proliferative disease/lymphoma: clinicopathologic, serologic, and molecular analysis. Am J Hematol 2002;70(1):31–8.

116. Young LS, Murray PG. Epstein-Barr virus and onco-genesis: from latent genes to tumours. Oncogene 2003;22(33):5108–21.

117. Dogan A, Jaffe ES, Muller-Hermelink HK, et al. Angioimmunoblastic T-cell lymphoma and other nodal lymphomas of T-follicular helper cell origin. In: Swerdlow SH, Harris NL, Jaffe ES, et al, editors. WHO classification of tumours of haematopoietic and lymphoid tissues. Lyon (France): IARC; 2017. p. 407–12.

118. Weiss LM, Strickler JG, Dorfman RF, et al. Clonal T-cell populations in angioimmunoblastic lymphadenopathy and angioimmunoblastic lymphadenopathy-like lymphoma. Am J Pathol 1986;122(3):392–7.

119. Hawley RC, Cankovic M, Zarbo RJ. Angioimmuno-blastic T-cell lymphoma with supervening Epstein-Barr virus-associated large B-cell lymphoma. Arch Pathol Lab Med 2006;130(11):1707–11.

120. Brauninger A, Spieker T, Willenbrock K, et al. Survival and clonal expansion of mutating "forbidden" (immunoglobulin receptor-deficient) Epstein-Barr virus-infected b cells in angioimmunoblastic t cell lymphoma. J Exp Med 2001;194(7):927–40.

121. Kuppers R. Somatic hypermutation and B cell receptor selection in normal and transformed human B cells. Ann N Y Acad Sci 2003;987:173–9.

122. Huang Y, Moreau A, Dupuis J, et al. Peripheral T-cell lymphomas with a follicular growth pattern are derived from follicular helper T cells (TFH) and may show overlapping features with angioim-munoblastic T-cell lymphomas. Am J Surg Pathol 2009;33(5):682–90.

123. Streubel B, Vinatzer U, Willheim M, et al. Novel t(5;9)(q33;q22) fuses ITK to SYK in unspecified peripheral T-cell lymphoma. Leukemia 2006;20(2): 313–8.

124. Hasserjian RP, Harris NL. NK-cell lymphomas and leukemias: a spectrum of tumors with variable manifestations and immunophenotype. Am J Clin Pathol 2007;127(6):860–8.

125. Ho FC, Srivastava G, Loke SL, et al. Presence of Epstein-Barr virus DNA in nasal lymphomas of B and 'T' cell type. Hematol Oncol 1990;8(5):271–81.

126. Chan J, Quintanilla-Martinez L, Ferry JA. Extrano-dal NK/T-cell lymphoma, nasal type. In: Swerdlow SH, Campo E, Jaffe ES, et al, editors. WHO classification of tumors of hematopoietic and lymphoid tissues. Lyon (France): IARC; 2017. p. 368–71.

127. Noguchi T, Ikeda K, Yamamoto K, et al. Antisense oligodeoxynucleotides to latent membrane protein 1 induce growth inhibition, apoptosis and Bcl-2 suppression in Epstein-Barr virus (EBV)-transformed B-lymphoblastoid cells, but not in EBV-positive natural killer cell lymphoma cells. Br J Haematol 2001;114(1):84–92.

128. Sun L, Zhao Y, Shi H, et al. LMP1 promotes nasal NK/T-cell lymphoma cell function by eIF4E via NF-kappaB pathway. Oncol Rep 2015;34(6): 3264–71.

129. Takada H, Imadome KI, Shibayama H, et al. EBV induces persistent NF-kappaB activation and contributes to survival of EBV-positive neoplastic T- or NK-cells. PLoS One 2017;12(3):e0174136.

130. Takahara M, Kis LL, Nagy N, et al. Concomitant increase of LMP1 and CD25 (IL-2-receptor alpha) expression induced by IL-10 in the EBV-positive NK lines SNK6 and KAI3. Int J Cancer 2006; 119(12):2775–83.

131. Au WY, Pang A, Choy C, et al. Quantification of circulating Epstein-Barr virus (EBV) DNA in the diagnosis and monitoring of natural killer cell and EBV-positive lymphomas in immunocompetent patients. Blood 2004;104(1):243–9.

132. Chan J, Jaffe ES, Ko YH. Aggressive NK-cell leukaemia. In: Swerdlow SH, Campo E, Jaffe ES, et al, editors. WHO classification of tumors of hematopoietic and lymphoid tissues. Lyon (France): IARC; 2017. p. 353–5.

133. Zhang Q, Jing W, Ouyang J, et al. Six cases of aggressive natural killer-cell leukemia in a Chinese population. Int J Clin Exp Pathol 2014;7(6): 3423–31.

134. Gao J, Behdad A, Ji P, et al. EBV-negative aggressive NK-cell leukemia/lymphoma: a clinical and pathological study from a single institution. Mod Pathol 2017;30(8):1100–15.

135. Chan JK. Natural killer cell neoplasms. Anat Pathol 1998;3:77–145.

136. Cheung MM, Chan JK, Wong KF. Natural killer cell neoplasms: a distinctive group of highly aggressive lymphomas/leukemias. Semin Hematol 2003; 40(3):221–32.

137. Nava VE, Jaffe ES. The pathology of NK-cell lymphomas and leukemias. Adv Anat Pathol 2005; 12(1):27–34.

138. Rezk SA, Huang Q. Extranodal NK/T-cell lymphoma, nasal type extensively involving the bone marrow. Int J Clin Exp Pathol 2011;4(7):713–7.

139. Nakashima Y, Tagawa H, Suzuki R, et al. Genome-wide array-based comparative genomic hybridization of natural killer cell lymphoma/leukemia: different genomic alteration patterns of aggressive NK-cell leukemia and extranodal Nk/T-cell lymphoma, nasal type. Genes Chromosomes Cancer 2005;44(3):247–55.

140. Grywalska E, Rolinski J. Epstein-Barr virus-associated lymphomas. Semin Oncol 2015;42(2): 291–303.

141. Yoshii M, Ishida M, Hodohara K, et al. Systemic Epstein-Barr virus-positive T-cell lymphoproliferative disease of childhood: report of a case with review of the literature. Oncol Lett 2012;4(3):381–4.

142. Quintanilla-Martinez L, Kumar S, Fend F, et al. Fulminant EBV(+) T-cell lymphoproliferative disorder following acute/chronic EBV infection: a distinct clinicopathologic syndrome. Blood 2000;96(2): 443–51.

143. Suzuki K, Ohshima K, Karube K, et al. Clinicopathological states of Epstein-Barr virus-associated T/NK-cell lymphoproliferative disorders (severe chronic active EBV infection) of children and young adults. Int J Oncol 2004;24(5):1165–74.

144. Pileri S, Sng I, Nakamura S, et al. Peripheral T-cell lymphoma, NOS. In: Swerdlow SH, Campo E, Jaffe ES, et al, editors. WHO classification of tumors of hematopoietic and lymphoid tissues. Lyon (France): IARC; 2017. p. 403–7.

145. Weisenburger DD, Savage KJ, Harris NL, et al. Peripheral T-cell lymphoma, not otherwise specified: a report of 340 cases from the International Peripheral T-cell Lymphoma Project. Blood 2011; 117(12):3402–8.

146. Yang L, Aozasa K, Oshimi K, et al. Epstein-Barr virus (EBV)-encoded RNA promotes growth of EBV-infected T cells through interleukin-9 induction. Cancer Res 2004;64(15):5332–7.

147. Liebowitz D. Epstein-Barr virus and a cellular signaling pathway in lymphomas from immunosuppressed patients. N Engl J Med 1998;338(20): 1413–21.

148. Dupuis J, Emile JF, Mounier N, et al. Prognostic significance of Epstein-Barr virus in nodal peripheral T-cell lymphoma, unspecified: a Groupe d'Etude des Lymphomes de l'Adulte (GELA) study. Blood 2006;108(13):4163–9.

149. Mori A, Takao S, Pradutkanchana J, et al. High tumor necrosis factor-alpha levels in the patients with Epstein-Barr virus-associated peripheral T-cell proliferative disease/lymphoma. Leuk Res 2003;27(6): 493–8.

150. Said J, Rosenwald A, Harris NL. Lymphomas associated with HIV infection. In: Swerdlow SH, Campo E, Jaffe ES, et al, editors. WHO classification of tumors of hematopoietic and lymphoid tissues. Lyon (France): IARC; 2017. p. 449–52.

151. Linke-Serinsoz E, Fend F, Quintanilla-Martinez L. Human immunodeficiency virus (HIV) and Epstein-Barr virus (EBV) related lymphomas, pathology view point. Semin Diagn Pathol 2017; 34(4):352–63.

152. Carbone A, Cesarman E, Spina M, et al. HIV-associated lymphomas and gamma-herpesviruses. Blood 2009;113(6):1213–24.

153. Carbone A, Gloghini A, Dotti G. EBV-associated lymphoproliferative disorders: classification and treatment. Oncologist 2008;13(5):577–85.

154. Carbone A, Gloghini A. AIDS-related lymphomas: from pathogenesis to pathology. Br J Haematol 2005;130(5):662–70.

155. Carbone A. Emerging pathways in the development of AIDS-related lymphomas. Lancet Oncol 2003;4(1):22–9.

156. Krause J. AIDS-related non-Hodgkin's lymphomas. Microsc Res Tech 2005;68(3–4):168–75.

157. Goedert JJ. The epidemiology of acquired immunodeficiency syndrome malignancies. Semin Oncol 2000;27(4):390–401.

158. Sugita Y, Muta H, Ohshima K, et al. Primary central nervous system lymphomas and related diseases: pathological characteristics and discussion of the differential diagnosis. Neuropathology 2016;36(4): 313–24.

159. Gottschalk S, Rooney CM, Heslop HE. Post-transplant lymphoproliferative disorders. Annu Rev Med 2005;56:29–44.

160. Morscio J, Tousseyn T. Recent insights in the pathogenesis of post-transplantation lymphoproliferative disorders. World J Transplant 2016;6(3):505–16.

161. Swerdlow SH, Chadburn A, Fery JA. Post-transplant lymphoproliferative disorders. In: Swerdlow SH, Harris NL, Jaffe ES, et al, editors. WHO classification of tumors of hematopoietic and lymphoid tissues. Lyon (France): IARC; 2016. p. 453–62.

162. Gibson SE, Swerdlow SH, Craig FE, et al. EBV-positive extranodal marginal zone lymphoma of mucosa-associated lymphoid tissue in the post-transplant setting: a distinct type of posttransplant lymphoproliferative disorder? Am J Surg Pathol 2011;35(6):807–15.

163. Thompson MP, Kurzrock R. Epstein-Barr virus and cancer. Clin Cancer Res 2004;10(3):803–21.

164. Capello D, Rossi D, Gaidano G. Post-transplant lymphoproliferative disorders: molecular basis of disease histogenesis and pathogenesis. Hematol Oncol 2005;23(2):61–7.

165. Timms JM, Bell A, Flavell JR, et al. Target cells of Epstein-Barr-virus (EBV)-positive post-transplant lymphoproliferative disease: similarities to EBV-positive Hodgkin's lymphoma. Lancet 2003; 361(9353):217–23.

166. Gonzalez-Farre B, Rovira J, Martinez D, et al. In vivo intratumoral Epstein-Barr virus replication is associated with XBP1 activation and early-onset post-transplant lymphoproliferative disorders with prognostic implications. Mod Pathol 2014; 27(12):1599–611.

167. Brink AA, Dukers DF, van den Brule AJ, et al. Presence of Epstein-Barr virus latency type III at the single cell level in post-transplantation lymphoproliferative disorders and AIDS related lymphomas. J Clin Pathol 1997;50(11):911–8.

168. Nelson BP, Wolniak KL, Evens A, et al. Early post-transplant lymphoproliferative disease: clinicopathologic features and correlation with mTOR signaling pathway activation. Am J Clin Pathol 2012;138(4):568–78.

169. Gaulard P, Harris NL, Sundstrom C, et al. Other iatrogenic immunodeficiency-associated lymphoproliferative disorders. In: Swerdlow SH, Campo E, Jaffe ES, et al, editors. WHO classification of tumors of hematopoietic and lymphoid tissues. Lyon (France): IARC; 2017. p. 462–4.

170. Salloum E, Cooper DL, Howe G, et al. Spontaneous regression of lymphoproliferative disorders in patients treated with methotrexate for rheumatoid arthritis and other rheumatic diseases. J Clin Oncol 1996;14(6):1943–9.

171. Wolfe F, Michaud K. The effect of methotrexate and anti-tumor necrosis factor therapy on the risk of lymphoma in rheumatoid arthritis in 19,562 patients during 89,710 person-years of observation. Arthritis Rheum 2007;56(5):1433–9.

172. Nakanishi R, Ishida M, Hodohara K, et al. Occurrence of Epstein-Barr virus-associated plasmacytic lymphoproliferative disorder after antithymocyte globulin therapy for aplastic anemia: a case report with review of the literature. Int J Clin Exp Pathol 2014;7(4):1748–54.

173. Wondergem MJ, Stevens SJ, Janssen JJ, et al. Monitoring of EBV reactivation is justified in patients with aplastic anemia treated with rabbit ATG as a second course of immunosuppression. Blood 2008;111(3):1739, [author reply: 1739–40].

174. Mackey AC, Green L, Liang LC, et al. Hepatosplenic T cell lymphoma associated with infliximab use in young patients treated for inflammatory bowel disease. J Pediatr Gastroenterol Nutr 2007; 44(2):265–7.

175. Deepak P, Sifuentes H, Sherid M, et al. T-cell non-Hodgkin's lymphomas reported to the FDA AERS with tumor necrosis factor-alpha (TNF-alpha) inhibitors: results of the REFURBISH study. Am J Gastroenterol 2013;108(1):99–105.

176. Hoshida Y, Xu JX, Fujita S, et al. Lymphoproliferative disorders in rheumatoid arthritis: clinicopathological analysis of 76 cases in relation to methotrexate medication. J Rheumatol 2007; 34(2):322–31.

177. Baecklund E, Smedby KE, Sutton LA, et al. Lymphoma development in patients with autoimmune and inflammatory disorders–what are the driving forces? Semin Cancer Biol 2014;24:61–70.

178. Yamada K, Oshiro Y, Okamura S, et al. Clinicopathological characteristics and rituximab addition to cytotoxic therapies in patients with rheumatoid arthritis and methotrexate-associated large B lymphoproliferative disorders. Histopathology 2015; 67(1):70–80.

179. van Krieken JH, Elenitoba-Johnson KS, Jaffe ES. Lymphoproliferative diseases associated with primary immune disorders. In: Swerdlow SH, Harris NL, Jaffe ES, et al, editors. WHO classification of tumors of hematopoietic and lymphoid tissues. Lyon (France): IARC; 2017. p. 444–8.

180. van Krieken JH. Lymphoproliferative disease associated with immune deficiency in children. Am J Clin Pathol 2004;122(Suppl):S122–7.

181. Gilmour KC, Gaspar HB. Pathogenesis and diagnosis of X-linked lymphoproliferative disease. Expert Rev Mol Diagn 2003;3(5):549–61.

Human Immunodeficiency Virus-Associated Lymphoproliferative Disorders

Amy J. Lilly, MD, Yuri Fedoriw, MD*

KEYWORDS

- HIV • HIV-associated Lymphoma • Epstein-Barr virus • B-cell lymphoma

Key Points

- Infection with HIV continues to be associated with an increased risk of lymphoma development, and HIV has both direct and indirect roles in lymphomagenesis.
- HIV-associated lymphomas tend to be high-grade, mature B-cell neoplasms and present at an earlier median age compared with those in the HIV-negative population.
- Antiretroviral therapy has significantly changed the distribution of lymphomas arising in HIV-infected persons, with an associated steady increase in the incidence of Classic Hodgkin lymphoma.

ABSTRACT

HIV infection is associated with an increased risk for developing B-cell lymphoproliferative disorders. The spectrum of disease differs in HIV-infected versus HIV-uninfected persons, with aggressive B-cell non-Hodgkin lymphomas constituting a higher proportion of all lymphoproliferative disorders in the HIV-positive population. Although antiretroviral therapy (ART) has significantly changed the landscape of lymphomas arising in HIV-infected persons, population growth and aging are reflected in the steady increase in non–AIDS-defining cancers. In the ART era, outcomes for HIV-infected lymphoma patients are similar to those of HIV-negative patients. This article reviews the diagnostic features and summarizes current biologic understanding of HIV-associated lymphomas.

OVERVIEW

HIV infection is associated with an increased risk for developing B-cell lymphoproliferative disorders, including bona fide malignant lymphomas as well as polyclonal and virally driven expansions. Although the introduction of antiretroviral therapy (ART) in the United States was associated with an early and marked decrease in the incidence of HIV lymphomas that plateaued in the late 1990s, improvements in overall survival, population growth, and aging resulted in an increased disease prevalence and steady rise in incidence of in non–AIDS-defining cancers, including Classic Hodgkin lymphoma (CHL).[1–3]

The spectrum of lymphoproliferative disorders differs in HIV-infected versus HIV-uninfected persons, with aggressive B-cell non-Hodgkin lymphomas (NHLs) constituting a higher proportion of all lymphoproliferative disorders in the HIV-positive population. In terms of cellular ontogeny, the lymphomas arising in the setting of HIV infection, as a whole, tend to represent proliferations of more mature and near terminally differentiated B-cells. This is reflected in the immunoblastic to plasmablastic morphology of many HIV-associated lymphomas.[4,5] Even CHL, which has shown a steadily increasing incidence since ART initiation, arises from germinal center (GC)

Disclosure Statement: The authors have nothing to disclose.
Department of Pathology and Laboratory Medicine, University of North Carolina School of Medicine, CB #7525, Chapel Hill, NC 27599-7525, USA
* Corresponding author.
E-mail address: yuri.fedoriw@unchealth.unc.edu

Surgical Pathology 12 (2019) 771–782
https://doi.org/10.1016/j.path.2019.03.005

surgpath.theclinics.com

B cells with crippled immunoglobulin processing and synthesis.[6]

The pathogenesis of HIV-associated lymphomas is complex, and the specific aberrations, to the degree to which they are understood, are largely beyond the scope of this review. Nonetheless, understanding the principles of lymphomagenesis aids in conceptualization of diagnosis and classification of HIV-associated lymphomas; they are summarized in **Fig. 1**.[7–10] HIV infection results in chronic B-cell activation both directly from HIV virions bearing CD40L and HIV proteins, including gp120, p17, and TAT, and indirectly through altered cytokine production and release. Normally, activation and antigen presentation trigger proliferation, maturation, and somatic hypermutation necessary for the development of mature and specifically targeted B cells. Because the process is far from efficient, a majority of activated B cells (ABCs) undergo apoptosis in the GC. In the setting of HIV, dysregulation of systemic immunity with accompanied defects of immunosurveillance mechanisms is permissive for B-cell transformation by other viral agents. Chronic activation in combination with Epstein-Barr virus (EBV) induced immortalization and a dysregulated local immune environment (inverted CD4:CD8 ratio is an immune risk phenotype that is associated with altered immune function, immune senescence, and chronic inflammation) strongly selects for malignant transformation. EBV-associated and human herpes virus 8 (HHV-8)–associated lymphomas are far more frequent in the HIV-infected population. Overall, the increased lymphomagenic pressures in the context of HIV are reflected in a younger age of disease presentation compared with similar tumors arising in HIV-uninfected persons.

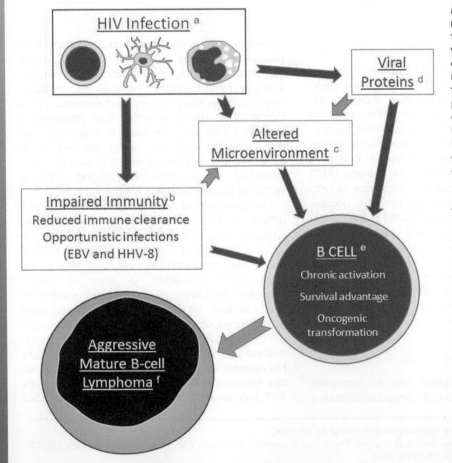

Fig. 1. HIV-associated lymphomagenesis. [a] HIV infects and develops reservoirs in body-wide CD4 T cells, dendritic cells, and macrophages. This infection results in chronic production and release of viral proteins, impaired immunity, and changes in the structure and composition of the microenvironment. [b] Impaired immunity not only results in a decreased ability to target and eliminate neoplastic cells but also is permissive for neoplastic transformation by the oncogenic viruses EBV and HHV-8. [c] HIV infection changes the lymphoid microenvironment via direct infection and stimulation of cells that shape the microenvironment (eg, macrophages) and indirectly by altering the cytokine milieu via dysregulation of the immune system. [d] Viral proteins are produced, which act on both B cells and cells of the microenvironment. [e] The combination of these various driving forces favors neoplasm development due to chronic B cell activation within a pro-oncogenic environment. [f] Because these neoplasms arise from a state of chronic activation, they tend to be mature B-cell neoplasms with plasmacytoid morphology.

This article reviews the salient clinical and diagnostic features of lymphomas arising in HIV-infected individuals and provides practical assistance to distinguish between lymphoma subtypes.

DIFFUSE LARGE B-CELL LYMPHOMA

Diffuse large B-cell lymphoma (DLBCL) is the most common type of NHL both in the general population and in HIV-infected patients. It encompasses a heterogeneous group of high-grade B-cell neoplasms that are diagnostically and prognostically subdivided based on immunohistochemical and molecular studies.[7]

DLBCL classically arises in the elderly (median age seventh decade) as a rapidly enlarging tumor mass involving lymph nodes in 60% of cases and/or various extranodal sites (gastrointestinal [GI] tract, bone, testes, spleen, tonsils, salivary glands, thyroid, liver, kidneys, and adrenal glands).[7] Approximately half of cases present as stage I or stage II disease with or without B symptoms. In HIV-infected patients, DLBCL is more likely to be extranodal, with primary sites including the central nervous system (CNS), GI tract, bone marrow, and liver.[7,11] HIV-associated DLBCL presents more frequently as stage III or stage IV and is 10 times more likely associated with EBV compared with the general population (30% vs 3%).[11] With the initiation of ART, the incidence of DLBCL has decreased, largely due to the sharp reduction in primary CNS lymphoma (PCNSL).[12]

There are 2 classically recognized morphologic subtypes of DLBCL, centroblastic and immunoblastic. Cells of the centroblastic variant are medium to large with large oval-shaped, vesicular nuclei; multiple nucleoli; and scant basophilic cytoplasm. Immunoblastic variants have cells with more abundant basophilic cytoplasm, an eccentrically placed nucleus, and 1 prominent nucleolus (**Fig. 2**). A majority of DLBCLs occurring in the general population show centroblastic morphology, whereas the immunoblastic variant is more common in the HIV population, especially those with higher degrees of immunosuppression, and is associated with high EBV positivity (80%–90%).[4,5] With the advent of ART, the relative proportion of immunoblastic DLBCLs has decreased, and DLBCLs arising in well-controlled HIV infection tend to have a centroblastic morphology and lower frequency of EBV positivity (30%–40%).[5]

There are numerous prognostic subtypes of de novo DLBCL; the primary classification scheme is based on cell of origin (COO) classification relating to GC and post-GC expression profiles. DLBCLs with a GC phenotype have a better

prognosis compared with those with a post-GC, ABC type.[13–15] Immunohistochemical algorithms are widely used as surrogates for COO classification in clinical practice.[16–19] The prognostic implications, however, in the setting of HIV infection are less clear. DLBCLs arising in HIV-infected patients have an inverted COO distribution (60% GC and 40% ABC) compared with the general population (40% GC and 60% ABC), and COO designation has no association with progression free or overall survival in HIV-infected patients.[11] Proliferation index may have prognostic significance when interpreted in the context of treatment modality. For example, 1 author reported that a high proliferation index (Ki-67 > 90%) may be associated with better overall and progression free survival when patients are treated with a continuous infusion regimen.[20]

In the ART era, HIV-associated DLBCL lymphoma is a curable disease with outcomes after standard chemotherapy similar to those of HIV-negative patients when controlled for stage of disease and performance score.[12] HIV patients, however, still tend to present with high-stage disease and lower performance scores.

PCNSL is a specific type of DLBCL deserving attention in a discussion of HIV-associated lymphomas. This neoplasm arises in severely immunocompromised patients (>90% of patients with a CD4 count <200; 60%–70% of these with a CD4 count <50), tends to have immunoblastic morphology, is almost universally EBV positive, and has an aggressive clinical course.[11] The development of PCNSL often is a harbinger of death. It presents late in the course of HIV infection in patients that have had severe and prolonged immunosuppression. Most die within months of diagnosis due to opportunistic infections. Treatment modalities include whole-brain radiation, intrathecal methotrexate, and initiation and/or maximization of ART. No standard therapy exists, however, and patients usually are enrolled in a clinical trial. Fortunately, the incidence of this entity has dramatically decreased in the post-ART era.[12]

BURKITT LYMPHOMA

Burkitt lymphoma (BL) is an aggressive, high-grade B-cell neoplasm characterized by a c-MYC translocation with 1 of 3 partner genes: immunoglobulin heavy chain on chromosome 14 (most common), kappa light chain on chromosome 2, or lambda light chain on chromosome 22.[7] Histologically, BL has the classic starry sky pattern composed of intermediate-sized cells with basophilic cytoplasm, oval nuclei, distinct

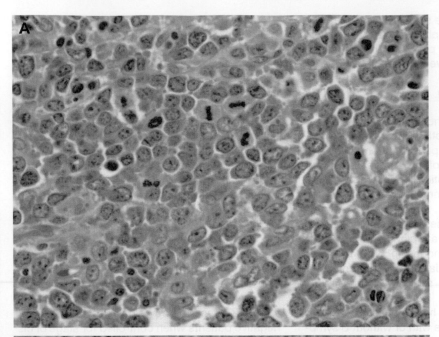

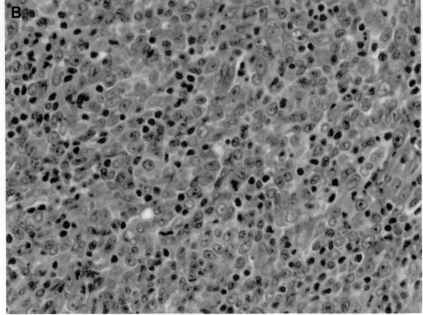

Fig. 2. Morphologic subtypes of DLBCL. (*A*) Centroblastic morphology is identified by the large oval-shaped vesicular nuclei with multiple nucleoli and scant cytoplasm. (*B*) Immunoblastic (or plasmablastic) morphology is identified by eccentrically placed nuclei with a single prominent nucleolus and increased cytoplasm (hematoxylin-eosin, original objective magnification ×40).

nucleoli, frequent mitoses, apoptotic debris, and scattered tingible body macrophages (**Fig. 3**). Clinical subtypes of disease include endemic, sporadic, and HIV-associated BL. Compared with the sporadic cases, HIV-associated cases are more frequently associated with EBV and demonstrate extranodal involvement. In addition, HIV-associated cases are more likely to exhibit plasmacytoid features (abundant cytoplasm, eccentric nuclei, central prominent nucleoli,

pleomorphism in nuclear size, and cytoplasmic immunoglobulin expression). By immunohistochemistry (IHC), BL shows expression of pan–B-cell antigen markers, CD10, and Bcl-6, and are consistently negative for Bcl-2, with near 100% Ki-67 staining.[4]

HIV-associated BL tends to present early in the course of HIV infection and is seen more frequently in young patients with intermediate to high CD4 counts (>250 cells/μL). Curiously, BL is not

Fig. 3. BL. Characteristic features, including proliferation of generally uniform, intermediate-sized neoplastic cells with a starry sky pattern (hematoxylin-eosin, original objective magnification ×40).

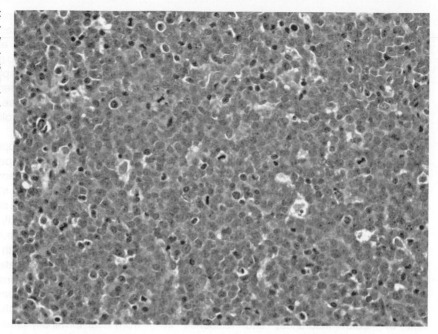

associated with other forms of immunosuppression, suggesting a significant role of HIV in its lymphomagenesis. Translocation of c-MYC with 1 of the 3 main partner genes requires a double-stranded DNA break combined with close proximity to enable erroneous rejoining during DNA repair. Normally, physical separation of the genes in the nucleus prevents this occurrence. During HIV infection, however, virally secreted protein, TAT, facilitates the relocalization of c-MYC so that it is adjacent to 1 of the 3 main partner genes, increasing the probability of a translocation. In addition, TAT can interact with RB2/p130, a primary controller of the G0 to G1 transition in the cell cycle, and inhibit its physiologic control of cell cycle progression. The combination of c-MYC overexpression and RB2/p130 dysfunction acts synergistically in the development of BL. Infection with EBV further supports, but is not necessary for, lymphomagenesis in this setting.[21–23]

In the pre-ART era, HIV-associated BL had a dismal prognosis. Most patients received inadequate chemotherapy doses due to a high degree of immunosuppression and treatment intolerance. In the post-ART era, the ability to treat and control these neoplasms has greatly improved and 1-year survival rates have increased up to 85%.[22]

CLASSIC HODGKIN LYMPHOMA

CHL is unique among the HIV-associated lymphomas in that it has shown an increased incidence in the post-ART era. Well-controlled HIV

disease may select for this neoplasm because the incidence of these neoplasms is highest among those with intermediate CD4 cell counts (225–249 cells/μL), undetectable HIV viral loads, long-standing infection (median of 13 years), and exposure to ART. CHL arising in the HIV population tends to be widespread at presentation (stage III or IV in 60%–80%) with frequent constitutional symptoms, extranodal disease, and poor clinical performance scores. COO studies have shown that the Hodgkin/Reed-Sternberg (H/RS) cells are derived from late GC or post-GC B cells carrying somatically hypermutated immunoglobulin heavy chain variable region genes that have escaped apoptosis.[5,11]

CHLs arising in HIV-infected patients share most histopathologic features with cases in the HIV-uninfected population.[7] The neoplastic H/RS cells are scattered in a background of a mixed inflammatory infiltrate and variable degrees of fibrosis. In contrast to the general population, where nodular sclerosis is the most common subtype, there is a larger proportion of mixed cellularity (25%–55%) and lymphocyte-depleted (5%–20%) subtypes in HIV-associated CHL. HIV-associated cases more frequently show a fibrohistiocytic stromal background, large confluent areas of necrosis, and a sarcomatoid pattern associated with an increased number of CD163+ spindle-shaped macrophages.[24] The H/RS cells show the archetypal expression of CD30 by IHC and frequently are positive for CD15, show faint positivity for PAX5, and are negative for CD45 and

CD20 in both populations. Unlike HIV-negative cases, the neoplastic cells in HIV-associated cases are almost universally positive for EBV by in situ hybridization for EBV-encoded RNAs (EBERs). In addition, there are subtle microenvironment differences, including increased number of CD8-positive T cells, resulting in an inversion of the CD4:CD8 ratio in HIV-associated CHL. In addition, there are lower numbers of CD56[+] (natural killer [NK]) cells and CD57[+] cells (terminally differentiated T cells and mature NK cells) infiltrating the HIV-infected cases.[25]

In the pre-ART era, CHL-HIV patients achieved a complete response in less than 50% of cases. This has increased to more than 80%, with a 5-year survival greater than 75%. HIV patients with CHL have the same overall and progression-free survival rates as HIV-negative patients after adjusting for stage and socioeconomic factors. Unfortunately, HIV patients may be less likely to receive chemotherapy (risk factors include black race, lack of health insurance, and residence in high-poverty area) and have a higher mortality due to other HIV-related factors. The standard treatment regimen in these patients is optimized ART and standard combination chemotherapy.[1,4,6,26,27]

PLASMABLASTIC LYMPHOMA

Plasmablastic lymphoma (PBL) is a high-grade neoplasm composed of cells resembling B immunoblasts with a plasma cell immunophenotype. Its original description was a clinically aggressive oral cavity lesion seen primarily in HIV-infected males.[28] Despite this classic association, PBL is now known to arise in extraoral sites and HIV-negative patients who are either immunosuppressed (eg, post-transplant patients or elderly patients with immunosenescence) or immunocompetent and can arise in the setting of previously existing lymphoproliferative or autoimmune disorder.[29,30]

PBL accounts for approximately 2% of HIV-related lymphomas compared with less than 0.1% of lymphomas in the general population.[7,29,30] In both populations, PBL shows a male predominance, presents at a high stage, and has an aggressive clinical course. In HIV patients, PBL develops at a younger age (median age approximately 40 years) compared with the general population (median age approximately 60 years) and more frequently arises in the oral cavity.

Although the pathogenesis of PBL is not fully defined, it is believed that the neoplasm arises from near terminally differentiated B cells, whose development is corrupted by a combination of MYC rearrangements, loss of p53, EBV infection, and immunodeficiency.

PBL is primarily an extranodal disease presenting most commonly in the oral cavity (48%) followed by the GI tract (12%) and skin (6%).[29] It also has been reported in the genitourinary tract, bone, nasal cavity, paranasal sinuses, CNS, liver, lungs, and orbit.[7] Histologically, PBL has a diffuse starry sky growth pattern and shows a morphologic range from immunoblastic to markedly plasmacytic (**Fig. 4**). The immunoblastic predominant

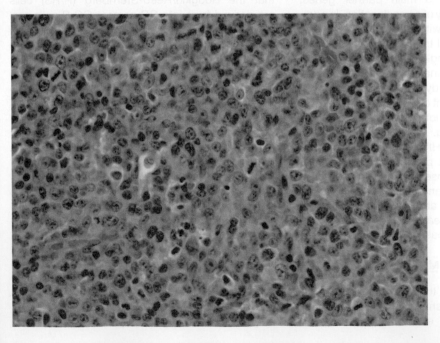

Fig. 4. PBL. Large abnormal lymphoid cells with characteristics plasmacytoid morphology (hematoxylin-eosin, original objective magnification ×40).

subtype is associated more frequently with HIV infection and tumor location in the oral, nasal, and paranasal sinuses and is easily mistaken for DLBCL.[28] The plasmacytic subtype tends to arise in lymph nodes and extranodal sites away from the oral cavity.

In general, PBL shows expression of plasma cell markers (CD38, CD138, CD79a, IRF-4/MUM-1, BLIMP-1, and cytoplasmic immunoglobulin), lacks expression of the B-cell markers (CD19, CD20, and PAX-5), and has weak reactivity to CD45. PBLs have a high proliferation index (Ki-67 >80%), and MYC positivity is seen in greater than 50% of cases. EBER is positive in 70% of cases overall and approximately 100% of HIV-associated cases. Variations from the plasmablast phenotype do occur, including aberrant expression of CD2, CD4, and CD56. CD56 expression complicates diagnosis and distinction from plasmacytomas becomes challenging.[31] Because a majority of PBL harbor MYC rearrangements (or MYC amplification in a minor subset) and EBV positivity in HIV-infected individuals, however, distinction from true plasma cell neoplasms is possible.[7]

PBL is a difficult diagnosis to make due to its rarity and broad morphologic spectrum. The primary and most challenging differential consideration is with plasmablastic plasma cell neoplasms, including extramedullary plasmacytoma and plasma cell myeloma, because these lesions can be morphologically and immunophenotypically identical to PBL.[31,32] The primary differentiating features between these lesions are their clinical presentation and behavior (Table 1). Note that extramedullary plasmacytoma may be indistinguishable from PBL, and the correct diagnosis is guided by clinical factors. It is essential to distinguish PBL and plasma cell neoplasms (PCN) because the clinical course and treatment of these entities are markedly different. Other diagnostic considerations include DLBCL with plasmacytoid morphology, ALK+ large B-cell lymphoma, extracavitary PEL, EBV+ DLBCL not otherwise specified, HHV8+ large B-cell lymphoma, and DLBCL associated with chronic infection. DLBCL with plasmacytoid morphology is CD20+ and is not associated with immunosuppression or EBV infection. ALK+ large B-cell lymphomas are negative for EBV, positive for ALK, and have an ALK gene rearrangement. Extracavitary PEL is positive for HHV-8. HHV-8+ DLBCL is positive for HHV-8 and usually negative for EBV.

Prognosis for PBL is poor, with overall survival in untreated patients of approximately 3 months to 4 months regardless of HIV status. When treated, some investigators have observed that HIV patients have a better clinical outcome than non-HIV patients; however, these findings are not reproducible.[33] There is no defined optimal therapy for these patients and treatment is based on case reports and case series. Favorable prognostic factors include low stage, clinical response to chemotherapy, age less than 60 years, oral location, and absence of MYC/IgH rearrangements. Poor prognostic indicators include MYC rearrangements, advanced stage, and poor performance status. It is unclear whether ART has an impact on prognosis. Prognosis has not changed in the post-ART era; however, spontaneous regression of PBL after ART initiation has been reported in the literature.[34]

PRIMARY EFFUSION LYMPHOMA

Primary effusion lymphoma (PEL) is a rare, aggressive B-cell neoplasm that accounts for 1% to 4% of HIV-associated lymphomas and less than 1% of non–HIV-associated lymphomas. It classically presents as a malignant pleural, pericardial, or peritoneal effusion in young to middle-aged (median age = 42 years) men with AIDS. It also arises, however, in HIV patients with normal CD4 counts, transplant patients, and elderly (median age = 73 years) patients living in HHV-8 endemic areas. The primary oncogenic driver in this neoplasm is latent infection by HHV-8, which produces numerous gene products that inhibit apoptosis, increase proliferation, and impart drug resistance. The primary oncogenic protein, latency-associated nuclear antigen 1 (LANA-1), also aids in diagnosis through immunohistochemical reactivity. Due to the association with HHV-8, one-third to one-half of patients develop Kaposi sarcoma, and some develop multicentric Castleman disease. EBV is present in 60% to 90% of these neoplasms but has no known pathogenic role.[35,36]

Grossly, PEL usually presents as a malignant effusion in the peritoneal, pleural, or pericardial cavity.[7] It can also primarily involve joint spaces and cerebral spinal fluid, however, and rarely can present as an extracavitary mass in the absence of a current or prior effusion. The most common tissue sites of extracavitary PEL are the skin, lungs, GI tract, CNS, and rarely lymph nodes.[37] Histologically, PEL is a high-grade process with variable morphologic appearances bridging those seen in large-cell immunoblastic lymphoma, PBL, and anaplastic large cell lymphoma. The large malignant cells have round to irregular nuclei, prominent nucleoli, and deeply basophilic cytoplasm with occasional vacuoles (Figs. 5 and 6). Some cells have a perinuclear hof imparting a

Table 1
Primary differential for plasmablastic lymphoma

	Plasmablastic Lymphoma	Extramedullary Plasmacytoma	Plasma Cell Myeloma
Clinical	Oral cavity BM[a] with diffuse disease Paraproteinemia (rare)	Isolated mass of head and neck	Bone marrow Paraproteinemia CRAB[b] symptoms
Morphology (plasmablastic to plasmacytic)		Spectrum: plasmablastic to plasmacytic	
IHC		Positive: CD38, CD138, MUM1 Aberrant expression: CD10, CD56 Negative: CD45, CD20, PAX-5 Light chain restricted High Ki-67 (>80%)	
EBV	Associated (EBER+ or high VL)	Rarely associated	
Prognosis	Aggressive	Less aggressive	
Treatment	Intensive chemotherapy		Immunomodulatory agents, steroids, protease inhibitors

[a] Bone marrow.
[b] Monoclonal paraproteinemia, hypercalcemia, renal dysfunction, anemia, and lytic bone lesion.
Abbreviations: BM, bone marrow; EBER, EBV encoded small RNA; VL, viral load.

Fig. 5. PEL. Cytology specimens of PEL have a characteristic high-grade morphology with large eccentric nuclei displaying marked pleomorphism, deep basophilic cytoplasm with a perinuclear hof, and scattered cytoplasmic vacuoles (Wright-Geimsa stain, original objective magnifications ×20 [*A*] and ×40 [*B*]).

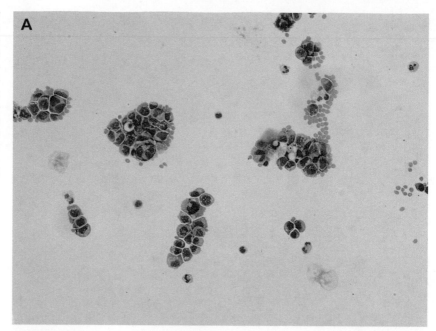

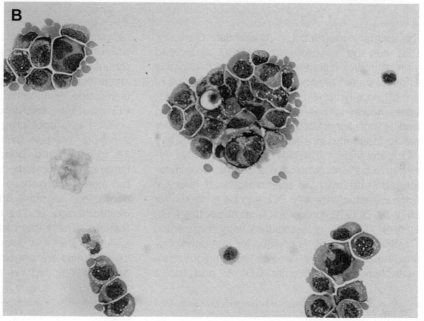

plasmacytoid appearance and occasional binucleated or multinucleated cells, resembling Reed-Sternberg cells, may be seen. Multiple mitoses and a high proliferation index are present.[7,35]

A diagnosis of PEL hinges on the identification of HHV-8 within the neoplastic cells. IHC shows characteristic nuclear staining with LANA-1 and, although less frequently available, reactivity for virally produced interleukin 6. PEL cells are positive for CD45 but are negative for pan–B-cell and T-cell markers (CD19, CD20, CD79a, surface and cytoplasmic Ig, CD3, CD4, and CD8). In keeping with their post-GC nature, they are positive for markers of lymphocyte activation (CD30, CD38, CD71, EMA, and HLA-DR) and markers of plasma cell differentiation (CD38, CD138, and MUM-1/IRF-4). EBER shows EBV positivity in a majority of cases.[7,36]

The differential considerations for PEL are broad, and accurate diagnosis requires knowledge of the clinical presentation, morphology, and HHV-8 infection status. Refer to **Table 2** for

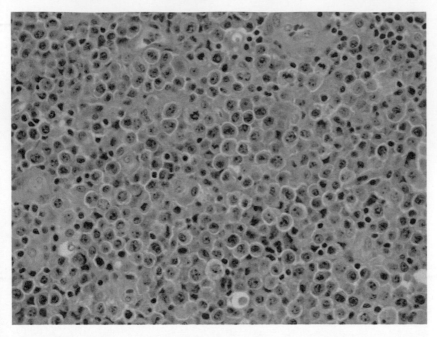

Fig. 6. Extracavitary PEL. Although the degree of atypia and distinct morphologic features seen in classic PEL (see **Fig. 5**) are less evident in this extracavitary lesion, high-grade plasmacytoid features are seen that should raise this diagnostic consideration (hematoxylin-eosin, original objective magnification ×40).

the primary morphologic differential. Clinically, PEL can be mistaken for DLBCL associated with chronic inflammation or HHV-8–negative effusion-based lymphoma due to the presence of a malignant lymphoid effusion. Each of these entities, however, has a particular clinical setting and is not associated with HHV-8. The former arises in elderly Japanese patients with a history of tuberculosis.[38] The latter arises in elderly HIV-negative patients who have a chronic fluid overloaded state, such as congestive heart failure.[39] Immunohistochemically, PEL can be mistaken for HHV-8+ DLBCL. In contrast to extracavitary PEL, HHV-8+ DLBCL is associated with multicentric Castleman disease; is positive for immunoglobulins, especially IgM, as well as lambda light chain restriction; is negative for CD138; and has a

nonmutated immunoglobulin gene.[36] In general, when an HIV-positive patient presents with a malignant effusion, or when an AIDS or severely immunocompromised patient presents with a high-grade lymphoma, PEL and extracavitary PEL must be considered.

PEL has a poor prognosis with few long-term survivors, median overall survival of less than 12 months, and poor response to standard lymphoma chemotherapy. Treatment, guided by expert consensus instead of randomized controlled studies, includes ART, intensive chemotherapy, and treatment of opportunistic infections. The impact of ART is lower than that seen in other HIV-associated lymphomas, and clinical trials are ongoing to test targeted therapies that may improve survival in these patients.

Table 2
Morphologic mimics of primary effusion lymphoma*

	Primary Effusion Lymphoma	Plasmablastic Lymphoma	Plasmablastic Diffuse Large B-cell Lymphoma or Burkitt Lymphoma	Anaplastic Myeloma	Carcinoma or Mesothelioma
Clinical	Effusion or extracavitary	Oral cavity	Variable	Bone marrow	Effusion and prior history
IHC	CD38/138+ LANA-1+	CD38/138+	CD19/CD20+	CD38/138+	CD138+ Specific to primary
HHV-8	Positive	Negative	Negative	Negative	Negative

* Morphologic features can be overlapping among these entities.
  Morphology: Immunoblastic, plasmablastic, or anaplastic.

Poor prognostic factors include poor performance status, absence of ART before PEL diagnosis, and involvement of more than 1 body cavity. Patients with extracavitary PEL have a slightly better survival compared with patients with classic PEL.[40]

SUMMARY

HIV infection and accompanied immune dysregulation significantly increase the risk of lymphoma development. The landscape of lymphomas arising in HIV-infected persons has changed dramatically since the advent and further refinement of ART, with CHL largely responsible for the increased recent incidence of disease. Most HIV-associated lymphomas share diagnostic features with those arising in the HIV-negative population, whereas others more uniquely develop in the setting of HIV infection. Appreciating underlying disease biology and the spectrum of lymphomas arising in this setting can assist in accurate classification and improved care for patients with HIV-associated lymphoma.

REFERENCES

1. Shiels MS, Pfeiffer RM, Gail MH, et al. Cancer burden in the HIV-infected population in the United States. J Natl Cancer Inst 2011;103(9):753–62.
2. Besson C, Goubar A, Gabarre J, et al. Changes in AIDS-related lymphoma since the era of highly active antiretroviral therapy. Blood 2001;98(8):2339–44.
3. Gopal S, Patel MR, Yanik EL, et al. Temporal trends in presentation and survival for HIV-associated lymphoma in the antiretroviral therapy era. J Natl Cancer Inst 2013;105(16):1221–9.
4. Chadburn A, Abdul-Nabi AM, Teruya BS, et al. Lymphoid proliferations associated with human immunodeficiency virus infection. Arch Pathol Lab Med 2013;137(3):360–70.
5. Mahe E, Ross C, Sur M. Lymphoproliferative lesions in the setting of HIV infection: a five-year retrospective case series and review. Patholog Res Int 2011; 2011:618760.
6. Olszewski AJ, Castillo JJ. Outcomes of HIV-associated Hodgkin lymphoma in the era of antiretroviral therapy. AIDS 2016;30(5):787–96.
7. Swerdlow SH, International Agency for Research on Cancer. WHO classification of tumours of haematopoietic and lymphoid tissues. Revised 4th edition. Lyon (France): International Agency for Research on Cancer (IARC) press; 2017.
8. Arvey A, Ojesina AI, Pedamallu CS, et al. The tumor virus landscape of AIDS-related lymphomas. Blood 2015;125(20):e14–22.
9. Pantanowitz L, Carbone A, Dolcetti R. Microenvironment and HIV-related lymphomagenesis. Semin Cancer Biol 2015;34:52–7.
10. Taylor JG, Liapis K, Gribben JG. The role of the tumor microenvironment in HIV-associated lymphomas. Biomark Med 2015;9(5):473–82.
11. Chadburn A, Chiu A, Lee JY, et al. Immunophenotypic analysis of AIDS-related diffuse large B-cell lymphoma and clinical implications in patients from AIDS Malignancies Consortium clinical trials 010 and 034. J Clin Oncol 2009;27(30):5039–48.
12. Besson C, Lancar R, Prevot S, et al. Outcomes for HIV-associated diffuse large B-cell lymphoma in the modern combined antiretroviral therapy era. AIDS 2017;31(18):2493–501.
13. Alizadeh AA, Eisen MB, Davis RE, et al. Distinct types of diffuse large B-cell lymphoma identified by gene expression profiling. Nature 2000; 403(6769):503–11.
14. Lenz G, Wright GW, Emre NC, et al. Molecular subtypes of diffuse large B-cell lymphoma arise by distinct genetic pathways. Proc Natl Acad Sci U S A 2008;105(36):13520–5.
15. Wright G, Tan B, Rosenwald A, et al. A gene expression-based method to diagnose clinically distinct subgroups of diffuse large B cell lymphoma. Proc Natl Acad Sci U S A 2003;100(17):9991–6.
16. Hans CP, Weisenburger DD, Greiner TC, et al. Confirmation of the molecular classification of diffuse large B-cell lymphoma by immunohistochemistry using a tissue microarray. Blood 2004; 103(1):275–82.
17. Meyer PN, Fu K, Greiner TC, et al. Immunohistochemical methods for predicting cell of origin and survival in patients with diffuse large B-cell lymphoma treated with rituximab. J Clin Oncol 2011; 29(2):200–7.
18. Choi WW, Weisenburger DD, Greiner TC, et al. A new immunostain algorithm classifies diffuse large B-cell lymphoma into molecular subtypes with high accuracy. Clin Cancer Res 2009;15(17): 5494–502.
19. Muris JJ, Meijer CJ, Vos W, et al. Immunohistochemical profiling based on Bcl-2, CD10 and MUM1 expression improves risk stratification in patients with primary nodal diffuse large B cell lymphoma. J Pathol 2006;208(5):714–23.
20. Miller TP, Grogan TM, Dahlberg S, et al. Prognostic significance of the Ki-67-associated proliferative antigen in aggressive non-Hodgkin's lymphomas: a prospective Southwest Oncology Group trial. Blood 1994;83(6):1460–6.
21. Bellan C, Lazzi S, De Falco G, et al. Burkitt's lymphoma: new insights into molecular pathogenesis. J Clin Pathol 2003;56(3):188–92.
22. Bibas M, Antinori A. EBV and HIV-related lymphoma. Mediterr J Hematol Infect Dis 2009;1(2):e2009032.

23. Germini D, Tsfasman T, Klibi M, et al. HIV Tat induces a prolonged MYC relocalization next to IGH in circulating B-cells. Leukemia 2017;31(11):2515–22.

24. Thompson LD, Fisher SI, Chu WS, et al. HIV-associated Hodgkin lymphoma: a clinicopathologic and immunophenotypic study of 45 cases. Am J Clin Pathol 2004;121(5):727–38.

25. Carbone A, Gloghini A, Caruso A, et al. The impact of EBV and HIV infection on the microenvironmental niche underlying Hodgkin lymphoma pathogenesis. Int J Cancer 2017;140(6):1233–45.

26. Besson C, Canioni D, Lepage E, et al. Characteristics and outcome of diffuse large B-cell lymphoma in hepatitis C virus-positive patients in LNH 93 and LNH 98 Groupe d'Etude des Lymphomes de l'Adulte programs. J Clin Oncol 2006;24(6):953–60.

27. Chadburn A. Immunodeficiency-associated lymphoid proliferations (ALPS, HIV, and KSHV/HHV8). Semin Diagn Pathol 2013;30(2):113–29.

28. Delecluse HJ, Anagnostopoulos I, Dallenbach F, et al. Plasmablastic lymphomas of the oral cavity: a new entity associated with the human immunodeficiency virus infection. Blood 1997;89(4):1413–20.

29. Castillo JJ, Bibas M, Miranda RN. The biology and treatment of plasmablastic lymphoma. Blood 2015; 125(15):2323–30.

30. Morscio J, Dierickx D, Nijs J, et al. Clinicopathologic comparison of plasmablastic lymphoma in HIV-positive, immunocompetent, and posttransplant patients: single-center series of 25 cases and meta-analysis of 277 reported cases. Am J Surg Pathol 2014;38(7):875–86.

31. Harmon CM, Smith LB. Plasmablastic lymphoma: a review of clinicopathologic features and differential diagnosis. Arch Pathol Lab Med 2016;140(10): 1074–8.

32. Ahn JS, Okal R, Vos JA, et al. Plasmablastic lymphoma versus plasmablastic myeloma: an ongoing diagnostic dilemma. J Clin Pathol 2017;70(9): 775–80.

33. Vasquez JHJ, Quintana S. Clinicopathologic comparison of plasmablastic lymphoma in HIV-positive versus HIV-negative patients: single-center experience. Blood 2016;128(22):1864.

34. Loghavi S, Alayed K, Aladily TN, et al. Stage, age, and EBV status impact outcomes of plasmablastic lymphoma patients: a clinicopathologic analysis of 61 patients. J Hematol Oncol 2015;8:65.

35. Patel S, Xiao P. Primary effusion lymphoma. Arch Pathol Lab Med 2013;137(8):1152–4.

36. Shimada K, Hayakawa F, Kiyoi H. Biology and management of primary effusion lymphoma. Blood 2018, 132(18):1879–88.

37. Kim Y, Leventaki V, Bhaijee F, et al. Extracavitary/solid variant of primary effusion lymphoma. Ann Diagn Pathol 2012;16(6):441–6.

38. Aozasa K, Takakuwa T, Nakatsuka S. Pyothorax-associated lymphoma: a lymphoma developing in chronic inflammation. Adv Anat Pathol 2005;12(6): 324–31.

39. Alexanian S, Said J, Lones M, et al. KSHV/HHV8-negative effusion-based lymphoma, a distinct entity associated with fluid overload states. Am J Surg Pathol 2013;37(2):241–9.

40. Okada S, Goto H, Yotsumoto M. Current status of treatment for primary effusion lymphoma. Intractable rare Dis Res 2014;3(3):65–74.

Recent Advances in Cutaneous T-cell Lymphoma
Diagnostic and Prognostic Considerations

Margaret Cocks, MD, PhD[a], Pierluigi Porcu, MD[b],
Mark R. Wick, MD[c], Alejandro A. Gru, MD[d],*

KEYWORDS

- Cutaneous T-cell lymphoma • Mycosis fungoides • Sézary syndrome • Lymphomatoid papulosis
- Primary cutaneous anaplastic large cell lymphoma • Primary cutaneous lymphoma
- Prognostic parameters • Molecular diagnostics

Key Points

- Numerous updates in the understanding of cutaneous T-cell lymphomas have occurred since the 2017 revision of the World Health Organization classification of tumors of hematopoietic and lymphoid tissues.
- In mycosis fungoides (MF) and Sézary syndrome, new molecular alterations and new treatment options have been introduced, and prognostic indictors have been refined, especially pertaining to folliculotropic MF.
- Three new subtypes of lymphomatoid papulosis: type D, type E, and LyP with DUSP22/IRF4 translocation, have been described.
- Differentiating between primary cutaneous anaplastic large cell lymphoma (ALCL) from skin involvement by systemic ALCL remains a diagnostic challenge but may be aided with analysis of DUSP22/IRF4 translocations.
- The understanding of the rarer types of cutaneous T-cell lymphomas continues to grow, and an awareness of unique histologic features alongside appropriate ancillary testing, including immunohistochemistry, as well as clinicopathologic correlation is key to accurate diagnosis.

ABSTRACT

This review describes the latest advances in the diagnosis of cutaneous T-cell lymphoma focusing on the most clinically useful features introduced since the publication of the World Health Organization revision in 2017. Clinical entities described include mycosis fungoides, Sézary syndrome, lymphomatoid papulosis, primary cutaneous anaplastic large cell lymphoma, primary cutaneous gamma delta T-cell lymphoma, primary cutaneous acral CD8+ T-cell lymphoma, primary cutaneous CD4+ small/medium T-cell lymphoproliferative disorder, and hydroa-vacciniforme-like lymphoproliferative disorder. Distinguishing histologic clues to diagnosis are discussed, and important molecular advances are described. Key prognostic indicators that may assist clinicians with timely and appropriate management options are presented.

Disclosure Statement: The authors have nothing to disclose.
[a] Department of Pathology, University of Virginia, PO Box 800214, 1215 Lee Street, Hospital Expansion Building Room 2015, Charlottesville, VA 22908, USA; [b] Division of Medical Oncology and Hematopoietic Stem Cell Transplantation, Jefferson University, Suite 420A, 925 Chestnut Street, Philadelphia, PA 19107, USA; [c] Department of Pathology, University of Virginia, PO Box 800214, 1215 Lee Street, Hospital Expansion Building Room 3020, Charlottesville, VA 22908, USA; [d] Department of Pathology, University of Virginia, PO Box 800214, 1215 Lee Street, Hospital Expansion Building Room 3018, Charlottesville, VA 22908, USA
* Corresponding author.
E-mail address: AAG4B@virginia.edu

Surgical Pathology 12 (2019) 783–803
https://doi.org/10.1016/j.path.2019.03.006

surgpath.theclinics.com

OVERVIEW

Cutaneous T-cell lymphomas (CTCL) continue to represent a significant diagnostic challenge. Resolving a diagnosis involves synthesizing varied clinical presentations with complex immunohistochemical findings as well as molecular data and ancillary testing, such as flow cytometry. The field is also ever changing, with new diagnostic and prognostic considerations flooding the literature, making sorting through the latest developments seem almost impossible. Tackling the difficulties of diagnosing and classifying CTCLs for the surgical pathologist can be a daunting task, but there are unique attributes to cutaneous hematopoietic lesions that can greatly aid diagnosis.

In 2017, the World Health Organization (WHO) published a major revision of the fourth edition of the classification of hematopoietic and lymphoid neoplasms and introduced several changes to the current classification and understanding of CTCLs (**Box 1**). Many of the subtypes described in the latest WHO revision are quite rare and may not be routinely encountered by the surgical pathologist; thus, a basic knowledge of the categories is the first step to diagnosis.

In this review, the authors describe the latest advances in CTCL diagnosis focusing on the most clinically useful features introduced since the publication of the WHO revision. The authors present distinguishing histologic clues to diagnosis, important molecular advances that may support histologic impressions as well as key prognostic indicators that may assist clinicians with timely and appropriate management options.

MYCOSIS FUNGOIDES AND SÉZARY SYNDROME

Mycosis fungoides (MF) is the most common form of CTCL and accounts for between 52% and 62% of all CTCL cases.[1] Clinically, it is characterized by erythematous cutaneous patches, plaques, or tumors that demonstrate significant morphologic overlap with nonmalignant inflammatory skin diseases, such as psoriasis and eczema. Histopathologic findings include the presence of an atypical population of epidermotropic lymphocytes with linear arrangement along the basement membrane zone. Superficial fibrosis is also present. An intraepidermal collection of lymphocytes (Pautrier microabscess) is present in a small percentage of cases (~20%–30%). MF can progress to involve lymph nodes and also have secondary peripheral blood involvement. Sézary syndrome (SS) is a rare leukemic form of CTCL and typically presents with erythroderma alongside measurable levels of malignant T cells in the peripheral blood.

When diagnosed early, MF carries a good prognosis with median survival often exceeding 10 years, but significant diagnostic delays are common, not least because of the entity's clinical similarity with benign cutaneous conditions.[2] Advanced MF and SS (described in detail in later discussion) carry a much more dismal prognosis with median survival ranging from 1 to 5 years. In recent years, new molecular findings have been introduced with the aim of improving diagnosis; however, these analyses have demonstrated the genomic landscape of MF and SS to be exceedingly complex, only to illustrate the heterogeneity of the disease.

Major advances have been published recently in relationship to the mutational landscape of MF and SS, in addition to the discovery of particular molecular rearrangements.[3–7] Choi and colleagues[8] found frequent deletions in chromatin-modifying genes (*ARID1A* [62.5%], *CTCF* [12.5%], and *DNMT3A* [42.5%]). *RB1* was deleted in 25% of samples. *CARD11* and *JAK2* amplification were seen in 22.5% and 12.5% of cases, respectively. *MYC* amplification was noted in 42.5% of samples. da Silva Almeida and colleagues[9] identified a median of 21 copy-number alterations per sample (range of 0–56) in SS, with characteristic recurrent gains

---

Box 1
Classification of cutaneous T-cell lymphomas (World Health Organization 2018)
Mycosis fungoides
Sézary syndrome
Primary cutaneous CD30-positive lymphoproliferative disorders
Lymphomatoid papulosis
Primary cutaneous anaplastic large cell lymphoma
Primary cutaneous gamma-delta T-cell lymphoma
Primary cutaneous CD8-positive aggressive epidermotropic cytotoxic T-cell lymphoma
Primary cutaneous acral CD8-positive T-cell lymphoma
Primary cutaneous CD4-positive small/medium T-cell lymphoproliferative disorder

in chromosome 7 (5/25, 20%), 8q (13/25, 52%), and 17q (2/25, 8%), as well as recurrent deletions involving tumor-suppressor genes in 17p13.1 (TP53; 13/25, 52%), 13q14.2 (RB1; 4/25, 16%), 10q23.3 (PTEN, 5/25; 20%), and 12p13.1 (CDKN1B; 5/25, 20%). Kiel and colleagues[5] showed numerous (n = 42) fusion genes, including TPR-MET, MYBL1-TOX, DNAJC15-ZMYM2, and EZH2-FOXP1, which, albeit not recurrent, could contribute to the pathogenesis of SS. Ungewickell and colleagues[10] found structural variation events (excluding copy-number gains) in pathways related to T-cell survival and proliferation in 11% of patients with MF or SS. Interestingly, the structural variants were largely mutually exclusive with the TNFR2 alterations. The structural variants included NFKB2 gene truncations in 5% (4/73) of cases with the deletion of a region whose loss is known to generate a truncated p100 protein with predicted proteasome-independent NF-κB2 nuclear localization as well as a deletion involving TRAF3 that would also be expected to increase noncanonical NF-κB signaling. A recurrent CTLA4-CD28 fusion was also discovered.

Scarisbrick and colleagues[11] identified several important prognostic markers for MF based on data evaluating 1275 patients from with advanced MF and SS. Their univariable analysis showed higher stage (stage IV), age greater than 60 years, absence of folliculotropism (atypical lymphocytes invading the follicular epithelium), large-cell transformation, an elevated white blood count, and elevated lactate dehydrogenase (LDH) levels were adverse prognostic markers. Multivariable analysis showed that stage IV disease, age greater than 60, large cell transformation, and elevated serum LDH were independent prognostic variables for worse survival. Large cell transformation is defined as the presence of more than 25% large cells in the infiltrate or large cell nodules (large cells being defined as cells more than 4 times the size of a normal lymphocyte).[12,13]

MF has traditionally been staged using the Mycosis Fungoides Cooperative Group staging system developed in the 1970s. This system relies on TNM features to give stages from IA to IVB. This system was later revised by the International Society for Cutaneous Lymphoma and the Cutaneous Lymphoma Task Force of the European Organisation for the Research and Treatment of Cancer to include blood involvement (B), which is particularly important when staging SS.

Folliculotropic mycosis fungoides (FMF) was recognized as a distinct variant of CTCL in the 2008 and 2017 revision of the WHO classification. This subtype is a fairly common subtype of MF, accounting for nearly 18% of MF diagnoses in an international registry of early-stage MF patients.[14] It is characterized by unique clinicopathologic features that distinguish it from classic MF, including a folliculotropic neoplastic infiltrate, head and neck localization with preference for eyebrow involvement, and concurrent alopecia. Other characteristic features include the presence of grouped follicular papules (Fig. 1), alopecia, acneiform and cystic lesions, and frequent pruritus and secondary bacterial infections. Several studies over the years have found that FMF has a worse prognosis when compared with classic MF.[15,16] A study of 49 cases of FMF found that 10-year disease-specific survival was only 26%, compared with 61% to 84% for classic MF (tumor stage and plaque stage).[15] Furthermore, patients with FMF are less responsive to traditional first-line classic MF therapies.

The poor prognostic power of FMF has recently been contested with several papers suggesting that FMF is much more complex than previously thought. Hodak and colleagues[17] sought to clarify this diagnostic category by examining FMF in 34 patients at a single medical center. Based on their data, they further divided FMF into 2 discrete diagnostic categories with measurable distinct biologic behaviors: early stage and advanced stage (Figs. 2 and 3). Advanced stage lesions were more likely to involve the head or neck, had more pruritus, had heavier perifollicular infiltrates, were deeper, and had higher numbers of eosinophils. Other studies seem to support these findings.[18] The difference in these conclusions has largely been attributed to the failure of these earlier studies to stratify patients based on MF stage. When patients were matched for age, sex, and stage, folliculotropism did not affect overall survival, but rather male sex, older age, and stage greater than IB were predictors of poor survival.[18]

A large case series of interstitial MF has also been published. Originally described by Shapiro and Pinto[19] in 1994 as a rare histopathologic pattern of MF, this variant is characterized by long, linear aggregates of dermal lymphocytes splaying collagen fibers most often involving the entire dermis. Immunohistochemical stains often reveal a cytotoxic phenotype. Reggiani and colleagues[20] reviewed 21 cases of interstitial MF. Clinically, these lesions most often present as patches or plaques; however, no unique clinical morphologies have been attributed to the diagnosis, which remains purely a histopathological

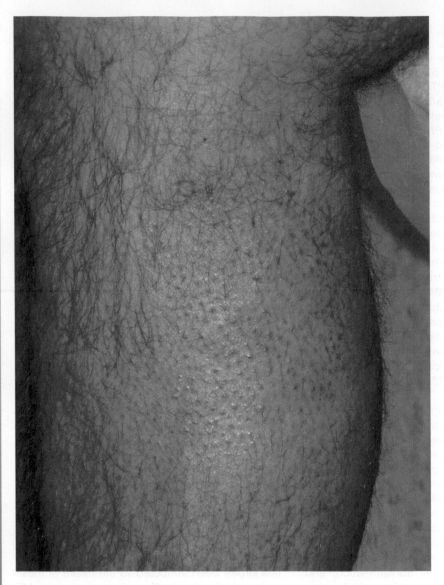

Fig. 1. FMF. Follicular papules in the leg. (*Courtesy of* Dr. Chauncey McHargue, Department of Dermatology, Henry Ford Health System, Detroit, MI)

variant (**Fig. 4**). Rarely does interstitial MF present as the only manifestation of disease but rather is often accompanied, preceded by or followed by a more conventional histopathologic diagnosis of MF.

New treatment options for MF have also emerged. Although early-stage disease is often treated effectively with topical therapies, such as topical steroids, psoralens plus UV-A light, narrow-band UV-B light, and topical cytotoxic drugs (eg, mechlorethamine), advanced cases do not respond well to this therapeutic approach.[21] Brentuximab vedotin (BV), a CD30 targeting antibody-drug conjugate, was recently approved by the Food and Drug Administration

(FDA) for the treatment of CD30-expressing CTCL, including MF. An initial phase 2 trial assessed the efficacy of BV in 28 patients with advanced MF/SS expressing CD30 and found a 54% overall response rate (ORR) with a median time to response of 12 weeks and a median duration of response of 32 weeks, independent of the degree of CD30 expression.[22] Another phase 2 trial of 32 patients with relapsed or refractory MF/SS showed an ORR of 70% and found a lower likelihood of global response in patients with CD30 expression less than 5%.[23] A randomized phase 3 trial comparing BV versus physician's medication choice (ALCANZA study) in advanced stage MF showed a major advantage in global

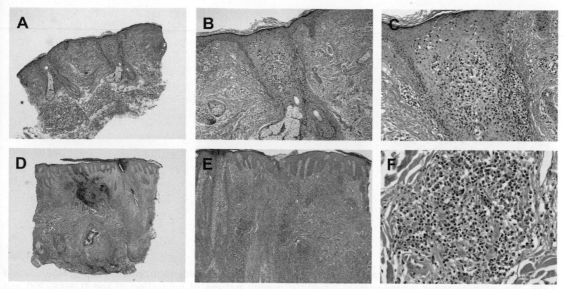

Fig. 2. FMF, early stage (*A–C*) and advanced stage (*D–F*). The punch biopsy shows a perifollicular and intrafollicular lymphocytic infiltrate (*A* and *B*, H&E×20 and ×200). A closer inspection shows that the infiltrate is characterized by atypical cells with nuclear hyperchromasia, perinuclear halos, and cerebriform nuclei (*C*, H&E×400). In the case of advanced stage FMF, the infiltrate is deep, and there is rupture of the hair follicles (*D*, H&E×20). Marked perifollicular and intrafollicular infiltration is present, in addition to follicular mucinosis (*E*, H&E×40). The destruction of the hair follicles results in the presence of a mixture of eosinophils and plasma cells, a potential mimicker of a nonneoplastic process (*F*, H&E×400).

response (56.3% vs 12.5%) for BV, a fact that led to FDA approval.[24] Although the FDA indication acknowledges that CD30 expressing cases (>10% expression) benefit the most, cases with less than 10% expression can also be treated with BV (as long as they express CD30 in >1% cells).

The use of pathologic biomarkers in the treatment of cancer has created a major revolution in the modern pathology era, particularly given the

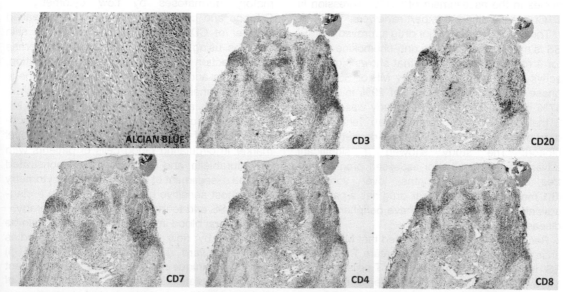

Fig. 3. FMF, immunophenotype. Alcian blue stain shows follicular mucinosis Alcian blue, ×100. The infiltrate is represented by CD3⁺ T cells (CD3, ×20). CD20 shows only sparse number of B cells in the dermis (CD20, ×20). The T cells show aberrant loss of CD7 (approximately 50% loss). (CD7, ×20) Most of the T cells are CD4⁺ (CD4, ×20), whereas CD8 (CD8, ×20) stains a much smaller population of T cells. The CD4:CD8 ratio is greater than 10:1.

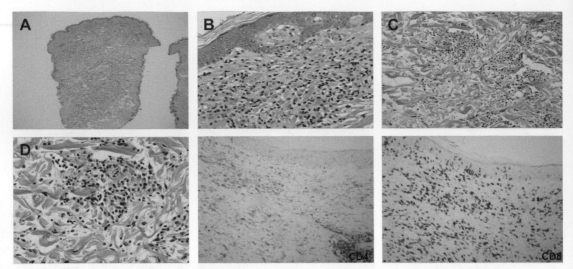

Fig. 4. MF, interstitial variant. Atypical lymphoid infiltrate with limited epidermotropism (*A* and *B*, H&E×20 and ×200). The infiltrate shows a predominant interstitial growth pattern of infiltration (*C* and *D*, H&E×200 and ×400). There appears to be a predominance of CD8⁺ (CD8, ×100) lymphocytes over CD4⁺ (CD4, ×100) T cells.

debate over the optimal expression levels to be used. A very interesting study by Rahbar and colleagues[25] showed major changes in levels of CD30 expression within different lesions, and even within the same lesion. Such study emphasizes a potential need for more than 1 biopsy in patients with advanced stage disease in order to optimize therapy. Another problem surrounding the use of tissue biomarkers is the interobserver variability. A recent study revealed major discrepancies in the assessment of CD30 expression in CTCL across different expert reviewers.[26]

The second recent major drug approved for MF/SS is mogamulizumab, an anti-chemokine receptor 4 monoclonal antibody that shows significant activity in treatment-refractory MF or SS with a phase 1/2 showing an ORR of 29% in MF and 47% in SS.[27] The MAVORIC study was a phase 3 trial comparing mogamulizumab versus standard of care vorinostat (a histone deacetylase inhibitor). The study showed a significant advantage in investigator-assessed progression-free survival (7.7 months) over vorinostat (3.1 months). This particular drug has a particular advantage in patients who have peripheral blood disease.[28]

Recent studies have suggested that MF and SS arise from distinct subsets of mature T cells, with SS deriving from central memory T cells, whereas MF evolves from skin-resident effector memory T cells.[29] However, erythrodermic MF and SS may be very difficult to distinguish clinically, especially when blood findings are subtle.[30] In SS, malignant cells can be identified using flow cytometry

because they often lack expression of CD26 and CD7, as well as other pan-T-cell markers, including CD2, CD3, and CD5. Distinguishing this flow cytometry pattern from some benign inflammatory dermatoses may be difficult because both can show similar patterns.[31] Recent studies have demonstrated new diagnostic opportunities. CD158k/KIR3DL2, a natural killer (NK) receptor, is a new molecular marker that can be used to distinguish SS from benign erythrodermic inflammatory dermatoses by flow cytometry.[32,33] Ortonne and colleagues[34] showed an increased number of CD158k/KIR3DL2 transcripts in skin samples using reverse transcription polymerase chain reaction (RT-PCR) techniques. In addition, Bensussan and colleagues found that peripheral blood malignant CD4⁺ T lymphocytes also express NKp46, an activating receptor found on NK lymphocytes, on their cell surface. A similar technique using RT-PCR was used to identify this novel marker in circulating blood cells of patients with SS. Hurabielle and colleagues[35] demonstrated that the assessment of KIR3DL2 by flow cytometry is the most sensitive method to establish a diagnosis of SS and to monitor response to therapy.

Peripheral blood involvement in SS may also be evaluated by flow cytometry using antibodies directed toward the T-cell receptor-β (TCR-β) chain, a technique that has been shown to detect a clonal population in between 79% and 100% of patients.[3,36] When tested on gated atypical populations, the method has been found to be more specific but less sensitive than PCR.[4] One advantage of this method is that unlike PCR it can provide a quantitative assessment of blood involvement and thus has been proposed as a means of determining tumor burden as well as monitoring response to therapy.[3] Currently, though, guidelines for appropriate utilization of TCR-β are not available, and it remains an expensive test, although suggestions for how to make the test more cost-efficient, such as targeting only specific subdomains before evaluating the entire repertoire, have been proposed.[5]

The molecular diagnosis of MF/SS is also being revolutionized by novel molecular techniques. Traditional methods to prove clonality for T cells have been based on the BIOMED-2 multiplex PCR assay that analyzes TCR gene rearrangements. High-throughput sequencing (next-generation sequencing [NGS]) has been shown to be more sensitive and specific for detection of clonal T cells, but at the same time at a higher cost.[6,7] Using high-throughput sequencing, Kirsch and colleagues[6] were able to detect distinctly expanded T-cell clones in 46/46 skin samples of patients with CTCL. Indeed, the investigators demonstrated clear differences between the clones of neoplastic and inflammatory skin conditions. Weng and colleagues[37] use NGS to evaluate minimal residual disease monitoring in a cohort of patients with MF/SS who underwent bone marrow transplantation. The assay had a sensitivity of detecting tumor cells at a level of 1/50,000 in peripheral blood mononuclear cells.[37] More recently, de Masson and colleagues[38] used the evaluation of tumor clone frequency (TCF), a marker of amount of clonal T cells by TCR-NGS, and found that cases with a TCF greater than 25 have a higher risk of disease progression. To this extent, NGS offers the possibility of quantifying disease, a feature that is not possible with standard molecular methods.

LYMPHOMATOID PAPULOSIS

Lymphomatoid papulosis is characterized by a waxing and waning course of chronic, recurrent, self-resolving papules (Fig. 5) and small nodules that are CD30[+] on histopathology.[39] It is important to remember that such patients have a higher risk of developing a second lymphoma, more typically MF and cutaneous anaplastic large cell lymphoma (C-ALCL). A recent study by Duvic and colleagues[39] followed retrospectively a cohort of 180 patients with LyP and observed that 52% of those developed a second malignancy. Approximately 61% of patients developed MF and 26% developed anaplastic large cell lymphoma (ALCL). Traditionally, 3 main types of LyP have been recognized: type A (histiocytic variant), type B (MF-like), and type C (ALCL-like). The new WHO revision now includes 3 new types: type D, type E, and LyP with *DUSP22/IRF4* translocation. A small subset of cases of LyP can show focal dissemination to the lymph nodes adjacent to the skin lesions. Such finding is important, because some of these cases have been misdiagnosed as classic Hodgkin lymphoma.[40] Type D was first described by Magro and colleagues[41] in 2006 with a larger case series presented by Saggini and colleagues[42] in 2010, who also proposed the now accepted "type D" designation. Clinically, all patients present with classic LyP lesions; however,

Fig. 5. Lymphomatoid papulosis. Classic small papules on the extremities.

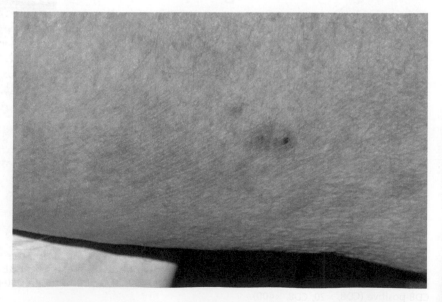

histology shows large numbers of medium-sized pleomorphic lymphocytes infiltrating the epidermis with a pagetoid reticulosis (PR)-like pattern combined with a cytotoxic phenotype (BetafF1$^+$, CD3$^+$, CD4$^-$, CD8$^+$, and either TIA-1, perforin, and/or Granzyme B) (**Fig. 6**). The important differential to keep in mind is primary cutaneous aggressive epidermotropic CD8$^+$ cytotoxic T-cell lymphoma (Berti lymphoma), which, unlike type D LyP, has an aggressive course and very poor prognosis. These 2 entities are differentiated clinically: the former shows infiltrative patches, plaques, and ulcers with mucosal involvement and a relative progressive course, without the self-remitting character seen in LyP. Another important differential diagnosis is PR, a localized variant of MF, which may have CD8$^+$ and CD30$^+$ epidermotropic cells that also express cytotoxic antigens. Clinically, the lesions of PR have a predilection for acral sites and have the more typical features of patches and plaques with or without ulceration. PR has an exquisite clinical response to radiotherapy.

A fifth type of LyP, type E or angioinvasive LyP, has also now been described. The clinical features of type E LyP include papulonodular lesions that rapidly evolve into large ulcerations that often develop a hemorrhagic necrotic crust with an escharlike appearance.[43] Spontaneous regression of lesions occurs but often with scar formation. The differential diagnosis for the clinical presentation includes pyoderma gangrenosum, ulcerative herpes infection or Orf disease, and vasculitis. On histology, this LyP subtype is characterized by dermal angiocentric infiltrates of small-, medium-, and large-sized pleomorphic cells that infiltrate the walls of small- and medium-sized dermal and subcutaneous blood vessels (**Fig. 7**). Thrombosis is also a common feature. Immunohistochemical stains show the perivascular and/or intratumoral lymphocytes express CD30 and CD8 with variable expression of TIA-1.[43] It is essential to exclude primary cutaneous anaplastic large cell lymphoma (PC-ALCL), which can also exhibit angiocentric infiltrates and a CD30$^+$/CD8$^+$ immunoprofile. Clinical correlation with multiple versus solitary lesions as well as resolution and recurrence are essential because the latter diagnosis has a much graver prognosis.

Lymphomatoid papulosis with *DUSP22/IRF4* translocations has a characteristic combination of both epidermal and dermal involvement by the neoplastic infiltrate. The pronounced epidermotropism is a feature typical of this subtype of LyP and also shared by type D LyP. However, the latter lacks a significant dermal component. In addition to CD30 expression, the cases with *DUSP22/IRF4* translocation have a dual staining pattern of CD30 expression (dim in the epidermis and strong in the dermal portion). Another distinctive feature of this LyP subtype is the marked decreased expression of cytotoxic markers (TIA-1, granzyme B, and perforin).[44]

A separate subtype (type "F") with prominent follicular involvement has been proposed by different investigators.[45,46] However, most accept that folliculotropism is an element that can be seen in the classic subtypes of LyP (A, B, and C). The importance of this subgroup is the distinction of

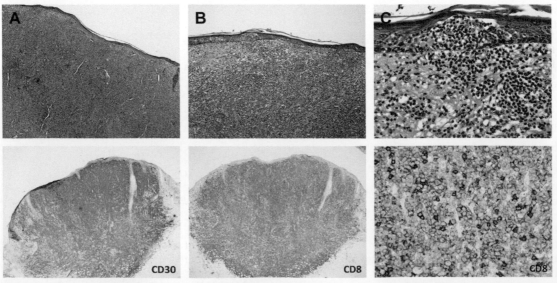

Fig. 6. Lymphomatoid papulosis, type D. A dense dermal infiltrate is present (*A*, H&E×40). The infiltrate shows prominent epidermotropism (*B* and *C*, H&E×100 and ×400). The infiltrate is CD30-positive (CD30, ×20) and CD8-positive (CD8, ×20; CD8, ×400).

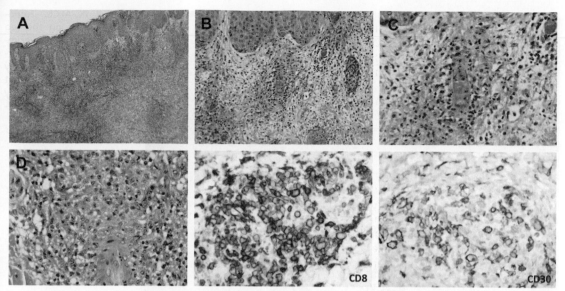

Fig. 7. LYP, type E? A dense perivascular infiltrate is present (*A* and *B*, H&E×40 and ×200). The infiltrate is angio-centric and shows vasculitic changes (*C* and *D*, H&E×400). The atypical infiltrate is positive for both CD8 (CD8, ×400) and CD30 (CD30, ×400).

LyP and FMF, which has a more aggressive clinical behavior.

PRIMARY CUTANEOUS ANAPLASTIC LARGE CELL LYMPHOMA

ALCLs are a group of CD30-positive non-Hodgkin lymphomas that fall into 3 diagnostic entities per WHO classification: PC-ALCL, and systemic ALCL, which can be either anaplastic lymphoma kinase (ALK) positive or negative. PC-ALCL is limited to skin involvement, has an excellent prognosis, and is usually ALK negative. Clinically, patients present with a rapidly growing solitary ulcerated nodule that can undergo partial or complete spontaneous regression (**Fig. 8**). Extracutaneous involvement occurs in about 10% of cases and is usually limited to regional lymph nodes. PC-ALCL has long-term survival rates of greater than 90%.[47] Pathology shows sheetlike infiltrates of atypical lymphocytes often with large, pleomorphic cells that have reniform or horseshoe-shaped cells that are designated as "hallmark" cells (**Fig. 9**). Greater than 75% of cells must express CD30 and also usually express CD4 and demonstrate variable expression of other T-cell markers (CD2, CD3, and CD5) and other cytotoxic proteins. Some cases can be CD8 positive, and the less common phenotype includes cases that are negative for both CD4 and CD8. CD43 is typically positive in most cases, whereas EM epithelial membrane antigen (EMA) A is negative. Some cases have a so-called null phenotype

(characterized by loss of most of the T-cell antigens). The latter is more common in systemic ALK⁻ ALCL, but less common in PC-ALCL.

Distinguishing PC-ALCL from skin involvement by systemic ALK⁻ ALCL remains a diagnostic challenge and appears to be based on adequate staging procedures, excluding the possibility of lymph node involvement. However, strong and diffuse expression of EMA should raise concern for a systemic process.[48] Molecular similarities between ALK⁻ ALCL and C-ALCL are seen. Feldman and colleagues[49] were the first to demonstrate recurrent *DUSP22/IRF4* translocations in PC-ALCL in approximately 30% of patients. A similar percentage is seen in systemic ALK⁻ ALCL. Subsequent studies confirmed this finding with *IRF4* locus gene rearrangement seen in 20% to 75% of PC-ALCL.[50–52] Fluorescence in situ hybridization for *DUSP22-IRF4* locus is thought to have 99% specificity and 90% positive predictive value for PC-ALCL.[51] Although the presence of *DUSP22/IRF4* rearrangements may be useful, they are also present in about 30% of ALK⁻ ALCL as well as in some cases of lymphomatoid papulosis.[44,53] In addition, a recent study suggested that *DUSP22* rearrangements do not help in differentiating between transformed MF and PC-ALCL.[54] Furthermore, the diagnosis of PC-ALCL is not compatible with a current or previous diagnosis of MF because this may represent MF with large cell transformation. Interestingly, among PC-ALCL with *DUSP22/IRF4*, a significant subset of cases shows an intravascular growth

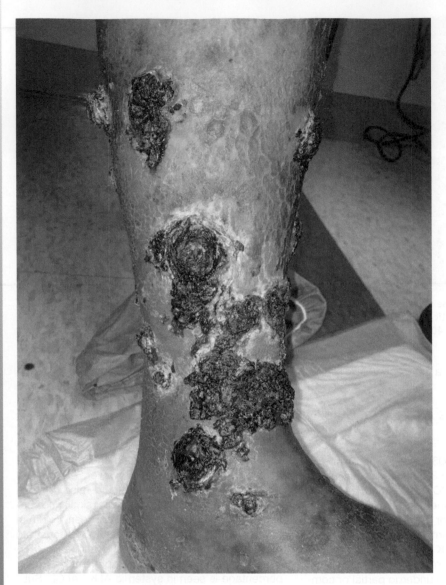

Fig. 8. PC-ALCL. Tumorous lesions on the leg are present with overimposed infection. (Courtesy of Dr. Chauncey McHargue, Department of Dermatology, Henry Ford Heatlh System, Detroit, MI).

pattern.[55] Most cases of PC-ALCL with *DUSP22/IRF4* show a peculiar epidermotropic pattern and a biphasic pattern of CD30 expression (with strong expression in the dermis and weak among the epidermotropic lymphocytes). Another characteristic immunophenotypic feature of ALCL is the absence of cytotoxic marker expression, particularly TIA-1 (the same ones described for LyP with *DUSP22/IRF4*). The outcome of PC-ALCL with *DUSP22* is excellent. More recently, the molecular biology of DUSP22⁺ tumors has been elucidated and shows a genetic signature that is linked to the upregulation of CD58 and HLA class II molecules, and downregulation of programmed death 1 (PD-1) and programmed death ligand 1 (PD-L1) expression, a feature that makes such tumors uniquely

susceptible to the immune system attack, by being unable to escape the attack of the host T cells.[56] A third and more uncommon group of PC-ALCL shows a *TP63* translocation. Only 2 cases with isolated skin involvement have been described, both of which show a more aggressive clinical course, an unusual feature in the disease, and a similar feature to what is seen in systemic ALK⁻ ALCL with such translocation.[57] Last, the authors recently reported the association of ALK⁻ ALCL involving the skin, in association with immunodeficiency, Epstein-Barr virus (EBV) expression, and a peculiar *BRAF V600E* mutation, confirmed by Sanger sequencing and immunohistochemistry.[58]

Several cases of ALK-positive PC-ALCL have been reported in the literature, but this remains a

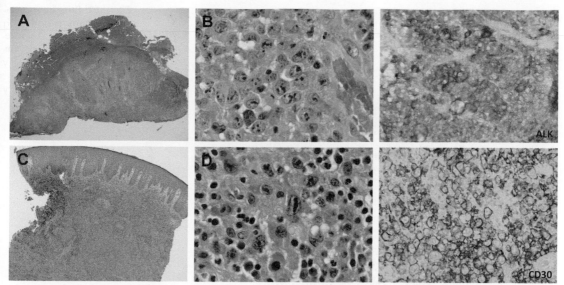

Fig. 9. PC-ALCL. The lesion shows surface ulceration and a dense malignant dermal infiltrate (*A*, H&E×20). Numerous hallmark cells in the dermis are present (*B*, H&E×600). ALK immunostain is positive in the tumor cells with an unusual pattern (cytoplasmic and granular) suggestive of a variant translocation. Another example of PC-ALCL with hallmark cells and a rich background of acute inflammation (*C* and *D*, H&E×20 and ×600). The malignant cells are diffusely positive for CD30 (CD30, ×400).

controversial diagnostic entity.[59,60] A recent review of the 21 cases described to date found the diagnosis was made in a much younger cohort of patients with a median age at diagnosis of ALK-positive PC-ALCL of 23.5 years compared with the sixth decade for ALK⁻ ALCL.[59] Many cases of cutaneous-limited ALK⁺ ALCL have been reported in the pediatric age group, following insect bites.[61]

PRIMARY CUTANEOUS GAMMA DELTA T-CELL LYMPHOMA

Primary cutaneous gamma delta T-cell lymphoma (PCGD-TCL) was first introduced in the 2008 revision of the WHO but was made a permanent category in 2017. Originally thought to be a subtype of subcutaneous panniculitis-like T-cell lymphoma, PCGD-TCL was subsequently separated from that entity by the characteristic expression of TCR-gamma in the neoplastic cells, and a very aggressive clinical behavior. PCGD-TCL is extremely rare, accounting for less than 1% of cutaneous lymphomas, and has an aggressive course with 5-year survival rates ranging from 20% to 30%.[62,63] Clinically, patients may present with either deep panniculitis-like features and disseminated indurated plaques that often ulcerate and have necrosis (**Fig. 10**), or with a clinical picture resembling MF.[63,64] Mucosal sites may or may not be involved. Pathologic findings include

3 main patterns of involvement: subcutaneous, dermal, and epidermotropic (**Fig. 11**). The first 2 subtypes are the most common and are often described together. Angioinvasion and angionecrosis are also frequent. The tumor cells often infiltrate the adipose tissue with a typical adipocyte rimming. In some cases, hemophagocytosis can also be seen in the skin biopsies. On immunohistochemistry, atypical lymphocytes are CD3⁺, TCR-gamma⁺, TCR-delta⁺,[65] CD4⁻, BF-1⁻, and CD8⁻, with variable expression of CD30 (**Fig. 12**). The classic phenotype shows CD56⁺ as well as variable loss of pan-T-cell markers. Often there is also expression of at least 1 cytotoxic marker (eg,.TIA-1, perforin, and granzyme B).[63] TCR clonality is detected in most cases.

The largest series of PCGD-TCL was published in 2012 by Guitart and colleagues.[63] This series studied 53 cases of PCGD-TCL. The subset of patients presenting with MF-like features clinically appeared to have a better prognosis. Unlike MF, on histology, these cases did not demonstrate Pautrier microabscesses and had many scattered necrotic keratinocytes. A subset of cases (4/53) has EBV positivity. Kash and colleagues[66] observed a phenotypic switch between indolent patch phase skin lesions and ulcerated lesions. Gamma/delta cells were not activated in the former cases with minimal or absent TIA-1 and granzyme B expression with increased expression of these markers in latter lesions.

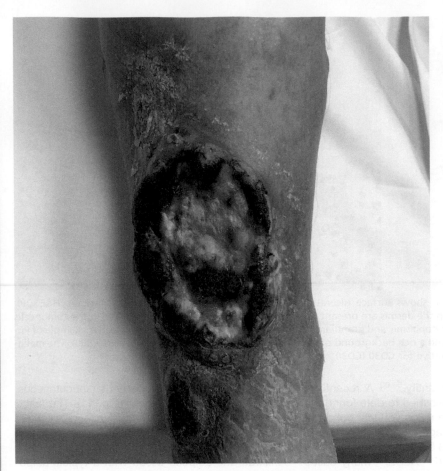

Fig. 10. Primary cutaneous gamma-delta T-cell lymphoma. A large ulcerated tumor in the leg is present.

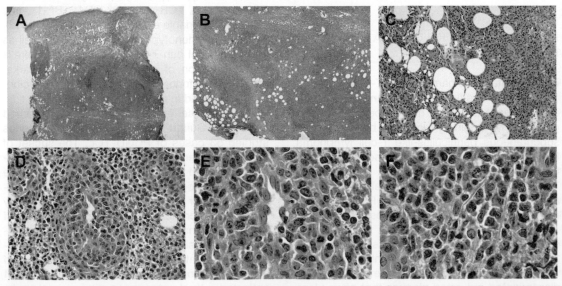

Fig. 11. Primary cutaneous gamma-delta T-cell lymphoma. A dense dermal infiltrate is noted with extension into the adipose tissue (*A* and *B*, H&E×20 and ×40). Adipocyte rimming by the neoplastic cells is seen (*C*, H&E×200). Marked angiotropism is typical of this tumor (*D* and *E*, H&E×400 and ×600). The malignant cells are medium to large with marked nuclear pleomorphism (*F*, H&E×600).

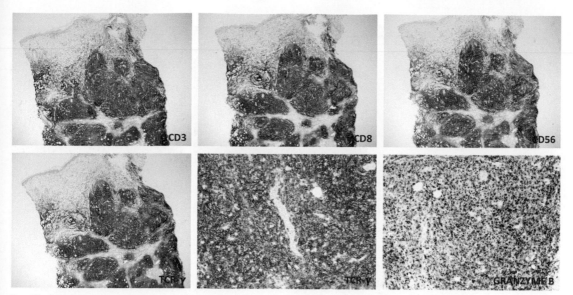

Fig. 12. Primary cutaneous gamma-delta T-cell lymphoma, immunophenotype. The neoplastic cells are positive for CD3 (CD3 ×20), CD8 (CD8, ×20), CD56 (CD56, ×20) TCR-gamma (TCR-gamma, ×20 and ×200), and granzyme B (granzyme B, ×200).

Merrill and colleagues[67] recently showed that PCGD-TCL may in fact be a more heterogeneous group of lymphomas than previously thought by examining the pathology and behavior of epidermal subtypes versus dermal/subcutaneous subtypes. Histologically, these subtypes differ in that the former has prominent epidermotropism by atypical lymphocytes that is often accompanied by adnexotropism, low cellularity, and small- to medium-size cells. Epidermal variants were more likely to demonstrate interface changes. The overall immunophenotypes were similar, although dermal/subcutaneous PCGD-TCL was more likely to be CD56+. Patients with epidermal type PCGD-TCL also had better overall survival and lower mortality from disease. The group does highlight the potential coexistence of different histopathologic patterns in the same patient and the need for multiple biopsies from different involved sites.

Another problem in the diagnosis of PCGD-TCL has been the use of TCR-gamma expression as a defining marker for the disease. More recently, expression of TCR-gamma has been reported to occur in a variety of neoplastic and reactive dermatologic conditions, including lymphomatoid papulosis,[68,69] T-lymphoblastic lymphoma/leukemia,[70] pityriasis lichenoides,[71] and arthropod bite reactions.[72]

PRIMARY CUTANEOUS ACRAL CD8+ T-CELL LYMPHOMA

Primary cutaneous acral CD8+ T-cell lymphoma is a new provisional entity in the 2016 WHO.

Originally described by Petrella and colleagues[73] in 2007 as a cutaneous lymphoma with indolent behavior occurring primarily on the ear, this new diagnostic category has now been expanded to include indolent CD8+ lymphoid proliferations at peripheral sites, including the nose, hands, and feet.[74,75] Patients present with slow-growing, usually solitary nodules or plaques that on histology show a diffuse proliferation of intermediate-sized CD8+ T cells with irregular, lymphoblast-like nuclei involving the dermis and the subcutis (**Fig. 13**). A grenz zone is usually present, and epidermotropism is not seen. The atypical cells are positive for CD3, CD8, TCR-βF1, CD68 (dotlike), and TIA-1 and negative for CD4, CD30, CD56, granzyme B, and EBV with a low Ki-67 proliferation index (<10%).[73] There is variable loss of other T-cell antigens. TCR rearrangement studies are most often monoclonal. Clinically, patients are often older than 50 years and predominantly men. Although relapses limited to cutaneous involvement have been reported, progression to systemic disease is extraordinarily rare. Surgery or local radiotherapy is often sufficient treatment modalities to achieve complete remission. Single reports of extension to extracutaneous sites and progression to a more aggressive subtype of lymphoma have been described.[76,77]

PRIMARY CUTANEOUS CD4+ SMALL/MEDIUM T-CELL LYMPHOPROLIFERATIVE DISORDER

In the 2016 WHO revision, primary cutaneous CD4+ small/medium pleomorphic T-cell

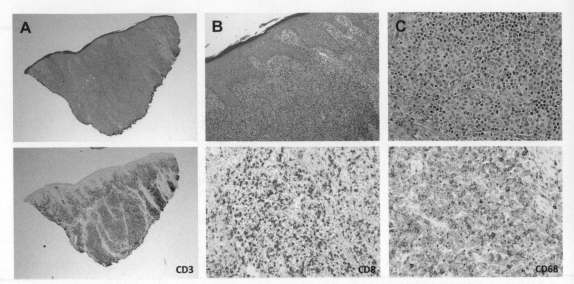

Fig. 13. Primary cutaneous acral CD8-positive T-cell lymphoma. Very dense and diffuse dermal infiltrate with very limited epidermotropism (*A* and *B*, H&E×20 and ×100). The infiltrate is composed of small- to medium-sized lymphocytes (*C*, H&E×400). The infiltrate is positive for CD3 (CD3, ×20), partially for CD8 (CD8, ×200), and shows a characteristic staining pattern for CD68 (CD68, ×200), with perinuclear dotlike immunoreactivity.

lymphoma has been reclassified as primary cutaneous CD4+ small/medium pleomorphic T-cell lymphoproliferative disorder (PCSMP-TLPD). Clinically, patients usually have a solitary plaque or tumor predominantly on the face (**Fig. 14**), neck, or upper trunk, but less commonly there may be more than 1 lesion.[78,79] It accounts for 2% to 3% of cutaneous lymphomas.

This entity is characterized by small- to medium-size pleomorphic CD4+ lymphocytes with a Ki67 proliferation index of less than 30%. Occasional larger cells are present, but they are always the minority of the infiltrate (**Fig. 15**). The latter is based in the dermis and may have a nodular or bandlike distribution often with a grenz zone separating it from the epidermis. Focal epidermotropism or extension to the subcutaneous fat may also occur. A mixed inflammatory infiltrate of plasma cells, eosinophils, and histiocytes may be present as well. Numerous variants, including granulomatous and folliculotropic patterns, have been discussed in the literature.[79] The pleomorphic cells are always CD3+, CD4+, CD8−CD30−. Helpful immunohistochemical findings include positivity for PD-1, B-cell lymphoma 6, C-X-C motif chemokine ligand 13, inducible costimulator, and CD10, compatible with a T-follicular helper phenotype (**Fig. 16**).[80] These lesions often have a rich reactive B-cell background with CD20 staining representing 10% to 60% of the infiltrate. Clonal TCR gene rearrangement has been detected in approximately 60% of cases, a

helpful diagnostic clue differentiating PSCMP-TLPD from reactive or pseudolymphomas.[78,81] Another helpful clue may be nuclear expression of NFATc1, although this finding has not yet validated.[82]

The change in its classification from "lymphoma" to "lymphoproliferative disorder" was prompted by the fairly indolent course and favorable prognosis of the disease but also because the malignant potential of this entity remains uncertain. It has been suggested that PCSMP-TLPD may represent a limited clonal response to an unknown stimulus and therefore does not fulfill criteria for malignancy.[83] PCSMP-TLPD generally has a favorable prognosis and indolent behavior. A systematic review of the availably English language literature found a 5-year survival rate of 98.4% among reported cases, particularly in cases whereby only solitary lesions were present, whereas other studies suggest these range from 60% to 80%.[84–86] The original series from Garcia-Herrera and colleagues revealed a subset of patients (5/24) with a more aggressive clinical course: such patients invariably had a higher Ki67 (>30%) and would be excluded from the current WHO classification using the modern criteria.

HYDROA VACCINIFORME-LIKE LYMPHOPROLIFERATIVE DISORDER

Hydroa vacciniforme-like lymphoproliferative disorder (HV-LPD) was recognized as a distinct

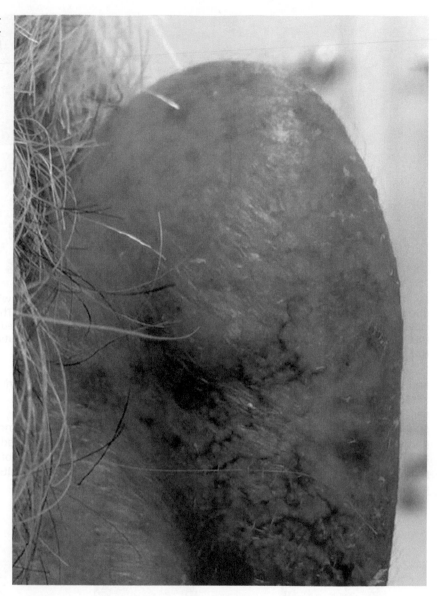

Fig. 14. Primary cutaneous CD4⁺ small/medium T-cell LPD. Small nodule on the ear.

entity in the 2008 WHO revision, under 2 separate categories: hydroa vacciniforme (HV) and HV-like lymphoma. Because it is very difficult to predict clinically and pathologically which patients will go on to develop lymphoma, the term lymphoproliferative disorder was adopted in the update of the last classification. It is an EBV-associated CTCL observed in children and young adults of Latin American or Asian ethnicity. Children most commonly present with persistent facial edema with necrotic areas that often develop into vacciniforme or pitted scars (**Fig. 17**). Microscopic examination shows epidermal necrosis A relationship with classic HV has been described. Classic HV is a rare photodermatosis that usually begins in childhood. Patients develop itchiness and stinging after sun exposure, which then develops into an erythematous rash. Eventually, this rash progresses into papules that may vesiculate, crust over, and then leave a pitted scar. Histology shows a dense perivascular lymphocytic infiltrate, spongiosis, and varying degrees of epidermal necrosis (**Fig. 18**).[87] Immunophenotypically, HV-LPD shows a T-cell or NK-cell phenotype. All cases show expression of EBV. Expression of cytotoxic markers is also typical, and the Ki67 is variable. CD30 expression is more common in those cases with an NK-cell phenotype.

An association between HV and EBV has been demonstrated using in situ hybridization.[88] Two clinical forms of HV have been described: classic

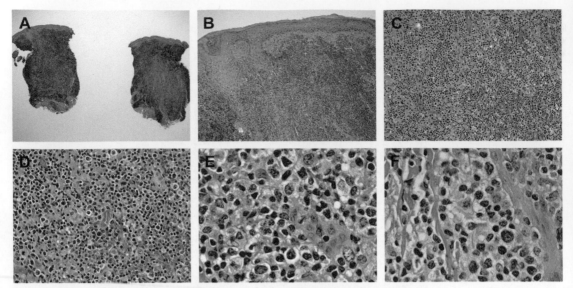

Fig. 15. Primary cutaneous CD4⁺ small/medium T-cell LPD. Diffuse dermal infiltrate with a superficial and deep distribution and lack of associated epidermotropism (*A* and *B*, H&E×20 and ×100). The infiltrate displays a variable amount of cellular pleomorphism but is largely composed of small- and medium-sized cells (*C* and *D*, H&E×200 and ×400). Closer inspection also shows the presence of a smaller population of large cells (*E* and *F*, H&E×600).

and atypical or systemic. The classic variant occurs in children on sun-exposed areas and is self-limited. Atypical HV can be seen in sun-protected areas, is associated with high-grade fever and liver damage, and may progress to EBV-positive T-cell lymphoma.[89] Data on the progression rate of HV to HV-like lymphoma are mixed and range from 17% to 75% in the literature.[87,90,91] Similarly, there are no clear clinical or pathologic features that predict progression.

Hypersensitivity to mosquito bites (HMB) is another EBV-associated T/NK LPD that has been considered part of a spectrum alongside the subtypes of HV. HMB results in intense local skin reactions and systemic symptoms,

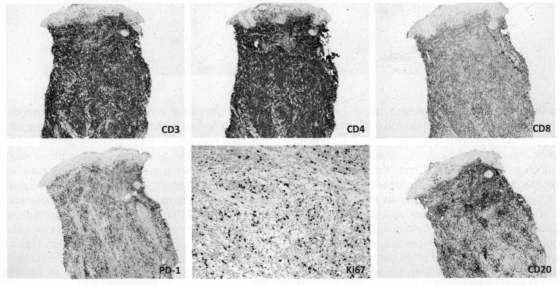

Fig. 16. Primary cutaneous CD4⁺ small/medium T-cell LPD. The infiltrate is composed of CD3⁺ (CD3, ×20) T cells. Most of the T cells are CD4⁺ (CD4, ×20), whereas CD8 (CD8, ×20) stains a much smaller population of cells. PD-1 (PD-1, ×20) shows positive staining in a large proportion of cells. Ki67 (Ki-67, ×200) is very low (<10%). CD20 (CD20, ×20) shows a rich background of nonneoplastic B cells.

Fig. 17. HV-like LPD. A papulovesicular eruption with scarring on the face is present.

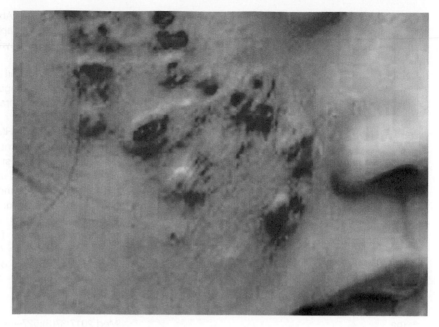

including high fever, lymphadenopathy, hepatosplenomegaly, and hemophagocytic syndrome, usually in response to mosquito bites, other insect bites, or vaccination.[92,93] These patients may also develop HV-like eruptions. Serologic studies reveal these patients have an increased percentage of circulating NK cells that are EBV infected. Miyake and colleagues[92] examined this spectrum of EBV-associated T/NK LPDs and found that in cases of systemic HV and HMB, onset after age 9 was associated with increased mortality, whereas sex and the presence of particular clinical symptoms, such as splenomegaly, fever, and lymphadenopathy, were not. This team also identified a molecular marker BZLF1 as a potential prognosticator of

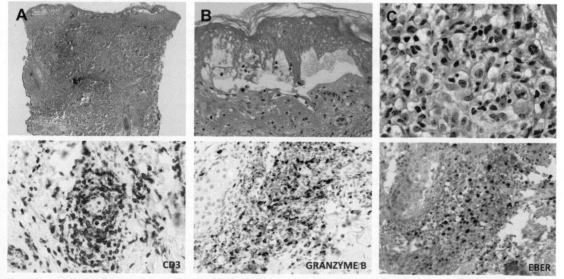

Fig. 18. HV-like LPD. Perivascular and periadnexal atypical lymphocytic infiltrate is present (*A*, H&E×20). Areas of transepidermal necrosis are noted (*B*, H&E×200). The infiltrate is composed of medium and occasional large cells, many of which have abundant finely granular cytoplasm (*C*, H&E×600). The infiltrate is positive for CD3 (CD3, ×400), granzyme B (Granzyme B, ×400), and EBER (EBER, ×400).

poor prognosis. BZLF1 messenger RNA expression was only observed in cases of systemic HV or HMB, whereas classic HV cases were negative for this marker and had the best prognosis overall.

SUMMARY

CTCLs demonstrate a variety of unique immuno-morphologic and molecular profiles. As the subtleties of each diagnosis undergo further refinement, the understanding of biologic behavior and prognosis also improves. Knowledge of these histologic variants alongside appropriate use of ancillary testing is key for both accurate diagnosis and ensuring adequate treatment.

REFERENCES

1. Fujii K. New therapies and immunological findings in cutaneous T-cell lymphoma. Front Oncol 2018;8: 198.
2. Olsen E, Vonderheid E, Pimpinelli N, et al. Revisions to the staging and classification of mycosis fungoides and Sezary syndrome: a proposal of the International Society for Cutaneous Lymphomas (ISCL) and the cutaneous lymphoma task force of the European Organization of Research and Treatment of Cancer (EORTC). Blood 2007;110(6): 1713–22.
3. Feng B, Jorgensen JL, Jones D, et al. Flow cytometric detection of peripheral blood involvement by mycosis fungoides and Sezary syndrome using T-cell receptor Vbeta chain antibodies and its application in blood staging. Mod Pathol 2010;23(2): 284–95.
4. Gibson JF, Huang J, Liu KJ, et al. Cutaneous T-cell lymphoma (CTCL): current practices in blood assessment and the utility of T-cell receptor (TCR)-Vbeta chain restriction. J Am Acad Dermatol 2016; 74(5):870–7.
5. Kiel MJ, Sahasrabuddhe AA, Rolland DC, et al. Genomic analyses reveal recurrent mutations in epigenetic modifiers and the JAK-STAT pathway in Sézary syndrome. Nat Commun 2015;6:8470.
6. Kirsch IR, Watanabe R, O'Malley JT, et al. TCR sequencing facilitates diagnosis and identifies mature T cells as the cell of origin in CTCL. Sci Transl Med 2015;7(308):308ra158.
7. Sufficool KE, Lockwood CM, Abel HJ, et al. T-cell clonality assessment by next-generation sequencing improves detection sensitivity in mycosis fungoides. J Am Acad Dermatol 2015; 73(2):228–36.e2.
8. Choi J, Goh G, Walradt T, et al. Genomic landscape of cutaneous T cell lymphoma. Nat Genet 2015; 47(9):1011–9.
9. da Silva Almeida AC, Abate F, Khiabanian H, et al. The mutational landscape of cutaneous T cell lymphoma and Sézary syndrome. Nat Genet 2015; 47(12):1465–70.
10. Ungewickell A, Bhaduri A, Rios E, et al. Genomic analysis of mycosis fungoides and Sezary syndrome identifies recurrent alterations in TNFR2. Nat Genet 2015;47(9):1056–60.
11. Scarisbrick JJ, Prince HM, Vermeer MH, et al. Cutaneous lymphoma international consortium study of outcome in advanced stages of mycosis fungoides and Sezary syndrome: effect of specific prognostic markers on survival and development of a prognostic model. J Clin Oncol 2015;33(32):3766–73.
12. Kadin ME, Hughey LC, Wood GS. Large-cell transformation of mycosis fungoides-differential diagnosis with implications for clinical management: a consensus statement of the US cutaneous lymphoma consortium. J Am Acad Dermatol 2014; 70(2):374–6.
13. Pulitzer M. Cutaneous T-cell lymphoma. Clin Lab Med 2017;37(3):527–46.
14. Scarisbrick JJ, Quaglino P, Prince HM, et al. The PROCLIPI international registry of early-stage mycosis fungoides identifies substantial diagnostic delay in most patients. Br J Dermatol 2018, [Epub ahead of print].
15. van Doorn R, Scheffer E, Willemze R. Follicular mycosis fungoides, a distinct disease entity with or without associated follicular mucinosis: a clinico-pathologic and follow-up study of 51 patients. Arch Dermatol 2002;138(2):191–8.
16. Gerami P, Rosen S, Kuzel T, et al. Folliculotropic mycosis fungoides: an aggressive variant of cutaneous T-cell lymphoma. Arch Dermatol 2008; 144(6):738–46.
17. Hodak E, Amitay-Laish I, Atzmony L, et al. New insights into folliculotropic mycosis fungoides (FMF): a single-center experience. J Am Acad Dermatol 2016;75(2):347–55.
18. Giberson M, Mourad A, Gniadecki R. Folliculotropism does not affect overall survival in mycosis fungoides: results from a single-center cohort and meta-analysis. Dermatology 2017;233(4):320–5.
19. Shapiro PE, Pinto FJ. The histologic spectrum of mycosis fungoides/Sézary syndrome (cutaneous T-cell lymphoma). A review of 222 biopsies, including newly described patterns and the earliest pathologic changes. Am J Surg Pathol 1994;18(7):645–67.
20. Reggiani C, Massone C, Fink-Puches R, et al. Interstitial mycosis fungoides: a clinicopathologic study of 21 patients. Am J Surg Pathol 2016;40(10):1360–7.
21. Willemze R, Hodak E, Zinzani PL, et al. Primary cutaneous lymphomas: ESMO clinical practice guidelines for diagnosis, treatment and follow-up. Ann Oncol 2018;29(Supplement_4):iv30–40.

22. Duvic M, Tetzlaff MT, Gangar P, et al. Results of a phase II trial of brentuximab vedotin for CD30+ cutaneous T-cell lymphoma and lymphomatoid papulosis. J Clin Oncol 2015;33(32):3759–65.

23. Kim YH, Tavallaee M, Sundram U, et al. Phase II investigator-initiated study of brentuximab vedotin in mycosis fungoides and Sezary syndrome with variable CD30 expression level: a multi-institution collaborative project. J Clin Oncol 2015;33(32):3750–8.

24. Prince HM, Kim YH, Horwitz SM, et al. Brentuximab vedotin or physician's choice in CD30-positive cutaneous T-cell lymphoma (ALCANZA): an international, open-label, randomised, phase 3, multicentre trial. Lancet 2017;390(10094):555–66.

25. Rahbar Z, Li S, Tavallaee M, et al. Variability in the expression of immunohistochemical markers: implications for biomarker interpretation in cutaneous T-cell lymphoma. J Invest Dermatol 2018;138(5):1204–6.

26. Gru AA, Kim J, Pulitzer M, et al. The use of central pathology review with digital slide scanning in advanced-stage mycosis fungoides and Sezary syndrome: a multi-institutional and international pathology study. Am J Surg Pathol 2018;42(6):726–34.

27. Duvic M, Pinter-Brown LC, Foss FM, et al. Phase 1/2 study of mogamulizumab, a defucosylated anti-CCR4 antibody, in previously treated patients with cutaneous T-cell lymphoma. Blood 2015;125(12):1883–9.

28. Kim YH, Bagot M, Pinter-Brown L, et al. Mogamulizumab versus vorinostat in previously treated cutaneous T-cell lymphoma (MAVORIC): an international, open-label, randomized, controlled phase 3 trial. Lancet Oncol 2018;19(9):1192–204.

29. Campbell JJ, Clark RA, Watanabe R, et al. Sezary syndrome and mycosis fungoides arise from distinct T-cell subsets: a biologic rationale for their distinct clinical behaviors. Blood 2010;116(5):767–71.

30. Nagler AR, Samimi S, Schaffer A, et al. Peripheral blood findings in erythrodermic patients: importance for the differential diagnosis of Sezary syndrome. J Am Acad Dermatol 2012;66(3):503–8.

31. Harmon CB, Witzig TE, Katzmann JA, et al. Detection of circulating T cells with CD4+CD7− immunophenotype in patients with benign and malignant lymphoproliferative dermatoses. J Am Acad Dermatol 1996;35(3 Pt 1):404–10.

32. Moins-Teisserenc H, Daubord M, Clave E, et al. CD158k is a reliable marker for diagnosis of Sezary syndrome and reveals an unprecedented heterogeneity of circulating malignant cells. J Invest Dermatol 2015;135(1):247–57.

33. Bahler DW, Hartung L, Hill S, et al. CD158k/KIR3DL2 is a useful marker for identifying neoplastic T-cells in Sezary syndrome by flow cytometry. Cytometry B Clin Cytom 2008;74(3):156–62.

34. Ortonne N, Le gouvello S, Mansour H, et al. CD158K/KIR3DL2 transcript detection in lesional skin of patients with erythroderma is a tool for the diagnosis of Sézary syndrome. J Invest Dermatol 2008;128(2):465–72.

35. Hurabielle C, Thonnart N, Ram-Wolff C, et al. Usefulness of KIR3DL2 to diagnose, follow-up, and manage the treatment of patients with Sezary syndrome. Clin Cancer Res 2017;23(14):3619–27.

36. Morice WG, Kimlinger T, Katzmann JA, et al. Flow cytometric assessment of TCR-Vbeta expression in the evaluation of peripheral blood involvement by T-cell lymphoproliferative disorders: a comparison with conventional T-cell immunophenotyping and molecular genetic techniques. Am J Clin Pathol 2004;121(3):373–83.

37. Weng WK, Armstrong R, Arai S, et al. Minimal residual disease monitoring with high-throughput sequencing of T cell receptors in cutaneous T cell lymphoma. Sci Transl Med 2013;5(214):214ra171.

38. de Masson A, O'Malley JT, Elco CP, et al. High-throughput sequencing of the T cell receptor beta gene identifies aggressive early-stage mycosis fungoides. Sci Transl Med 2018;10(440), [pii: eaar5894].

39. Wieser I, Oh CW, Talpur R, et al. Lymphomatoid papulosis: treatment response and associated lymphomas in a study of 180 patients. J Am Acad Dermatol 2016;74(1):59–67.

40. Eberle FC, Song JY, Xi L, et al. Nodal involvement by cutaneous CD30-positive T-cell lymphoma mimicking classical Hodgkin lymphoma. Am J Surg Pathol 2012;36(5):716–25.

41. Magro CM, Crowson AN, Morrison C, et al. CD8+ lymphomatoid papulosis and its differential diagnosis. Am J Clin Pathol 2006;125(4):490–501.

42. Saggini A, Gulia A, Argenyi Z, et al. A variant of lymphomatoid papulosis simulating primary cutaneous aggressive epidermotropic CD8+ cytotoxic T-cell lymphoma. Description of 9 cases. Am J Surg Pathol 2010;34(8):1168–75.

43. Kempf W, Kazakov DV, Scharer L, et al. Angioinvasive lymphomatoid papulosis: a new variant simulating aggressive lymphomas. Am J Surg Pathol 2013;37(1):1–13.

44. Karai LJ, Kadin ME, Hsi ED, et al. Chromosomal rearrangements of 6p25.3 define a new subtype of lymphomatoid papulosis. Am J Surg Pathol 2013;37(8):1173–81.

45. Dore E, Swick BL, Link BK, et al. Follicular lymphomatoid papulosis with follicular mucinosis: a clinicopathologic study of 3 cases with literature review and conceptual reappraisal. J Cutan Pathol 2017;44(4):360–6.

46. Kempf W, Kazakov DV, Baumgartner HP, et al. Follicular lymphomatoid papulosis revisited: a study of 11 cases, with new histopathological findings. J Am Acad Dermatol 2013;68(5):809–16.

47. Savage KJ, Harris NL, Vose JM, et al. ALK− anaplastic large-cell lymphoma is clinically and immunophenotypically different from both ALK+ ALCL and peripheral T-cell lymphoma, not otherwise specified: report from the International Peripheral T-Cell Lymphoma Project. Blood 2008;111(12): 5496–504.

48. Xing X, Feldman AL. Anaplastic large cell lymphomas: ALK positive, ALK negative, and primary cutaneous. Adv Anat Pathol 2015;22(1):29–49.

49. Feldman AL, Law M, Remstein ED, et al. Recurrent translocations involving the IRF4 oncogene locus in peripheral T-cell lymphomas. Leukemia 2009; 23(3):574–80.

50. Pham-Ledard A, Prochazkova-Carlotti M, Laharanno E, et al. IRF4 gene rearrangements define a subgroup of CD30-positive cutaneous T-cell lymphoma: a study of 54 cases. J Invest Dermatol 2010;130(3):816–25.

51. Wada DA, Law ME, Hsi ED, et al. Specificity of IRF4 translocations for primary cutaneous anaplastic large cell lymphoma: a multicenter study of 204 skin biopsies. Mod Pathol 2011;24(4):596–605.

52. Kiran T, Demirkesen C, Eker C, et al. The significance of MUM1/IRF4 protein expression and IRF4 translocation of CD30(+) cutaneous T-cell lymphoproliferative disorders: a study of 53 cases. Leuk Res 2013;37(4):396–400.

53. Parrilla Castellar ER, Jaffe ES, Said JW, et al. ALK-negative anaplastic large cell lymphoma is a genetically heterogeneous disease with widely disparate clinical outcomes. Blood 2014;124(9):1473–80.

54. Fauconneau A, Pham-Ledard A, Cappellen D, et al. Assessment of diagnostic criteria between primary cutaneous anaplastic large-cell lymphoma and CD30-rich transformed mycosis fungoides; a study of 66 cases. Br J Dermatol 2015;172(6):1547–54.

55. Samols MA, Su A, Ra S, et al. Intralymphatic cutaneous anaplastic large cell lymphoma/lymphomatoid papulosis: expanding the spectrum of CD30-positive lymphoproliferative disorders. Am J Surg Pathol 2014;38(9):1203–11.

56. Luchtel RA, Dasari S, Oishi N, et al. Molecular profiling reveals immunogenic cues in anaplastic large cell lymphomas with DUSP22 rearrangements. Blood 2018;132(13):1386–98.

57. Vasmatzis G, Johnson SH, Knudson RA, et al. Genome-wide analysis reveals recurrent structural abnormalities of TP63 and other p53-related genes in peripheral T-cell lymphomas. Blood 2012; 120(11):2280–9.

58. Gru AA, Williams E, Junkins-Hopkins JM. An immune suppression-associated EBV-positive anaplastic large cell lymphoma with a BRAF V600E mutation. Am J Surg Pathol 2019;43(1):140–6.

59. Geller S, Canavan TN, Pulitzer M, et al. ALK-positive primary cutaneous anaplastic large cell lymphoma: a case report and review of the literature. Int J Dermatol 2018;57(5):515–20.

60. Bhattacharjee R, Vinay K, Chatterjee D, et al. Comments concerning "ALK positive primary cutaneous anaplastic large cell lymphoma: a case report and review of the literature". Int J Dermatol 2018;57(10): e83–5.

61. Lamant L, Pileri S, Sabattini E, et al. Cutaneous presentation of ALK-positive anaplastic large cell lymphoma following insect bites: evidence for an association in five cases. Haematologica 2010; 95(3):449–55.

62. Toro JR, Liewehr DJ, Pabby N, et al. Gamma-delta T-cell phenotype is associated with significantly decreased survival in cutaneous T-cell lymphoma. Blood 2003;101(9):3407–12.

63. Guitart J, Weisenburger DD, Subtil A, et al. Cutaneous γδ T-cell lymphomas: a spectrum of presentations with overlap with other cytotoxic lymphomas. Am J Surg Pathol 2012;36(11):1656–65.

64. Damasco F, Akilov OE. Rare cutaneous T-cell lymphomas. Hematol Oncol Clin North Am 2019;33(1): 135–48.

65. Pulitzer M, Geller S, Kumar E, et al. T-cell receptor-δ expression and γδ+ T-cell infiltrates in primary cutaneous γδ T-cell lymphoma and other cutaneous T-cell lymphoproliferative disorders. Histopathology 2018;73(4):653–62.

66. Kash N, Massone C, Fink-Puches R, et al. Phenotypic variation in different lesions of mycosis fungoides biopsied within a short period of time from the same patient. Am J Dermatopathol 2016;38(7): 541–5.

67. Merrill ED, Agbay R, Miranda RN, et al. Primary cutaneous T-cell lymphomas showing gamma-delta (γδ) phenotype and predominantly epidermotropic pattern are clinicopathologically distinct from classic primary cutaneous γδ T-cell lymphomas. Am J Surg Pathol 2017;41(2):204–15.

68. Morimura S, Sugaya M, Tamaki Z, et al. Lymphomatoid papulosis showing γδ T-cell phenotype. Acta Derm Venereol 2011;91(6):712–3.

69. Rodriguez-Pinilla SM, Ortiz-Romero PL, Monsalvez V, et al. TCR-gamma expression in primary cutaneous T-cell lymphomas. Am J Surg Pathol 2013;37(3): 375–84.

70. Wei EX, Leventaki V, Choi JK, et al. γδ T-cell acute lymphoblastic leukemia/lymphoma: discussion of two pediatric cases and its distinction from other mature γδ T-cell malignancies. Case Rep Hematol 2017;2017:5873015.

71. King RL, Yan AC, Sekiguchi DR, et al. Atypical cutaneous γδ T cell proliferation with morphologic

features of lymphoma but with clinical features and course of PLEVA or lymphomatoid papulosis. J Cutan Pathol 2015;42(12):1012–7.

72. Gru A, et al, in press.

73. Petrella T, Maubec E, Cornillet-Lefebvre P, et al. Indolent CD8-positive lymphoid proliferation of the ear: a distinct primary cutaneous T-cell lymphoma? Am J Surg Pathol 2007;31(12):1887–92.

74. Greenblatt D, Ally M, Child F, et al. Indolent CD8(+) lymphoid proliferation of acral sites: a clinicopathologic study of six patients with some atypical features. J Cutan Pathol 2013;40(2):248–58.

75. Kluk J, Kai A, Koch D, et al. Indolent CD8-positive lymphoid proliferation of acral sites: three further cases of a rare entity and an update on a unique patient. J Cutan Pathol 2016;43(2):125–36.

76. Alberti-Violetti S, Fanoni D, Provasi M, et al. Primary cutaneous acral CD8 positive T-cell lymphoma with extra-cutaneous involvement: a long-standing case with an unexpected progression. J Cutan Pathol 2017;44(11):964–8.

77. Beggs SM, Friedman BJ, Kornreich D, et al. Primary cutaneous CD8+ T-cell lymphoma, an indolent and locally aggressive form mimicking paronychia. Am J Dermatopathol 2018;40(4):e52–6.

78. Beltraminelli H, Leinweber B, Kerl H, et al. Primary cutaneous CD4+ small-/medium-sized pleomorphic T-cell lymphoma: a cutaneous nodular proliferation of pleomorphic T lymphocytes of undetermined significance? A study of 136 cases. Am J Dermatopathol 2009;31(4):317–22.

79. Gru AA, Wick MR, Eid M. Primary cutaneous CD4+ small/medium T-cell lymphoproliferative disorder-clinical and histopathologic features, differential diagnosis, and treatment. Semin Cutan Med Surg 2018;37(1):39–48.

80. Rodriguez Pinilla SM, Roncador G, Rodriguez-Peralto JL, et al. Primary cutaneous CD4+ small/medium-sized pleomorphic T-cell lymphoma expresses follicular T-cell markers. Am J Surg Pathol 2009;33(1):81–90.

81. Grogg KL, Jung S, Erickson LA, et al. Primary cutaneous CD4-positive small/medium-sized pleomorphic T-cell lymphoma: a clonal T-cell lymphoproliferative disorder with indolent behavior. Mod Pathol 2008;21(6):708–15.

82. Magro CM, Momtahen S. Differential NFATc1 expression in primary cutaneous CD4+ small/ medium-sized pleomorphic t-cell lymphoma and other forms of cutaneous T-cell lymphoma and pseudolymphoma. Am J Dermatopathol 2017; 39(2):95–103.

83. Swerdlow SH, Campo E, Pileri SA, et al. The 2016 revision of the World Health Organization classification of lymphoid neoplasms. Blood 2016;127(20): 2375–90.

84. Salah E. Primary cutaneous CD4+ small/medium pleomorphic T-cell lymphoproliferative disorder: Where do we stand? A systematic review. J Dtsch Dermatol Ges 2019;17(2):123–36.

85. Williams VL, Torres-Cabala CA, Duvic M. Primary cutaneous small- to medium-sized CD4+ pleomorphic T-cell lymphoma: a retrospective case series and review of the provisional cutaneous lymphoma category. Am J Clin Dermatol 2011;12(6):389–401.

86. Willemze R, Jaffe ES, Burg G, et al. WHO-EORTC classification for cutaneous lymphomas. Blood 2005;105(10):3768–85.

87. Chen CC, Chang KC, Medeiros LJ, et al. Hydroa vacciniforme and hydroa vacciniforme-like T-cell lymphoma: an uncommon event for transformation. J Cutan Pathol 2016;43(12):1102–11.

88. Iwatsuki K, Xu Z, Takata M, et al. The association of latent Epstein-Barr virus infection with hydroa vacciniforme. Br J Dermatol 1999;140(4):715–21.

89. Iwatsuki K, Satoh M, Yamamoto T, et al. Pathogenic link between hydroa vacciniforme and Epstein-Barr virus-associated hematologic disorders. Arch Dermatol 2006;142(5):587–95.

90. Ruiz-Maldonado R, Parrilla FM, Orozco-Covarrubias ML, et al. Edematous, scarring vasculitic panniculitis: a new multisystemic disease with malignant potential. J Am Acad Dermatol 1995; 32(1):37–44.

91. Cho KH, Kim CW, Lee DY, et al. An Epstein-Barr virus-associated lymphoproliferative lesion of the skin presenting as recurrent necrotic papulovesicles of the face. Br J Dermatol 1996;134(4):791–6.

92. Miyake T, Yamamoto T, Hirai Y, et al. Survival rates and prognostic factors of Epstein-Barr virus-associated hydroa vacciniforme and hypersensitivity to mosquito bites. Br J Dermatol 2015;172(1):56–63.

93. Tatsuno K, Fujiyama T, Matsuoka H, et al. Clinical categories of exaggerated skin reactions to mosquito bites and their pathophysiology. J Dermatol Sci 2016;82(3):145–52.

Histiocytic and Dendritic Cell Neoplasms

Zenggang Pan, MD, PhD[a], Mina L. Xu, MD[a,b],*

KEYWORDS

- Disseminated juvenile xanthogranuloma • Erdheim-Chester disease
- Follicular dendritic cell sarcoma • Indeterminate dendritic cell tumor
- Interdigitating dendritic cell sarcoma • Histiocytic sarcoma • Langerhans cell histiocytosis

Key Points

- To describe the major clinicopathologic features of the histiocytic and dendritic neoplasms.
- To emphasize the differential diagnoses of each histiocytic and dendritic neoplasm.
- To summarize the important workup and pitfalls of each entity.

ABSTRACT

Histiocytic and dendritic cell neoplasms are very rare, belonging to a group that share morphologic, immunophenotypic, and ultra-structural characteristics of mature histiocytic/dendritic neoplasms. Histiocytic and dendritic cell neoplasms may arise de novo or in association with B-cell, T-cell, or myeloid neoplasms. Recent molecular findings, particularly the discoveries of the mutations in the RAS-RAF-MEK-ERK pathway, have greatly advanced the diagnosis and treatment options. Histiocytic and dendritic cell neoplasms may closely resemble each other, non-hematopoietic neoplasms, and even reactive processes. Therefore, it is essential to understand the clinicopathologic characteristics, differential diagnoses, and pitfalls of each entity.

LANGERHANS CELL HISTIOCYTOSIS

INTRODUCTION

Langerhans cell histiocytosis (LCH) is a neoplasm of Langerhans cells. It mostly occurs in pediatric patients, as solitary or multifocal lesions in the bone and adjacent soft tissue. Lymph node involvement is infrequent. LCH in the central nervous system (CNS) may induce diabetes insipidus. Primary pulmonary LCH is nearly always associated with smoking.

PATHOLOGIC FEATURES

In the bone and soft tissue, LCH shows a diffuse infiltration in a background rich in eosinophils. In the lymph node, LCH often presents with a sinusoidal infiltrative pattern in the early stage of disease (**Fig.** 1A); then, the tumor cells gradually spread into the paracortex and eventually replace the entire lymph node. LCH cells are typically large and epithelioid. The nuclei are round, ovoid, folded, or "coffee bean" shaped with fine chromatin and inconspicuous nucleoli (**Fig.** 1B). Frequent cells reveal characteristic longitudinal nuclear grooves. The cytoplasm is abundant and pale-pink staining. Scattered osteoclast-like giant cells are often present, particularly in the cases with bone or paraosseous soft tissue involvement. In general, there is no significant cytologic atypia, and the mitotic figures are variable.

Disclosure: The authors have no relationship with a commercial company that has a direct financial interest in subject matter or materials discussed in article or with a company making a competing product.

[a] Department of Pathology, Yale University School of Medicine, 310 Cedar Street, New Haven, CT 06510-3218, USA; [b] Department of Laboratory Medicine, Yale University School of Medicine, 310 Cedar Street, New Haven, CT 06510-3218, USA

* Corresponding author. Department of Pathology, Yale University School of Medicine, 310 Cedar Street, New Haven, CT 06510-3218.

E-mail address: mina.xu@yale.edu

Surgical Pathology 12 (2019) 805–829
https://doi.org/10.1016/j.path.2019.03.013

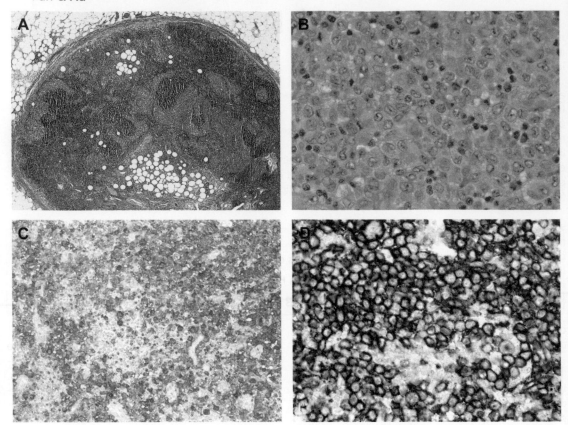

Fig. 1. Langerhans cell histiocytosis (LCH) in a lymph node. (*A*) Sinusoidal infiltration of tumor cells. (*B*) LCH cells with epithelioid cytology, "coffee bean" shaped nuclei, and occasional nuclear grooves. The tumor cells are positive for S100 (*C*) and CD1a (*D*).

Positive results on immunostaining for S100, CD1a, and langerin (CD207) are essential in the diagnosis of LCH (**Fig.** 1C, D). In addition, LCH cells express CD4, CD68, vimentin, and HLA-DR, whereas they are negative for other T-cell, B-cell and follicular dendritic cell markers. Under electron microscope, LCH has characteristic cytoplasmic Birbeck granules, which possess a tennis-racket or zipperlike shape. Langerin is an immunohistochemical surrogate marker of the Birbeck granules.

Rare cases of LCH can be transdifferentiated from acute lymphoblastic leukemias, acute myeloid leukemias, and mature B-cell or T-cell lymphomas and share the same genetic changes with the precursor lesions.[1–6] Indeed, clonal *IGH* or *TCR* gene rearrangements are detected in approximately 30% of LCH cases, including the de novo cases.

Most LCH cases have somatic mutations involving the RAS-RAF-MEK-ERK pathway, which result in constitutional activation of this oncogenic pathway.[7–9] The 2 most common mutations include *BRAF* V600E (50%–60% of cases) and *MAP2K1* (~25%), which are mutually exclusive.[10–12]

Immunohistochemical stain with VE1 antibody specifically targets the BRAF V600E mutant. In addition, *TP53* and *U2AF1* mutations have been detected in 17% and 19% of LCH cases, respectively, with the *TP53* mutations commonly associated with *BRAF* mutations.[13]

DIFFERENTIAL DIAGNOSIS

LCH must be differentiated from reactive Langerhans cell proliferation, Langerhans cell sarcoma, and other non-Langerhans cell histiocytic disorders, including Rosai-Dorfman disease (RDD), Erdheim-Chester disease (ECD), and histiocytic sarcoma. Reactive lymph nodes may have prominent paracortical Langerhans cell proliferation, which may resemble LCH. Features that aid in differentiating between these are summarized in the following table. In addition, cyclin D1 expression is helpful in separating LCH from reactive Langerhans cells.[14] In lymph nodes, both RDD and LCH commonly show a sinus infiltrative pattern with S100 expression. However, in contrast to LCH, the histiocytes in RDD are much larger with characteristic emperipolesis. Moreover, RDD lacks expression of CD1a and langerin.

ECD is a rare non-LCH and also commonly associated with *BRAF* V600E mutation.[8,15–19] Intriguingly, 12% to 19% cases of ECD have concurrent LCH, some of which are clonally related.[20,21] Morphologically, ECD contains lipid-laden macrophages and scattered Touton giant cells in a background with fibrosis and reactive plasma cells. The ECD histiocytes are negative for S100, CD1a, and langerin.

Histiocytic sarcoma often reveals at least focal sinusoidal infiltration in the lymph node, which may mimic LCH. However, the sarcoma cells display significantly more cytologic atypia and have no background eosinophils. Furthermore, histiocytic sarcoma is negative for LCH markers (S100, CD1a, and langerin).

Langerhans cell sarcoma is extremely rare and occurs in adults, with no documented transformation from LCH. Langerhans cell sarcoma shows significant cytologic atypia, markedly increased mitotic figures and apoptotic bodies, and coagulative necrosis (**Fig. 2**). Tumor cells express LCH markers albeit with variable positivity.

Metastatic melanoma in the lymph node may have a sinusoidal and/or paracortical infiltration pattern with a histiocyte-like cytology, resembling LCH with S100 positivity and *BRAF* mutations. However, melanoma lacks the background eosinophils or expression of CD1a and langerin, whereas melanocytic markers are commonly detectable, including HMB45, MEL-A, and SOX10.

DIAGNOSIS

Diagnosis of LCH is usually straight-forward based on the characteristic morphologic and immunophenotypic features. The large epithelioid LCH cells have ovoid nuclei and frequent nuclear grooves in a background rich in eosinophils. They are positive for S100, CD1a, and langerin.

PROGNOSIS

Clinically, LCH has a wide range of manifestations, and the prognosis depends on multiple factors, including age, location of involvement, and clinical stage. Localized congenital and neonatal LCH may regress, and primary pulmonary LCH is often indolent. Some localized cases can be managed with surgical excision, such as the ones from the skin, lymph node, and bone, whereas the systemic and CNS diseases are associated with an inferior prognosis and increased risk of death.

Key Features
LANGERHANS CELL HISTIOCYTOSIS

1. Large ovoid epithelioid histiocytes with nuclear grooves.

2. Abundant reactive eosinophils.

3. Sinusoidal infiltration in lymph node.

4. Positive for S100, CD1a, and langerin.

5. Cytoplasmic Birbeck granules ultrastructurally.

6. *BRAF* V600E mutation in 50% to 60% cases.

△△ **Differential Diagnosis**
REACTIVE LANGERHANS CELL HYPERPLASIA VERSUS NODAL LCH

	Reactive Langerhans Cell Hyperplasia	Nodal Langerhans Cell Histiocytosis
Distribution	Paracortical	Sinusoidal to paracortical
Pattern	Scattered, loose clusters	Cohesive clusters or sheets
Cytology	Bland, with occasional nuclear grooves	Atypical, epithelioid; increased mitoses, apoptosis and necrosis
Background Cells	Lymphocytes, histiocytes, and dendritic cells; no eosinophilia	Abundant eosinophils
CD1a, S100	Positive	Positive
Cyclin D1	Negative	Mostly positive
BRAF Mutation	Absent	50%–60%

Differential Diagnosis
LANGERHANS CELL HISTIOCYTOSIS

LCH vs	Helpful Distinguish Features
Reactive Langerhans cell proliferation in lymph node	• Paracortical pattern; no background eosinophilia. • Scattered or loose clusters. • Lack of cytologic atypia, as seen in LCH. • Negative cyclin D1 immunostaining. • No mutations in *BRAF* or *MAP2K1*.
Rosai-Dorfman disease	• Large histiocytes with emperipolesis. • No background eosinophilia. • Negative for CD1a and langerin. • Negative *BRAF* mutations.
Erdheim-Chester disease	• Lipid-laden macrophages and Touton giant cells. • Background with fibrosis and plasma cells, but no increased eosinophils. • Negative for S100, CD1a, and langerin.
Histiocytic sarcoma	• Histiocytic cytology with significant atypia. • Positive for CD4, CD14, CD45, CD68, and CD163. • Negative for S100, CD1a, and langerin.
Langerhans cell sarcoma	• Almost entirely confined to adults. • Marked cytologic atypia. • Increased mitoses, apoptosis, and necrosis. • Variably positive for S100, CD1a, and langerin. • Clinically aggressive with poor outcome.
Indeterminate cell tumor	• Variable cytology, from histiocytic to Langerhans cell appearing. • No background eosinophilia. • Positive for S100 and CD1a. • Negative for langerin.
Melanoma	• Lack of eosinophilia in the background. • Positive for S100 and melanocytic markers. • Negative for CD1a and langerin.

Pitfalls
LANGERHANS CELL HISTIOCYTOSIS

! Occasionally LCH does not have abundant background eosinophils.

! Prominent reactive paracortical Langerhans cell proliferation can be confused with LCH. However, the paracortical reactive Langerhans cells do not form solid clusters and have no associated eosinophilia. In addition, they lack overt cytologic atypia.

! Primary pulmonary LCH can be obscured by fibrosis and inflammation in the absence of eosinophilia. Therefore, immunostains with S100 and CD1a are recommended for peribronchial fibrosis after excluding other possibilities.

Fig. 2. Langerhans cell sarcoma with significant cytologic atypia, frequent mitotic figures, and coagulative necrosis.

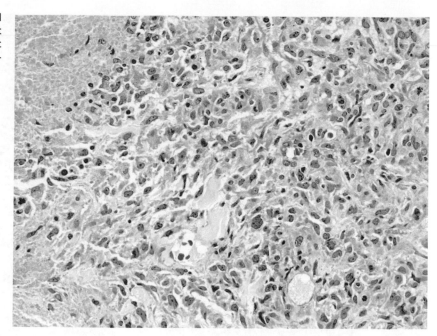

FOLLICULAR DENDRITIC CELL SARCOMA

INTRODUCTION

Follicular dendritic cells (FDC) are of mesenchymal origin, and the associated FDC sarcoma is rare with similar immunophenotype as normal FDC.[22,23] FDC sarcoma involves young to middle-aged patients, with a median age of ~ 50 years. Most cases occur in the lymph nodes, typically cervical nodes; ~30% of tumors are initially diagnosed in the extranodal sites. Clinically, FDC sarcoma mostly presents with a painless, slow-growing mass in the lymph node or soft tissue with no systemic symptoms. Approximately 10% to 20% of FDC sarcomas are associated with Castleman disease, mostly hyaline vascular type.[24] Recent studies with relatively small cohorts demonstrated that FDC sarcoma contains indolent T-lymphoblastic proliferations in ~45% of cases and is frequently associated with paraneoplastic autoimmune multiorgan syndrome.[25,26]

MICROSCOPIC FEATURES

FDC sarcoma displays a wide range of architectural patterns, including storiform, fascicular, whorled, and diffuse (**Fig. 3**A). The tumor cells possess ovoid to elongated bland nuclei with vesicular or granular chromatin, thin nuclear membrane, and a small but distinct nucleolus (**Fig. 3**B). They display indistinct cell borders and a moderate amount of pale-pink cytoplasm.

Characteristically, there are abundant reactive small lymphocytes admixed with the tumor cells (see **Fig. 3**B). In general, the FDC sarcoma has no significant cytologic atypia or prominent necrosis. The mitotic figures are typically infrequent at 0 to 10 mitoses per 10 high-power fields.

FDC sarcoma is positive for commonly used FDC markers, including CD21, CD23, and CD35 (**Fig. 3**C, D). CXCL13, podoplanin (D2-40), clusterin, vimentin, fascin, EGFR, and HLA-DR are usually positive, whereas stains for CD1a, CD3, CD20, CD30, CD34, CD45, CD79a, CD163, cytokeratin, S100, HMB45, MSA, lysozyme, and MPO are mostly negative. The proliferation rate by Ki67 staining is variable but typically low. FDC sarcoma is not associated with infection of human herpesvirus 8 or Epstein–Barr virus (EBV), except the cases occurring in the liver and spleen with inflammatory pseudotumor-like features (see section 4). FDC sarcomas have no clonal *IGH* or *TRG* gene rearrangements and are usually not transdifferentiated from B-cell or T-cell neoplasms. *BRAF* V600E mutation has been detected in ~19% of cases.[7]

DIFFERENTIAL DIAGNOSIS

The major differential diagnosis of FDC sarcoma includes inflammatory myofibroblastic tumor (IMT), interdigitating dendritic cell sarcoma, spindle cell thymoma, gastrointestinal stromal tumor, spindle cell carcinoma, and melanoma.

IMT has significant morphologic overlap with FDC sarcoma. IMT exhibits a mixed inflammatory

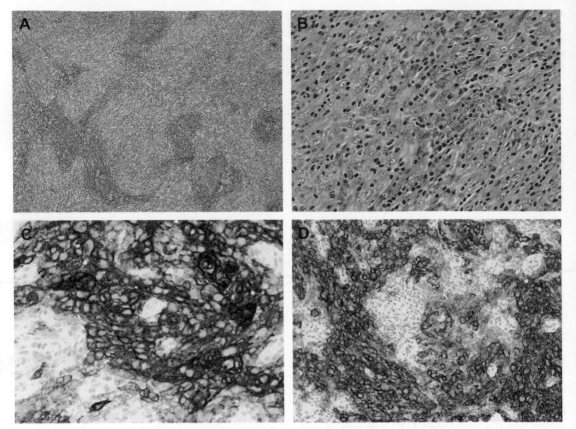

Fig. 3. FDC sarcoma. (*A*) Nodular proliferation of tumor cells with abundant lymphocytes between nodules. (*B*) Tumor cells have bland cytology with ovoid to elongated nuclei, indistinct cell borders, and a moderate amount of pale-pink cytoplasm. CD21 (*C*) and CD23 (*D*) are diffusely positive in the FDC sarcoma.

infiltrate of lymphocytes, plasma cells, eosinophils, and histiocyte, and the spindle cells are positive for smooth muscle actin but negative for FDC markers. Approximately 40% cases of IMT express ALK. Interdigitating dendritic cell sarcoma shows diffuse sheetlike distribution or characteristic interfollicular growth pattern. However, there are no prominent reactive lymphocytes in the tumor. Moreover, the tumor cells are positive for S100, but negative for FDC markers (CD21, CD23, and CD35). Spindle cell thymoma demonstrates spindle cell proliferation and admixed lymphocytes. However, the thymoma cells express cytokeratin but not FDC markers. Moreover, the lymphocytes in the background of thymoma are immature T cells, positive for CD1a, CD99, and terminal deoxynucleotidyl transferase (TdT).

Metastatic melanoma may have spindle cell cytology, but the tumor lacks prominent lymphocytic reaction. In addition, melanoma cells are positive for S100, SOX10, and HMB45, but negative for FDC markers. Spindle cell carcinoma

usually shows overt cytologic atypia and positivity of cytokeratin but not FDC markers, and clinical history of carcinoma is also helpful in establishing an accurate diagnosis.

IgG4-related sclerosing disease is a fibroinflammatory condition characterized by storiform fibrosis rich in fibroblasts, dense lymphoplasmacytic infiltrate, obliterative phlebitis, and significant increase in IgG4+ cells. IgG4-related disease may resemble FDC sarcoma morphologically, but it shows a mixed inflammatory background with abundant plasma cells, in addition to lymphocytes. Also, the fibroblasts in IgG4-related disease are negative for FDC markers.

DIAGNOSIS

Albeit a rare entity, diagnosis of FDC sarcoma requires characteristic morphologic features and utilization of multiple FDC markers, since antigen loss is not infrequent. Certainly, the aforementioned morphologic mimicries have to be excluded.

PROGNOSIS

FDC sarcoma is mostly low- to intermediate-grade and often managed by surgical excision with or without chemoradiotherapy. However, 40% to 50% patients experience local recurrences, and ~25% have distant metastases. Overall, approximately 20% of patients die of disease.

Key Features
FOLLICULAR DENDRITIC CELL SARCOMA

1. Associated with Castleman disease in 10% to 20% of FDC sarcomas.

2. Associated with indolent T-lymphoblastic proliferation (45%) and paraneoplastic autoimmune multiorgan syndrome.

3. Variable architectural patterns, including storiform, fascicular, whorled, and diffuse.

4. Bland spindle to ovoid cells with indistinct cell borders.

5. Abundant reactive small lymphocytes.

6. Positive for CD21, CD35, CD23, D2-40, clusterin, and fascin.

7. Negative for CD1a, cytokeratin, S100, HMB-45, and MSA.

Differential Diagnosis
FOLLICULAR DENDRITIC CELL SARCOMA

FDC Sarcoma vs	Helpful Distinguish Features
Inflammatory myofibroblastic tumor	• Mixed inflammatory infiltrate with lymphocytes, plasma cells, eosinophils, and histiocytes.
	• Positive for SMA and ALK (~40% of cases).
	• Negative for FDC markers.
Interdigitating dendritic cell sarcoma	• Interfollicular growth pattern.
	• Lack of abundant reactive lymphocytes.
	• Positive for S100.
	• Negative for FDC and melanocytic markers.
Spindle cell thymoma	• Spindle cells positive for cytokeratin but negative for FDC markers.
	• Immature T lymphocytes in the background with expression of CD1a and TdT.
Melanoma	• Lack of abundant reactive lymphocytes.
	• Positive for S100 and melanocytic markers.
	• Negative for FDC markers.
Gastrointestinal stromal tumor	• Lack of abundant lymphocytic infiltrates.
	• Positive for CD34, CD117, and DOG1.
	• Negative for FDC markers.
Spindle cell carcinoma	• Clinical history of carcinoma.
	• Positive for cytokeratin, but negative for FDC markers.
IgG4-related disease	• Mixed fibroinflammatory infiltrate with lymphocytes, plasma cells, and scattered eosinophils.
	• Obliterative phlebitis
	• Markedly increased IgG4+ cells.
	• Negative for FDC markers.

Pitfalls
FOLLICULAR DENDRITIC
CELL SARCOMA

! Rare large cell lymphomas may show spindle morphology with fibrosis and abundant reactive lymphocytes. Therefore, it is recommended that CD3, CD20, and CD45 be included during the initial workup for cases with morphologic features that suggest FDC sarcoma.

! FDC sarcoma may be overlooked and morphologically mimics reactive fibroblastic proliferation and spindle cell neoplasms.

INTERDIGITATING DENDRITIC CELL SARCOMA

INTRODUCTION

Interdigitating dendritic cells (IDCs) are T-cell–associated dendritic cells, which are localized in the paracortex of lymph node. They lack phagocytic activity but act to present antigens mostly to the paracortical T cells. Sarcoma of IDC origin is very rare, found primarily in adults with a median age of 56.5 years.[27,28] Most patients present with an asymptomatic mass in the lymph node or extranodal sites.

MICROSCOPIC FEATURES

Typically, IDC sarcoma shows a characteristic paracortical proliferation in sheet of fascicular, storiform, and whorled patterns with scattered residual lymphoid follicles (**Fig. 4**A). The tumor cells have round, ovoid, or spindled nuclei with bland or vesicular chromatin and a small to medium size nucleolus (**Fig. 4**B). Rare cells may have nuclear grooves. The cytoplasm is abundant and pale eosinophilic, with indistinct cell borders. Cytologic atypia varies from case to case. Mitotic figures are not significantly increased with less than 5 per 10 high-power fields. Large areas of coagulative necrosis are usually absent.

IDC sarcoma consistently expresses S100, fascin, and vimentin (**Fig. 4**C). The tumor cells are typically negative for FDC markers (CD21, CD23, CD35, and clusterin); histiocytic markers (CD163 and lysozyme); B-cell and T-cell markers; melanocytic markers (HMB45 and MITF); CD1a; CD30; CD34; langerin; and cytokeratin. *BRAF* V600E mutation and clonal *IGH* rearrangement have been detected in some cases.[29,30] Transdifferentiation to IDC sarcoma has been observed in diffuse large B-cell lymphoma and chronic lymphocytic leukemia/small lymphocytic lymphoma.[6,31]

DIFFERENTIAL DIAGNOSIS

Differential diagnosis of IDC sarcoma includes FDC sarcoma, spindle cell melanoma, spindle cell carcinoma, and high-grade lymphoma. In contrast to FDC sarcoma, IDC sarcoma often shows a paracortical proliferation with less reactive small lymphocytes, and the tumor cells are positive for S100 but not FDC markers (CD21, CD23, and CD35). Rare cases of metastatic carcinoma exhibits a spindle cell cytology, but it can be separated from IDC sarcoma based on the history of primary carcinoma elsewhere, expression of cytokeratin, and lack of S100 positivity. IDC sarcoma may be confused with more commonly encountered high-grade lymphomas, particularly the ones with convoluted nuclei, and utilization of lymphoid markers (CD3, CD20, and CD30) is helpful in distinguishing these entities.

To separate IDC sarcoma from spindle cell melanoma is very challenging due to similar morphologic and immunophenotypic features, including the expression of S100, MUM1, beta-catenin, SOX10, MITF, and P75; particularly, SOX10 positivity is noted in both entities.[32] Furthermore, both may harbor *BRAF* V600E mutations. Expression of CD68 (KP1)[33] and any evidence of transdifferentiation from clonally related lymphomas suggest IDC sarcoma.

DIAGNOSIS

IDC sarcoma is very rare, and the diagnosis relies on the typical morphologic features of paracortical infiltration, expression of S100, and exclusion of other more commonly encountered tumors, including melanoma, lymphoma, and carcinoma.

PROGNOSIS

IDC sarcoma exhibits aggressive clinical behavior. Patients are usually treated with local

Key Features
INTERDIGITATING DENDRITIC
CELL SARCOMA

1. Characteristic paracortical involvement.

2. Syncytial growth with indistinct cell borders.

3. Positive for S100, but negative for CD1a and FDC markers.

4. May be difficult to separate from spindle cell melanoma.

5. Some cases transdifferentiated from B-cell lymphomas.

excision, with radiotherapy and/or chemotherapy. However, local recurrence may occur and approximately 50% of patients die within 1 year after diagnosis.

INFLAMMATORY PSEUDOTUMOR-LIKE FOLLICULAR DENDRITIC CELL TUMOR

INTRODUCTION

Inflammatory pseudotumour-like FDC (IPT-FDC) tumor involves young to middle-aged patients with an average age of 54.5 years. There is a male predominance with a male-to-female ratio of ~2:1.[34–38] Characteristically, nearly all IPT-FDC tumors arise in the liver and spleen. Patients are usually asymptomatic or only present with abdominal discomfort or pain.

GROSS FEATURES

IPT-FDC tumor is mostly solitary and large, ranging from 2 cm to 22 cm (average 9.2 cm). Grossly, the tumor is round to ovoid and well circumscribed with pushing borders. The cut surface is tan and has irregular patches of hemorrhage and yellowish necrotic areas. Large lesions may have cystic changes and calcification (**Fig. 5**).

MICROSCOPIC FEATURES

Histologically, IPT-FDC tumor is well demarcated from the surrounding splenic or hepatic parenchyma. The bland spindle tumor cells can be arranged in storiform pattern, in fascicles or in solid sheets (**Fig. 6A–C**). The nuclei are ovoid or elongated with a thin nuclear membrane, fine chromatin, and small nucleoli. The cytoplasm is abundant and pale-pink with indistinct cell borders (see **Fig. 6C**). In some cases, there are scattered large, multinucleated atypical cells with coarsely condensed chromatin and prominent nucleoli (see **Fig. 6B**). Another characteristic feature is the presence of blood vessels with ectasia and abundant proteinaceous deposits in the vascular wall (see **Fig. 6A**). Admixed with the spindle cells are abundant plasma cells, lymphocytes, and scattered eosinophils.

Rare cases of granulomatous and eosinophil-rich variant of IPT-FDC tumor have been reported, containing abundant coalescent noncaseating epithelioid granulomas and/or prominent eosinophilic reaction with eosinophilic abscesses (**Fig. 7**).[39,40]

IPT-FDC tumor is variably positive for FDC markers, including CD21, CD23, CD35, clusterin, CNA.42, CXCL13, and D2-40. EBV is consistently detected in the spindle cells by in-situ hybridization (**Fig. 6D**), which is essentially diagnostic for this entity, particularly in the absence of strong FDC markers. The spindle cells are negative for anaplastic lymphoma kinase (ALK), desmin,

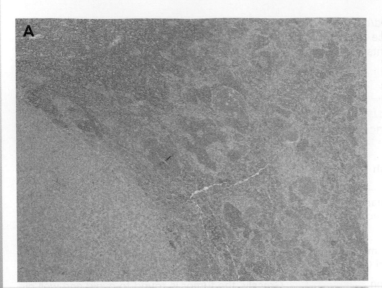

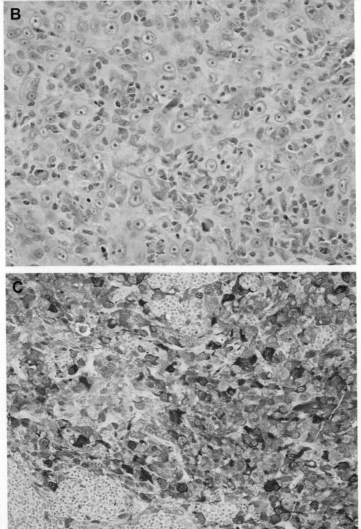

Fig. 4. IDC sarcoma with characteristic paracortical proliferation (*A*). The tumor cells have round or ovoid nuclei, abundant pale-pink cytoplasm, and indistinct cell borders (*B*). S100 is strongly positive in the lesional cells (*C*).

Fig. 5. IPT-FDC tumor. Image study showing a large solid and cystic lesion in the spleen with focal calcification.

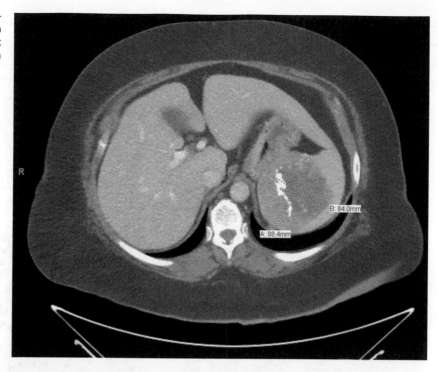

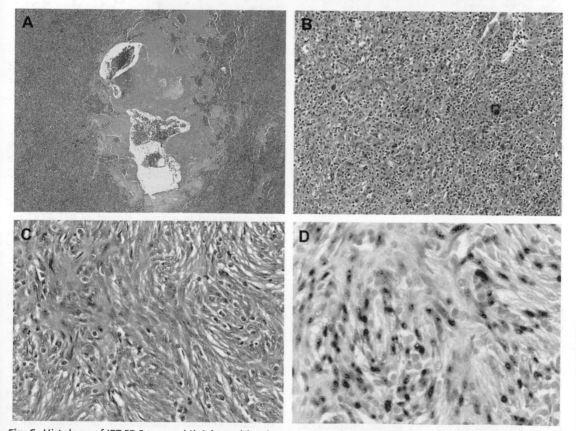

Fig. 6. Histology of IPT-FDC tumor. (*A*) A large blood vessel with ectasia and abundant proteinaceous deposits in the vascular wall. (*B*) Diffuse infiltration of tumor cells with admixed inflammatory cells and scattered large, multinucleated atypical cells. (*C*) The spindle tumor cells are arranged in storiform pattern and in fascicles with ovoid or elongated nuclei, abundant cytoplasm, and indistinct cell borders. (*D*) Characteristic EBV infection in the spindle cells.

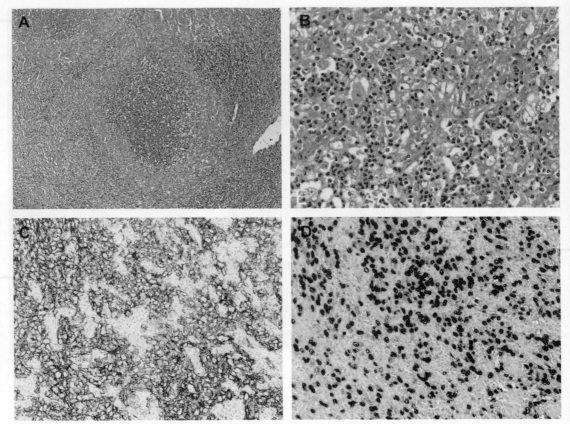

Fig. 7. Granulomatous and eosinophil-rich variant of IPT-FDC tumor. (*A*) Frequent large noncaseating epithelioid granulomas. (*B*) Large epithelioid cells in a background of abundant granulocytes. The tumor cells are positive for CD23 (*C*) and EBV infection (*D*).

caldesmon, CD1a, CD30, CD31, CD34, HMB45, and S100. IgG4+ cells are usually not increased in the tumor albeit presence of abundant plasma cells, but cases with increased IgG4+ cells have been reported.[41]

DIFFERENTIAL DIAGNOSIS

IPT-FDC tumor may closely mimic conventional FDC sarcoma, IMT, and IgG4-related sclerosing disease. In the spleen, it can be confused with sclerosing angiomatoid nodular transformation (SANT). In contrast to conventional FDC sarcoma, IPT-FDC tumor occurs in the spleen and/or liver with more mixed inflammatory cells, including plasma cells and granulocytes. In addition, EBER-ISH is always positive in the spindle cells of IPT-FDC tumor, which is diagnostic and helps separate this entity from the conventional FDC sarcoma. IMT also shows very similar morphologic features to IPT-FDC tumor; however, IMT is positive for SMA and ALK (~40% of cases) with no evidence of EBV infection.

IgG4-related sclerosing disease may involve biliary tract and liver but rarely occurs in the spleen. Morphologically, it is similar to IPT-FDC tumor with fibroblastic proliferation and lymphoplasmacytic infiltration. In addition, IgG4+ cells are increased in a small subset of IPT-FDC tumors.[41] Nevertheless, the clinical presentations (spleen or liver involvement) and detection of EBV in the spindle cells would lean toward IPT-FDC tumor.

SANT is a rare vascular lesion in the spleen, which shows a nodular growth pattern with a rich network of capillaries. There is a variable degree of fibrosis and macrophage collection. Although some FDC markers are variably positive in a subset of SANT cases, EBER-ISH is always negative.

IPT-FDC tumor may be confused with classic Hodgkin lymphoma with scattered large Hodgkin lymphoma-like cells, eosinophils, and presence of EBV infection, particularly on small needle core biopsies. However, the large atypical cells are negative for EBV, CD30, CD15, and PAX5. Nevertheless, an excisional biopsy or splenectomy should be recommended if the resulting workup is not sufficient for a diagnosis of classic Hodgkin lymphoma on a core biopsy.

DIAGNOSIS

Diagnosis of IPT-FDC tumor is based on the typical clinical presentations (hepatic and/or splenic mass lesion), morphology (spindle cell proliferation with mixed inflammatory background), positive FDC markers (CD21, CD23, and CD35), and particularly EBV infection on the spindle cells. However, rare cases may show epithelioid cytology, granulomatous reaction, and/or prominent eosinophilic infiltration, which place a great challenge for diagnosis. Therefore, EBER-ISH may be considered for the unusual spindle cell lesions in the liver and spleen.

PROGNOSIS

IPT-FDC tumor is mostly indolent with a low rate of local recurrence or metastasis. Reported splenic cases exhibited no recurrence or metastasis, whereas hepatic cases showed a low recurrence and metastasis rate. Surgical resection is usually sufficient for localized disease.

Key Features
IPT-FDC Tumor

1. Restricted to the spleen and liver.

2. Bland spindle cells in storiform pattern, fascicles, and solid sheets of proliferation.

3. Mixed lymphocytes, plasma cells, and eosinophils.

4. Blood vessels with ectasia and proteinaceous deposits.

5. Variably positive for FDC markers.

6. Consistently positive for EBV infection.

Differential Diagnosis
IPT-FDC Tumor

IPT-FDC Tumor vs	Helpful Distinguish Features
Conventional FDC sarcoma	• Rarely in the spleen and liver.
	• Predominantly lymphocytes in the background.
	• Uniformly positive for FDC markers.
	• Negative for EBV infection on the spindle cells.
Inflammatory myofibroblastic tumor	• Positive for SMA and ALK (~40% of cases).
	• Negative for FDC markers.
	• No evidence of EBV infection.
IgG4-related sclerosing disease	• Typically not occur in the spleen.
	• Presence of obliterative phlebitis.
	• Marked increase in IgG4+ cells and IgG4/IgG ratio.
	• Negative for FDC markers or EBV infection.
Sclerosing angiomatoid nodular transformation	• Nodular growth pattern.
	• Abundant capillaries, fibrosis, and macrophages.
	• Negative for FDC markers or EBV infection.
Classic Hodgkin lymphoma	• Large cells positive for CD15, CD30, and PAX5 (weak).
	• EBV, if positive, on the large atypical cells only.
	• Lack of EBV + spindle cells.

Pitfalls
IPT-FDC Tumor

! IPT-FDC tumor may mimic classic Hodgkin lymphoma with scattered large Hodgkin lymphoma-like cells, eosinophils, and positive EBER-ISH. However, the large atypical cells are negative for CD30, CD15, and PAX5. In addition, the EBV is detected on the spindle cells.

! The FDC markers can be weak or even negative in IPT-FDC tumor; however, the positive EBER-ISH is usually sufficient to establish the diagnosis with the typical clinical and morphologic features.

! Morphologically, IPT-FDC tumor can be very similar to FDC sarcoma, IMT, and IgG4-related sclerosing disease. EBER-ISH is essential for the differential diagnosis.

! IPT-FDC tumor may have prominent granulomatous and/or eosinophilic infiltration. Therefore, EBER-ISH is recommended for unusual hepatic and splenic cases with spindle cell proliferation.

HISTIOCYTIC SARCOMA

INTRODUCTION

Histiocytic sarcoma (HS) is a malignant neoplasm of mature histiocytes, which excludes myeloid sarcoma with monocytic differentiation and dendritic cell neoplasms.[42–44] HS may arise de novo or in association with B-cell lymphomas or myeloid neoplasms. Patients are usually adults with a median age of ~61 years and a slight male predilection.[42] Most cases involve extranodal locations, including skin, soft tissue, and gastrointestinal tract. Approximately 14% of cases occur in the lymph nodes. Clinical presentations range from localized mass lesion to systemic disease with B-symptoms.

PATHOLOGIC FEATURES

HS shows a diffuse infiltration in the soft tissue and a characteristic sinusoidal infiltrative pattern in the lymph nodes, liver, and spleen (**Fig. 8**A). The large tumor cells are mostly pleomorphic but often resemble mature histiocytes. The nuclei are oval and typically eccentrically placed with vesicular chromatin, large nucleoli, and occasional grooves (**Fig. 8**B). The cytoplasm is abundant, eosinophilic, and often foamy or vacuolated. Rarely, the tumor cells may display multinucleation and spindled cytology. In the background, there are variable numbers of reactive lymphocytes, plasma cells, benign histiocytes, and eosinophils.

HS expresses histiocytic markers, such as CD68, CD163, and lysozyme. In addition, CD4, CD45, HLA-DR, and α1-antitrypsin are usually positive. S100 is negative albeit focal reactivity can be seen in some cases. The tumor cells are typically negative for B-cell and T-cell markers, FDC markers (CD21, CD23, and CD35), Langerhans cell markers (langerin and CD1a), CD34, CD30, HMB45, MPO, and cytokeratins.

A subset of HS cases is positive for clonal *IGH* rearrangement. For the cases that have transdifferentiated from B-cell lymphomas, the neoplastic histiocytes retain the same genetic alterations in the prior B-cell lymphoma, including t(14;18).[6,45–49] *BRAF* V600E mutation has been detected in approximately 63% of HS cases.[7] Rare HS cases are associated with mediastinal non-seminomatous germ cell tumors and harbor an isochromosome 12p, identical to that seen in germ cell tumors.[50]

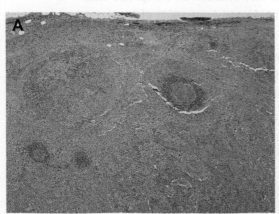
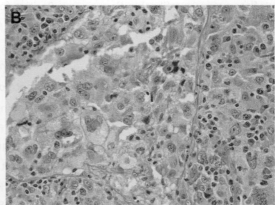

Fig. 8. Histiocytic sarcoma (HS). (*A*) HS reveals a characteristic sinusoidal infiltrative pattern in a lymph node. (*B*) The tumor cells have significant cytologic atypia but resemble mature histiocytes.

DIFFERENTIAL DIAGNOSIS

Anaplastic large cell lymphoma (ALCL), LCH, and metastatic carcinoma with anaplastic features may be reminiscent of HS, particularly the cases in the lymph node with a sinusoidal infiltrative pattern. ALCL is uniformly positive for CD30 with a variable expression of T-cell markers, whereas histiocytic markers (CD68, CD163, and lysozyme) are negative. LCH is typically accomplished with abundant eosinophils, and the tumor cells stain positive for CD1a, S100, and langerin, although CD4 and CD68 are often detected. Melanoma in the lymph node may primarily involve the sinuses with histiocytic cytology; however, melanoma cells are positive for S100, HMB45, and SOX10 but not histiocytic markers. Carcinoma with anaplastic features is positive for cytokeratin.

Myeloid sarcomas with monocytic differentiation can be confused with histiocytic sarcoma, but the blasts are much smaller than the HS cells with a higher nucleus-to-cytoplasm ratio. Reactive histiocytoses and storage diseases (ie, Gaucher disease and Niemann-Pick disease) may present with a marked histiocytic infiltration in the sinuses, but the benign histiocytes in these lesions lack cytologic atypia.

DIAGNOSIS

Mature histiocytic cytology with overt atypia and expression of histiocytic markers are essential for the diagnosis of HS. For cases with preceding or concurrent lymphomas, molecular genetic studies with PCR and FISH may be helpful to determine the clonal relationship between lymphomas and HS.

PROGNOSIS

HS is aggressive and most patients present at advanced clinical stage. The patients generally have a poor response to therapy with a median overall survival of 6 months.[42,43] A small subset of patients have localized disease, associated with a more favorable outcome. One case had an excellent response to MEK inhibition with trametinib and tyrosine kinase inhibition with imatinib.[51]

Key Features
HISTIOCYTIC SARCOMA

1. Mature histiocytic cytology with overt pleomorphism.

2. Sinusoidal infiltration in the lymph nodes.

---

3. Positive for histiocytic markers, CD68, CD163, and lysozyme.

4. Some cases associated with lymphoma and mediastinal germ cell tumor.

△△ Differential Diagnosis
HISTIOCYTIC SARCOMA

Histiocytic Sarcoma vs	Helpful Distinguish Features
Anaplastic large cell lymphoma	• Positive for CD30 and T-cell markers. • Negative for CD68, CD163, and lysozyme.
Langerhans cell histiocytosis	• Prominent reactive eosinophils. • Positive CD1a, S100, and langerin. • CD68 can be positive. • Negative for 163 and lysozyme.
Metastatic carcinoma	• Clinical history of carcinoma. • Positive for cytokeratin. • Negative for histiocytic markers.
Metastatic melanoma	• Positive for melanocytic markers, S100, HMB45, and SOX10. • Negative for histiocytic markers.
Myeloid sarcoma with monocytic differentiation	• Concurrent or subsequent involvement of blood and bone marrow. • Smaller size and higher N/C ratio.
Reactive histiocytoses and storage diseases	• Lack of overt cytologic atypia.

Pitfalls
HISTIOCYTIC SARCOMA

! HS may have highly pleomorphic or spindle cytology, mimicking pleomorphic or spindle cell sarcoma.

! HS may show a variable expression of S100.

! Clonal *IGH* or *TRG* gene rearrangements can be detected in de novo HS and cases dedifferentiated from lymphomas.

INDETERMINATE DENDRITIC CELL TUMOR

INTRODUCTION

Indeterminate dendritic cells are the precursors of Langerhans cells, and the associated indeterminate dendritic cell tumor (IDCT) is extraordinarily rare. IDCT shows similar immunophenotype to that of LCH but lacks Birbeck granules or expression of langerin.[52,53] It mostly occurs in the adults with a female predominance. Patients usually present with a solitary skin lesion or less commonly lesions in multiple sites.

MICROSCOPIC FEATURES

In the skin, IDCT shows a diffuse infiltration in the dermis and may extend into the subcutaneous tissue. The background contains reactive lymphocytes but no significant eosinophilic infiltrate. The cytology varies from histiocytic to Langerhans-like. The nuclei are usually bland and round, oval or irregular with occasional nuclear grooves and clefts (**Fig. 9**). Tumor cells contain abundant pale eosinophilic cytoplasm. Some cases contain multinucleated giant cells or show spindled cytology. Ultrastructurally, IDCT cells have complex interdigitating cell processes but no Birbeck granules or desmosomes.

IDCT is positive for S100 and CD1a, whereas langerin (CD207) is consistently absent. The tumor cells variably express CD4, CD45, CD56, CD68, and lysozyme. They are negative for B-cell and T-cell markers, FDC markers, CD30, CD163, and MPO. Transdifferentiation from follicular lymphoma was reported.[53] *BRAF* V600E mutation has also been detected in IDCT.[30]

DIFFERENTIAL DIAGNOSIS

The major differential diagnosis of IDCT is LCH. IDCT does not contain abundant reactive eosinophils, and importantly, the tumor cells are negative for langerin.

DIAGNOSIS

The diagnosis of IDCT relies on the morphology (histiocytic or Langerhans cell–like cytology) with expression of S100 and CD1a but not langerin.

PROGNOSIS

The clinical course of IDCT is variable. Some tumors may undergo spontaneous regression, whereas others show rapid progression.

Key Features
INDETERMINATE DENDRITIC CELL TUMOR

1. Histiocytic or Langerhans cell–like cytology.

2. Positive for S100 and CD1a.

3. Negative for langerin (CD207).

Differential Diagnosis
INDETERMINATE DENDRITIC CELL TUMOR

IDDC Tumor vs	Helpful Distinguish Features
Langerhans cell histiocytosis	• Abundant reactive eosinophils. • Positive for langerin, in addition to CD1a and S100.

Pitfalls
INDETERMINATE DENDRITIC CELL TUMOR

! IDTC may show langerhans cell–like cytology, which resembles LCH in conjunction with expression of CD1a and S100. Therefore, for an unusual histiocytic neoplasm with expression of CD1a and S100, it is recommended to add langerin staining, particularly in the case with no eosinophilic infiltrate.

ERDHEIM-CHESTER DISEASE

INTRODUCTION

ECD is a rare non-LCH characterized by multisystemic xanthomatous or xanthogranulomatous

Fig.   9. Indeterminate dendritic cell tumor. (*A*) Diffuse infiltration of tumor cells with scattered reactive lymphocytes. (*B*) Tumor cells are large in size and have bland nuclei and abundant cytoplasm.

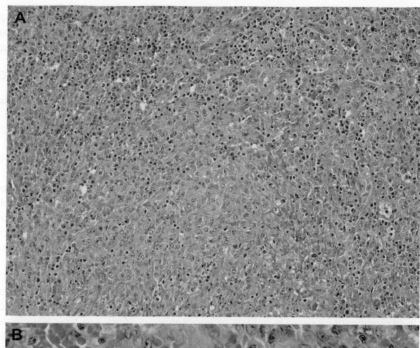

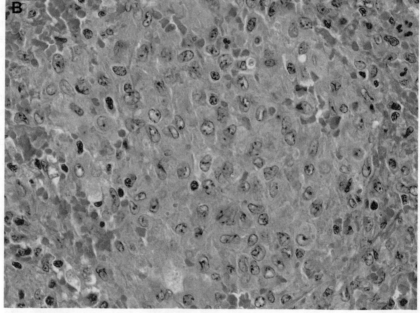

infiltrates of mature histiocytes in a background of inflammation and fibrosis.[54–61] ECD typically occurs in middle-aged to older patients (40–70 years, mean 55 years) with a male-to-female ratio of ~ 3:1. ECD can involve virtually every organ system, and the clinical symptoms depend on the extent and distribution of the disease. Notably, skeletal involvement is nearly always present and can be found in up to ~96% of ECD cases.[54] Extraosseous disorders include heart involvement,

exophthalmos, central diabetes insipidus, xanthelasmas, interstitial lung disease, renal failure, retroperitoneal fibrosis, and CNS infiltration.

RADIOLOGIC FEATURES

Bone involvement is noted in ~96% cases of ECD and shows characteristic symmetric diaphyseal and metaphyseal osteosclerosis of long bones within the lower extremities, which is best visualized by radiotracer uptake on bone scan (^{99}Technetium) and less sensitively by PET.[54] Abdominal imaging studies may show "coated aorta" with circumferential thickening of the aorta and "hairy kidney" due to infiltration of perinephric fat with fibrosis (**Fig. 10**). In the brain, ECD mostly affects the hypothalamic-pituitary axis with thickening and enhancement of the pituitary stalk.[62] In addition, patients may show meningeal involvement, as single or multiple dural masses or diffuse pachymeningeal thickening.

PATHOLOGIC FEATURES

ECD typically shows abundant foamy or lipid-laden histiocytes with background inflammatory cells and fibrosis.[63] The neoplastic histiocytes are often arranged into polymorphic xanthogranulomatous nests, and they have bland cytology with round or oval nuclei and abundant foamy cytoplasm (**Fig. 11**A, B). There is no tumor necrosis or significant increase in mitosis or apoptosis. Scattered Touton giant cells are often present.

ECD histiocytes express CD68, CD163, factor XIIIa, and fascin (**Fig. 11**C, D), whereas CD1a, S100, and langerin (CD207) are typically negative. The BRAF V600E mutant-specific antibody (VE1) may be used in assisting diagnosis of ECD. In addition, special stains with AFB, GMS, and PAS are often necessary to rule out mycobacterial and fungal infection.

Approximately 55% to 60% cases of ECD harbor *BRAF* V600E mutation.[8,15–19] The ECD cases with wild-type *BRAF* have additional mutations in the MAPK signaling pathways, including mutations in *PIK3CA* (10.9% of cases) and *NRAS* (3.7%).[64,65]

DIFFERENTIAL DIAGNOSIS

The major differential diagnoses of ECD include reactive and neoplastic histiocytic proliferations. Extranodal RDD reveals histiocytic infiltration, prominent fibrosis, and abundant plasma cells. However, in contrast to ECD histiocytes, the ones in RDD are much larger in size and have enlarged nuclei with prominent nucleoli. Characteristically, the RDD histiocytes contain viable intracytoplasmic lymphocytes, plasma cells, and/ or neutrophils, a unique phenomenon called "emperipolesis". Furthermore, S100 is positive in RDD but not ECD.

Both ECD and LCH commonly have *BRAF* V600E mutations. Approximately 12% to 19% of patients with ECD have concurrent LCH; these tumors are typically clonally related.[20,21] However, the LCH cells are epithelioid and have frequent nuclear grooves with increased mitoses and apoptosis. In addition, abundant eosinophils are commonly seen in the background of LCH. Immunostains for CD1a, S100, and langerin are positive in LCH but not ECD.

Similar to ECD, IgG4-related sclerosing disease contains prominent fibrosis and lymphoplasmacytic infiltration, but features of foamy histiocytes and xanthogranuloma are not present in IgG4-related disease.

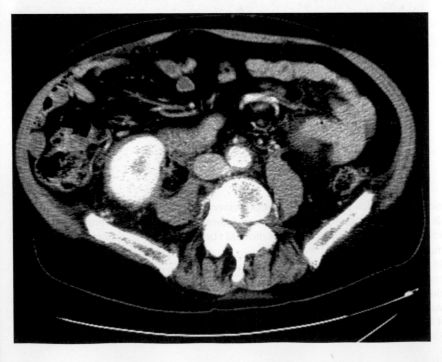

Fig. 10. Erdheim-Chester disease. A case with abdominal imaging studies shows characteristic "hairy kidney." (Courtesy from Dr. Liping Song, the Permanente Medical Group, CA).

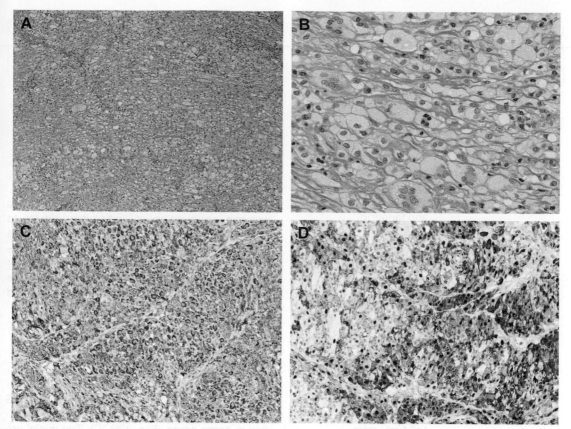

Fig. 11. Histology of ECD. (*A*) Abundant histiocytes in a background with fibrosis and inflammatory cells. (*B*) The neoplastic histiocytes have bland cytology with round or oval nuclei and abundant foamy cytoplasm. Scattered Touton giant cells are noted. CD68 (*C*) and factor XIIIa (*D*) are positive in the histiocytes.

Histiocytic and/or granulomatous reaction is also commonly noted in other conditions, including infection, inflammation, necrosis, and hemorrhage; therefore, it is essential to rule out the aforementioned causes with careful clinical correlation, morphologic evaluation, and ancillary studies (AFB and GMS special stains).

DIAGNOSIS

The consensus diagnostic criteria for ECD include (1) pathologic features: xanthogranulomatous lesions characterized by foamy histiocytes with admixed inflammation and fibrosis and (2) characteristic radiologic findings: skeletal findings of bilateral and symmetric abnormalities in the diaphyseal and metaphyseal regions of the long bones of the legs. In addition, the detection of mutations of *BRAF* and other genes in the MAPK signaling pathway is also helpful for the diagnosis.

PROGNOSIS

ECD can be managed with different approaches, including steroids, interferon alpha, recombinant interleukin 1R antagonist anakinra, and double

autologous HSCT.[66,67] Recent studies have demonstrated that vemurafenib, an inhibitor of BRAF V600E mutation, has shown dramatic and unprecedented clinical and radiographic responses of patients with ECD.[68–71] Overall, the 5-year survival is approximately 70%.

Key Features
ERDHEIM-CHESTER DISEASE

1. Characteristic symmetric diaphyseal and metaphyseal osteosclerosis of long bones, "coated aorta" and "hairy kidney."

2. Foamy and lipid-laden histiocytes, Touton giant cells.

3. Background fibrosis and reactive plasma cells.

4. Positive for CD68, CD163, and factor XIIIa.

5. Negative for CD1a, S100, and langerin.

6. *BRAF* V600E mutation in 55% to 60% of cases.

DISSEMINATED JUVENILE XANTHOGRANULOMA

INTRODUCTION

Disseminated juvenile xanthogranuloma (JXG) is a systemic proliferation of histiocytes, similar to those in the dermal JXG,[68,72] which excludes ECD in the current WHO classification. Disseminated JXG mostly occurs in children younger than 10 years and approximately 50% within the first year of life. The skin, mucosal surfaces, and soft tissues are most commonly affected.

PATHOLOGIC FEATURES

Disseminated JXG typically shows a diffuse histiocytic infiltrate. In the skin, the histiocytes are predominantly in the dermis (**Fig. 12**A). The JXG cells exhibit bland cytology and are slightly spindled in some cases (**Fig. 12**B, C). The nuclei are round or oval with no grooves. The cytoplasm of these cells is abundant, pale-pink, and often foamy or xanthomatous. Frequent Touton giant cells are present, particularly in the dermal cases. Older lesions reveal more fibrosis and mixed reactive cells, including neutrophils, lymphocytes, and eosinophils.

The immunophenotype of JXG cells is similar to that in the conventional histiocytes, with expression CD68, CD163, lysozyme, and factor XIIIa. Fascin and S100 can be detected in a small subset of cases. CD1a and langerin are negative. In contrast to ECD, disseminated JXG does not bear *BRAF* V600E or other mutations in the MAPK signaling pathway.[8,73]

DIFFERENTIAL DIAGNOSIS

The differential diagnosis of disseminated JXG includes xanthomatous changes in various reactive conditions, ECD, and LCH. Detailed clinical history, careful morphologic examination, and special stains (AFB and GMS) are essential to rule out reactive xanthomatous changes. ECD mostly affects adult patients, and most cases show mutations in the MAPK pathway. LCH cells are epithelioid with frequent nuclear grooves and abundant background eosinophils. In addition,

Fig. 12. Disseminated juvenile xanthogranuloma. (*A, B*) Extensive dermal infiltration of histiocytes with frequent Touton giant cells. (*C*) The neoplastic histiocytes exhibit bland cytology and have round or oval nuclei. The cytoplasm is abundant and foamy or xanthomatous.

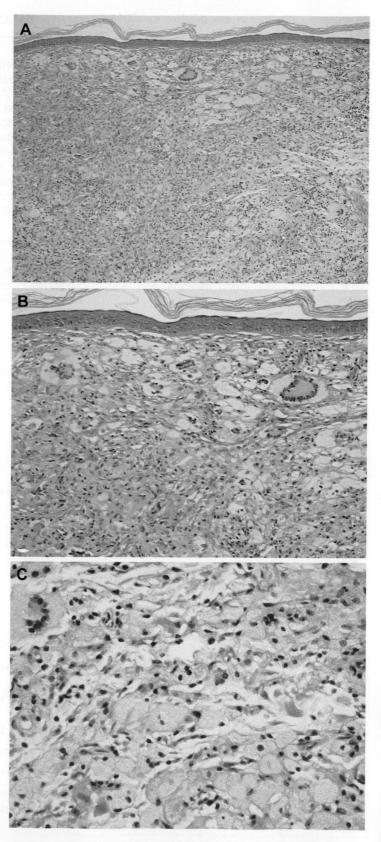

the lesional cells in LCH are positive for CD1a, S100, and langerin.

DIAGNOSIS

Diagnosis of disseminated JXG relies on the typical clinical presentations, morphologic features, and exclusion of other reactive xanthomatous diseases.

PROGNOSIS

Disseminated JXG is benign and some cases may slowly regress. However, it can be aggressive, particularly when lesions involve the central nervous system and other vital organs. It should be noted that some cases are associated with macrophage activation syndrome, which may result in cytopenias, organ damage, and even death.

OTHER HISTIOCYTIC AND DENDRITIC CELL NEOPLASMS

Fibroblastic reticular cell (FRC) tumor is very rare with hybrid features between epithelial and fibroblastic cells.[74] This tumor occurs in the lymph nodes, spleen, and soft tissue. FRC tumor has similar morphologic features to FDC or IDC sarcoma with different immunophenotype. The tumor cells are mostly positive for vimentin, epithelial markers (CK AE1/AE3, CK CAM5.2, CK8, and EMA), and muscle markers (SMA and desmin). Histiocytic and dendritic cell markers are negative, including CD68, lysosome, S100, CD1a, CD21, and CD23.

ALK + histiocytosis affects the patients in early infancy and commonly involves the skin and liver.[75] The clinical symptoms include hepatosplenomegaly, anemia, and thrombocytopenia. Morphologically, the histiocytes are large and the

---

Key Features
DISSEMINATED JUVENILE XANTHOGRANULOMA

1. Most patients within 10 years old.

2. Typically involves skin, mucosa, and soft tissue.

3. Foamy or xanthomatous histiocytes.

4. Frequent Touton cells and mixed inflammatory background.

5. Positive for histiocytic markers but negative for S100, CD1a, and langerin.

6. Lack of *BRAF* mutation.

Differential Diagnosis
DISSEMINATED JUVENILE XANTHOGRANULOMA

Disseminated JXG vs	Helpful Distinguish Features
Erdheim-Chester disease	• Occurs in middle-aged patients.
	• Nearly always involves bone with characteristic radiologic findings.
	• Most cases bear mutations in MAPK pathway, particularly *BRAF* V600E mutation.
Langerhans cell histiocytosis	• Epithelioid with frequent nuclear grooves.
	• Abundant background eosinophils.
	• Positive for CD1a, S100, and langerin.
	• *BRAF* mutation in 50%–60% of cases.
Reactive xanthomatous changes	• Rule out infection, inflammation, hemorrhage, and abnormal lipid metabolic conditions.

nuclei are markedly folded with fine chromatin and small nucleoli. The cytoplasm is abundant, pale eosinophilic, and often vacuolated. Characteristic ALK expression is detected in the neoplastic histiocytes with a cytoplasmic and membranous staining pattern, which may be associated with *ALK* rearrangement. In addition, the tumor cells express histiocytic markers (CD68, CD163, and lysozyme) and variable S100. CD1a and langerin are negative. This histiocytic lesion may regress slowly over many months. Therefore, it is recommended to frequently include ALK staining in the workup of pediatric histiocytic proliferation.

REFERENCES

1. Chen W, Wang J, Wang E, et al. Detection of clonal lymphoid receptor gene rearrangements in langerhans cell histiocytosis. Am J Surg Pathol 2010; 34(7):1049–57.

2. Ratei R, Hummel M, Anagnostopoulos I, et al. Common clonal origin of an acute B-lymphoblastic leukemia and a Langerhans' cell sarcoma: evidence for hematopoietic plasticity. Haematologica 2010; 95(9):1461–6.

3. West DS, Dogan A, Quint PS, et al. Clonally related follicular lymphomas and Langerhans cell neoplasms: expanding the spectrum of transdifferentiation. Am J Surg Pathol 2013;37(7):978–86.

4. Yohe SL, Chenault CB, Torlakovic EE, et al. Langerhans cell histiocytosis in acute leukemias of ambiguous or myeloid lineage in adult patients: support for a possible clonal relationship. Mod Pathol 2014; 27(5):651–6.

5. Schmitt-Graeff AH, Duerkop H, Vollmer-Kary B, et al. Clonal relationship between langerhans cell histiocytosis and myeloid sarcoma. Leukemia 2012;26(7): 1707–10.

6. Shao H, Xi L, Raffeld M, et al. Clonally related histiocytic/dendritic cell sarcoma and chronic lymphocytic leukemia/small lymphocytic lymphoma: a study of seven cases. Mod Pathol 2011;24(11): 1421–32.

7. Go H, Jeon YK, Huh J, et al. Frequent detection of BRAF(V600E) mutations in histiocytic and dendritic cell neoplasms. Histopathology 2014;65(2):261–72.

8. Haroche J, Charlotte F, Arnaud L, et al. High prevalence of BRAF V600E mutations in Erdheim-Chester disease but not in other non-Langerhans cell histiocytoses. Blood 2012;120(13):2700–3.

9. Haroche J, Cohen-Aubart F, Emile JF, et al. Dramatic efficacy of vemurafenib in both multisystemic and refractory Erdheim-Chester disease and Langerhans cell histiocytosis harboring the BRAF V600E mutation. Blood 2013;121(9):1495–500.

10. Chakraborty R, Hampton OA, Shen X, et al. Mutually exclusive recurrent somatic mutations in MAP2K1 and BRAF support a central role for ERK activation in LCH pathogenesis. Blood 2014;124(19):3007–15.

11. Roden AC, Hu X, Kip S, et al. BRAF V600E expression in Langerhans cell histiocytosis: clinical and immunohistochemical study on 25 pulmonary and 54 extrapulmonary cases. Am J Surg Pathol 2014; 38(4):548–51.

12. Brown NA, Furtado LV, Betz BL, et al. High prevalence of somatic MAP2K1 mutations in BRAF V600E-negative Langerhans cell histiocytosis. Blood 2014;124(10):1655–8.

13. McGinnis LM, Nybakken G, Ma L, et al. Frequency of MAP2K1, TP53, and U2AF1 mutations in BRAF-mutated langerhans cell histiocytosis: further characterizing the genomic landscape of LCH. Am J Surg Pathol 2018;42(7):885–90.

14. Chatterjee D, Vishwajeet V, Saikia UN, et al. CyclinD1 is useful to differentiate langerhans cell histiocytosis from reactive langerhans cells. Am J Dermatopathol 2018;41(3):188–92.

15. Cangi MG, Biavasco R, Cavalli G, et al. BRAFV600E-mutation is invariably present and associated to oncogene-induced senescence in Erdheim-Chester disease. Ann Rheum Dis 2015;74(8):1596–602.

16. Blombery P, Wong SQ, Lade S, et al. Erdheim-Chester disease harboring the BRAF V600E mutation. J Clin Oncol 2012;30(32):e331–2.

17. Cohen Aubart F, Emile JF, Maksud P, et al. Efficacy of the MEK inhibitor cobimetinib for wild-type BRAF Erdheim-Chester disease. Br J Haematol 2018; 180(1):150–3.

18. Emile JF, Charlotte F, Amoura Z, et al. BRAF mutations in Erdheim-Chester disease. J Clin Oncol 2013;31(3):398.

19. Nordmann TM, Juengling FD, Recher M, et al. Trametinib after disease reactivation under dabrafenib in Erdheim-Chester disease with both BRAF and KRAS mutations. Blood 2017;129(7):879–82.

20. Liersch J, Carlson JA, Schaller J. Histopathological and clinical findings in cutaneous manifestation of Erdheim-Chester disease and langerhans cell histiocytosis overlap syndrome associated with the BRAFV600E mutation. Am J Dermatopathol 2017; 39(7):493–503.

21. Hervier B, Haroche J, Arnaud L, et al. Association of both Langerhans cell histiocytosis and Erdheim-Chester disease linked to the BRAFV600E mutation. Blood 2014;124(7):1119–26.

22. Facchetti F, Lorenzi L. Follicular dendritic cells and related sarcoma. Semin Diagn Pathol 2016;33(5): 262–76.

23. Wu A, Pullarkat S. Follicular dendritic cell sarcoma. Arch Pathol Lab Med 2016;140(2):186–90.

24. Lin O, Frizzera G. Angiomyoid and follicular dendritic cell proliferative lesions in Castleman's disease of hyaline-vascular type: a study of 10 cases. Am J Surg Pathol 1997;21(11):1295–306.

25. Walters M, Pittelkow MR, Hasserjian RP, et al. Follicular dendritic cell sarcoma with indolent T-lymphoblastic proliferation is associated with paraneoplastic autoimmune multiorgan syndrome. Am J Surg Pathol 2018;42(12):1647–52.

26. Quesada AE, Young KH, Medeiros LJ, et al. Indolent T-lymphoblastic proliferation associated with low grade follicular dendritic cell sarcoma and Castleman disease. Pathology 2018;50(3):351–2.

27. Pokuri VK, Merzianu M, Gandhi S, et al. Interdigitating dendritic cell sarcoma. J Natl Compr Canc Netw 2015;13(2):128–32.

28. Saygin C, Uzunaslan D, Ozguroglu M, et al. Dendritic cell sarcoma: a pooled analysis including 462 cases with presentation of our case series. Crit Rev Oncol Hematol 2013;88(2):253–71.

29. Di Liso E, Pennelli N, Lodovichetti G, et al. Braf mutation in interdigitating dendritic cell sarcoma: a case report and review of the literature. Cancer Biol Ther 2015;16(8):1128–35.

30. O'Malley DP, Agrawal R, Grimm KE, et al. Evidence of BRAF V600E in indeterminate cell tumor and interdigitating dendritic cell sarcoma. Ann Diagn Pathol 2015;19(3):113–6.

31. Ochi Y, Hiramoto N, Yoshizato T, et al. Clonally related diffuse large B-cell lymphoma and interdigitating dendritic cell sarcoma sharing MYC translocation. Haematologica 2018;103(11):e553–6.

32. Stowman AM, Mills SE, Wick MR. Spindle cell melanoma and interdigitating dendritic cell sarcoma: do they represent the same process? Am J Surg Pathol 2016;40(9):1270–9.

33. Xue T, Jiang XN, Wang WG, et al. Interdigitating dendritic cell sarcoma: clinicopathologic study of 8 cases with review of the literature. Ann Diagn Pathol 2018;34:155–60.

34. Cheuk W, Chan JK, Shek TW, et al. Inflammatory pseudotumor-like follicular dendritic cell tumor: a distinctive low-grade malignant intra-abdominal neoplasm with consistent Epstein-Barr virus association. Am J Surg Pathol 2001;25(6):721–31.

35. Chen Y, Shi H, Li H, et al. Clinicopathological features of inflammatory pseudotumour-like follicular dendritic cell tumour of the abdomen. Histopathology 2016;68(6):858–65.

36. Ge R, Liu C, Yin X, et al. Clinicopathologic characteristics of inflammatory pseudotumor-like follicular dendritic cell sarcoma. Int J Clin Exp Pathol 2014;7(5):2421–9.

37. Kitamura Y, Takayama Y, Nishie A, et al. Inflammatory pseudotumor-like follicular dendritic cell tumor of the spleen: case report and review of the literature. Magn Reson Med Sci 2015;14(4):347–54.

38. Bui PL, Vicens RA, Westin JR, et al. Multimodality imaging of Epstein-Barr virus-associated inflammatory pseudotumor-like follicular dendritic cell tumor of the spleen: case report and literature review. Clin Imaging 2015;39(3):525–8.

39. Li XQ, Cheuk W, Lam PW, et al. Inflammatory pseudotumor-like follicular dendritic cell tumor of liver and spleen: granulomatous and eosinophil-rich variants mimicking inflammatory or infective lesions. Am J Surg Pathol 2014;38(5):646–53.

40. Kim HJ, Kim JE, Kang GH, et al. Inflammatory pseudotumor-like follicular dendritic cell tumor of the spleen with extensive histiocytic granulomas and necrosis: a case report and literature review. Korean J Pathol 2013;47(6):599–602.

41. Choe JY, Go H, Jeon YK, et al. Inflammatory pseudotumor-like follicular dendritic cell sarcoma of the spleen: a report of six cases with increased IgG4-positive plasma cells. Pathol Int 2013;63(5):245–51.

42. Kommalapati A, Tella SH, Go RS, et al. Predictors of survival, treatment patterns, and outcomes in histiocytic sarcoma. Leuk Lymphoma 2019;60(2):553–5.

43. Kommalapati A, Tella SH, Durkin M, et al. Histiocytic sarcoma: a population-based analysis of incidence, demographic disparities, and long-term outcomes. Blood 2018;131(2):265–8.

44. Skala SL, Lucas DR, Dewar R. Histiocytic sarcoma: review, discussion of transformation from B-cell lymphoma, and differential diagnosis. Arch Pathol Lab Med 2018;142(11):1322–9.

45. Mori M, Matsushita A, Takiuchi Y, et al. Histiocytic sarcoma and underlying chronic myelomonocytic leukemia: a proposal for the developmental classification of histiocytic sarcoma. Int J Hematol 2010;92(1):168–73.

46. Mehrotra S, Pan Z. Fine needle aspiration cytology of histiocytic sarcoma with dendritic cell differentiation: a case of transdifferentiation from low-grade follicular lymphoma. Diagn Cytopathol 2015;43(8):659–63.

47. Wang E, Papalas J, Hutchinson CB, et al. Sequential development of histiocytic sarcoma and diffuse large b-cell lymphoma in a patient with a remote history of follicular lymphoma with genotypic evidence of a clonal relationship: a divergent (bilineal) neoplastic transformation of an indolent B-cell lymphoma in a single individual. Am J Surg Pathol 2011;35(3):457–63.

48. Feldman AL, Arber DA, Pittaluga S, et al. Clonally related follicular lymphomas and histiocytic/dendritic cell sarcomas: evidence for transdifferentiation of the follicular lymphoma clone. Blood 2008;111(12):5433–9.

49. Waanders E, Hebeda KM, Kamping EJ, et al. Independent development of lymphoid and histiocytic malignancies from a shared early precursor. Leukemia 2016;30(4):955–8.

50. Shinoda H, Yoshida A, Teruya-Feldstein J. Malignant histiocytoses/disseminated histiocytic sarcoma with

hemophagocytic syndrome in a patient with mediastinal germ cell tumor. Appl Immunohistochem Mol Morphol 2009;17(4):338–44.

51. Voruz S, Cairoli A, Naveiras O, et al. Response to MEK inhibition with trametinib and tyrosine kinase inhibition with imatinib in multifocal histiocytic sarcoma. Haematologica 2018;103(1):e39–41.

52. Chen M, Agrawal R, Nasseri-Nik N, et al. Indeterminate cell tumor of the spleen. Hum Pathol 2012; 43(2):307–11.

53. Rezk SA, Spagnolo DV, Brynes RK, et al. Indeterminate cell tumor: a rare dendritic neoplasm. Am J Surg Pathol 2008;32(12):1868–76.

54. Diamond EL, Dagna L, Hyman DM, et al. Consensus guidelines for the diagnosis and clinical management of Erdheim-Chester disease. Blood 2014; 124(4):483–92.

55. Campochiaro C, Tomelleri A, Cavalli G, et al. Erdheim-Chester disease. Eur J Intern Med 2015; 26(4):223–9.

56. Cives M, Simone V, Rizzo FM, et al. Erdheim-Chester disease: a systematic review. Crit Rev Oncol Hematol 2015;95(1):1–11.

57. Haroche J, Arnaud L, Amoura Z. Erdheim-Chester disease. Curr Opin Rheumatol 2012;24(1):53–9.

58. Haroche J, Arnaud L, Cohen-Aubart F, et al. Erdheim-Chester disease. Rheum Dis Clin North Am 2013;39(2):299–311.

59. Haroche J, Cohen-Aubart F, Arnaud L, et al. Erdheim-Chester disease. Rev Med Interne 2014; 35(11):715–22.

60. Haroche J, Cohen-Aubart F, Charlotte F, et al. The histiocytosis Erdheim-Chester disease is an inflammatory myeloid neoplasm. Expert Rev Clin Immunol 2015;11(9):1033–42.

61. Haroche J, Papo M, Cohen-Aubart F, et al. Erdheim-Chester disease (ECD), an inflammatory myeloid neoplasia. Presse Med 2017;46(1):96–106.

62. Drier A, Haroche J, Savatovsky J, et al. Cerebral, facial, and orbital involvement in Erdheim-Chester disease: CT and MR imaging findings. Radiology 2010;255(2):586–94.

63. Ozkaya N, Rosenblum MK, Durham BH, et al. The histopathology of Erdheim-Chester disease: a comprehensive review of a molecularly characterized cohort. Mod Pathol 2018;31(4):581–97.

64. Emile JF, Diamond EL, Helias-Rodzewicz Z, et al. Recurrent RAS and PIK3CA mutations in Erdheim-Chester disease. Blood 2014;124(19):3016–9.

65. Diamond EL, Abdel-Wahab O, Pentsova E, et al. Detection of an NRAS mutation in Erdheim-Chester disease. Blood 2013;122(6):1089–91.

66. Hervier B, Arnaud L, Charlotte F, et al. Treatment of Erdheim-Chester disease with long-term high-dose interferon-alpha. Semin Arthritis Rheum 2012;41(6): 907–13.

67. Aouba A, Georgin-Lavialle S, Pagnoux C, et al. Rationale and efficacy of interleukin-1 targeting in Erdheim-Chester disease. Blood 2010;116(20): 4070–6.

68. Haroche J, Abla O. Uncommon histiocytic disorders: Rosai-Dorfman, juvenile xanthogranuloma, and Erdheim-Chester disease. Hematol Am Soc Hematol Educ Program 2015;2015:571–8.

69. Haroche J, Cohen-Aubart F, Emile JF, et al. Reproducible and sustained efficacy of targeted therapy with vemurafenib in patients with BRAF(V600E)-mutated Erdheim-Chester disease. J Clin Oncol 2015;33(5):411–8.

70. Oneal PA, Kwitkowski V, Luo L, et al. FDA approval summary: vemurafenib for the treatment of patients with Erdheim-Chester disease with the BRAFV600 mutation. Oncologist 2018;23(12):1520–4.

71. Vaglio A, Diamond EL. Erdheim-Chester disease: the "targeted" revolution. Blood 2017;130(11): 1282–4.

72. Vokuhl C, Oschlies I, Klapper W, et al. Histiocytic diseases in childhood and adolescence. Pathologe 2015;36(5):443–50.

73. Allen CE, Parsons DW. Biological and clinical significance of somatic mutations in Langerhans cell histiocytosis and related histiocytic neoplastic disorders. Hematol Am Soc Hematol Educ Program 2015;2015:559–64.

74. Goto N, Tsurumi H, Takami T, et al. Cytokeratin-positive fibroblastic reticular cell tumor with follicular dendritic cell features: a case report and review of the literature. Am J Surg Pathol 2015;39(4): 573–80.

75. Chan JK, Lamant L, Algar E, et al. ALK+ histiocytosis: a novel type of systemic histiocytic proliferative disorder of early infancy. Blood 2008;112(7):2965–8.

Bone Pathology for Hematopathologists

Deniz Peker, MD[1], Shi Wei, MD, PhD[1], Gene P. Siegal, MD, PhD*

KEYWORDS

- Plasmacytoma • Osteosarcoma • Osteomyelitis • Langerhans cell histiocytosis • Mastocytosis
- Rosai-Dorfman disease • Ewing sarcoma • Mesenchymal chondrosarcoma

Key Points

- Bone pathology can be challenging because the skeleton is a living tissue prone to developing a diverse array of neoplastic and non-neoplastic abnormalities.
- Differentiating plasmacytic disorders and osteoblastic tumors may be particularly difficult given the close resemblance of their histomorphology.
- Discriminating lymphoma/leukemia from small, blue, round cell tumors or some non-sarcoma bone lesions may also be problematic.

ABSTRACT

Bone pathology can be challenging because the skeleton is a living tissue prone to developing a diverse array of inflammatory, metabolic, genetic, reactive, circulatory, and neoplastic abnormalities. Several areas of bone pathology are particularly difficult or problematic for hematopathologists given the close resemblance of some hematologic entities to primary/metastatic bone lesions; examples include plasmacytic disorders versus osteoblastic tumors and lymphoma/leukemia versus round cell tumors of bone. This article provides a conceptual and practical overview of selective bone disorders commonly encountered in the differential diagnosis of hematologic diseases.

PLASMACYTOMA

OVERVIEW

Plasmacytoma is a rare solitary tumor characterized by a localized proliferation of monoclonal plasma cells without clinical evidence of plasma cell myeloma. The disease is divided into 2 types: solitary bone plasmacytoma (SBP), when the plasma cell proliferation originates in bone, and solitary extraosseous (extramedullary) plasmacytoma (SEP), when the tumor is located in extraosseous tissue. SBP accounts for approximately 1% to 2% of plasma cell dyscrasias[1] and its incidence is 40% higher than SEP.[2] The median age at diagnosis of plasmacytoma is 55 years to 60 years and it is slightly more common in men.[2] Plasmacytoma is more common in white populations followed by African American and other races[3] The most common location for SBP is the axial skeleton, including vertebrae, whereas SEP is frequently found in the oropharynx and nasopharynx.[4,5] Diagnosis of plasmacytoma requires a detailed clinical examination, laboratory work-up, imaging, and, as a gold standard, tissue diagnosis.

CLINICAL FINDINGS

The clinical symptoms vary depending on the involved site. Bone pain or spinal cord

Disclosure: Dr. Siegal has received partial support from the Haley's Hope Memorial Support Fund for Osteosarcoma Research at the University of Alabama at Birmingham and the Thomas Logan RAID Fund for Ewing's Sarcoma Research.

Department of Pathology, University of Alabama at Birmingham, 619 19th Street South, Birmingham, AL 35249, USA

[1]These authors contributed equally.

* Corresponding author.

E-mail address: gsiegal@uabmc.edu

compression is the most common clinical presentation in SBP. Soft tissue enlargement and compression-related symptoms, that is, airway obstruction, can be seen in SEP.

RADIOLOGIC FINDINGS

Imaging studies are important in detecting and characterizing plasmacytoma and to exclude plasma cell myeloma. On conventional skeleton radiography, plasmacytoma shows replacement of trabecular bone with partially conserved cortical bone.[6] In some cases, a multicystic appearance also may be seen.[7] Although conventional radiography is a helpful imaging tool in detecting bone lesions, its utility is limited in soft tissue involvement. Alone or in combination, CT, MRI, and PET typically are used to evaluate soft tissue lesions.

LABORATORY FINDINGS

A small monoclonal protein might be detectable in the serum and/or urine in a subset of patients, more commonly in SBP than SEP.[4] Free light chain ratio is abnormal in approximately half of patients.[8]

MICROSCOPIC FEATURES

Histologic examination of tissue shows infiltration of sheets of plasma cells without a significant lymphoid component (Fig. 1A, B). Clonality in plasma cells is determined based on kappa or lambda light chain restriction using immunohistochemistry, in situ hybridization, or flow cytometry. Detection of heavy chain and light chain gene rearrangement via polymerase chain reaction can be used to confirm plasma cell clonality. Neoplastic plasma cells are immunoreactive for select plasma cell markers, including CD38, CD138, and MUM1 (see Fig. 1C). CD79a expression often is seen in plasma cells with or without CD19 and CD20 coexpression. Aberrant expression of CD56 and CD117 also can be observed. Bone marrow clonal plasma cell infiltration should be less than 10% of total cellularity (and is typically zero) in the absence of lytic bone lesions and CRAB (hypercalcemia, renal insufficiency, anemia, and/or bone lesions) manifestations to rule out myeloma.[9]

DIFFERENTIAL DIAGNOSIS

- Plasma cell myeloma, requires clinical and laboratory criteria.
- Non-Hodgkin lymphomas; B-cell lymphomas, with marginal plasma cell differentiation that is, lymphoplasmacytic lymphoma; plasmablastic lymphoma; and marginal zone lymphoma. Plasmacytoma often demonstrates a phenotypic profile similar to myeloma with CD138 and bright CD38 expression. CD19, CD45, and surface light chain expression often indicate non-Hodgkin lymphoma rather than plasmacytoma whereas CD56 positivity

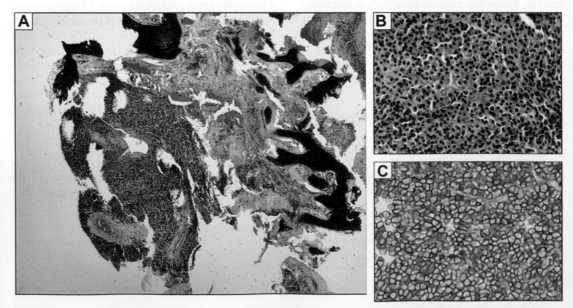

Fig. 1. Biopsy from a lytic bone lesion showing dense cellular infiltrate destroying bone (*A*) on routine hematoxylin-eosin stain (original magnification × 40) that is composed of mature plasma cells (*B*) (original magnification × 200). CD138 is diffusely positive in plasma cells (*C*) (original magnification × 200).

is seen almost exclusively in clonal plasma cell neoplasms.[10,11]

- Reactive conditions, including chronic osteomyelitis.

PROGNOSIS

Local recurrence and progression to myeloma define the prognosis in plasmacytoma.

Prognosis in plasmacytoma differs between SBP and SEP. Overall prognosis is less favorable in SBP due to a higher risk to evolve into myeloma.[4] Multiple parameters have been used to create a scoring system for plasmacytoma; however, none of these has been widely adopted. Many studies show that the tumor size and location are important risk factors.[4,12] Additionally, presence of bone marrow involvement is another important prognostic factor because studies showed that patients without marrow involvement have superior progression-free survival.[13] Similar to other plasma cell disorders, for example, myeloma, the serum free light chain ratio is an independent prognostic factor if it is outside of the normal range.[14]

TREATMENT

Plasmacytoma is a rare disease; as a result, there is no generally established treatment standard. Clonal plasma cells are sensitive to radiation therapy, enabling a significant response in patients to radiotherapy in many patients. Treatment should include all the involved tissue sites with generous margins because local recurrences may occur. Partial or complete surgical removal of tumor often is a part of the diagnostic work-up in many patients. Also, surgical procedures often are indicated in patients who need fixation of bone fractures, a decompressive laminectomy, spine stabilization, or removal of tumors obstructing the upper airway.[4,7] The role of chemotherapy is controversial.

OSTEOSARCOMA

OVERVIEW

Osteosarcoma is the most common nonhematopoietic primary malignant neoplasm of bone.[15] It has long been accepted that osteosarcoma has a bimodal age distribution; a majority of cases occur in childhood and adolescence and a smaller second incidence peak appears in the elderly, frequently with conditions known to predispose to osteosarcoma, including Paget disease and prior radiation. Recent studies have shown, however, that modern osteosarcomas do not have a second incidence peak but rather demonstrate a steady distribution rate after age 25, until the sixth decade when the incidence rate starts to decline.[16] The tumor can occur in any bone of the body, whereas the metaphyses of long bones (especially femur, tibia, and humerus) are the most common sites of involvement. A significant proportion of patients present with pain with or without a palpable mass. On imaging, there is almost always evidence of a destructive bony lesion, often with evidence of variable degree of new bone formation. There also may be an interrupted periosteal reaction associated with the lesion.

GROSS FEATURES

In contrast to many other tumor types, the standard of care for high-grade osteosarcomas after biopsy confirmation of diagnosis is neoadjuvant cytotoxic chemotherapy followed by surgical resection. Thus, gross examination is always performed on post-treatment specimens. In this regard, sampling of the tumor to assess chemotherapy response (percent tumor necrosis; Huvos grade) is carried out by taking 1 full cross-sectional slab of tumor at its greatest cross-sectional area.

Conventional osteosarcomas usually present as a large, gritty, intramedullary mass with variable degree of bone formation. Heavily mineralized tumors are typically tan-gray-white whereas cartilaginous component may be blue-gray to white and have a rubbery or myxoid texture. Areas of necrosis, hemorrhage, and cystic changes are not uncommon. Telangiectatic osteosarcomas characteristically have a dominant cystic architecture in the medullary space filled with blood. Small cell osteosarcomas are grossly indistinguishable from conventional osteosarcomas. High-grade surface osteosarcoma arises on the surface of bone.

Parosteal osteosarcoma and low-grade central osteosarcoma typically are gray-white masses with a firm and gritty texture affixed to the underlying cortex or arising within the intramedullary cavity, respectively. Arising from the cortical surface, periosteal osteosarcomas can be hard and tan-white. They usually are dominated by cartilaginous tissue/admixed with small amounts of tumor osteoid.

MICROSCOPIC FEATURES

The histologic hallmark of all osteosarcomas is the presence of tumor osteoid or bone produced by tumor cells, which is a dense, pink, amorphous material on hematoxylin-eosin–stained sections (Table 1). No minimal amount of neoplastic bone is required as sufficient to render a diagnosis.

Table 1
Key features of osteosarcoma

Osteoblastic osteosarcoma	Principal matrix: neoplastic bone
Chondroblastic osteosarcoma	Neoplastic bone and cartilage (variable amount, hyaline or myxoid)
Fibroblastic osteosarcoma	Neoplastic bone and spindle malignant cells (may be malignant fibrous histiocytoma-like)
Giant cell–rich osteosarcoma	Neoplastic bone and abundant non-neoplastic, osteoclast-type giant cells
Telangiectatic osteosarcoma	Malignant bone-forming tumor with large spaces filled with blood and separated by fibrous septa
Small cell osteosarcoma	Small, round, blue cells with neoplastic osteoid/bone formation
Parosteal osteosarcoma	Low-grade bone-forming tumor arising on the surface of bone
Periosteal osteosarcoma	Intermediate-grade, cartilage and bone-forming tumor arising on the surface of the bone
High-grade surface osteosarcoma	High-grade, malignant bone-forming tumor arising on the surface of the bone

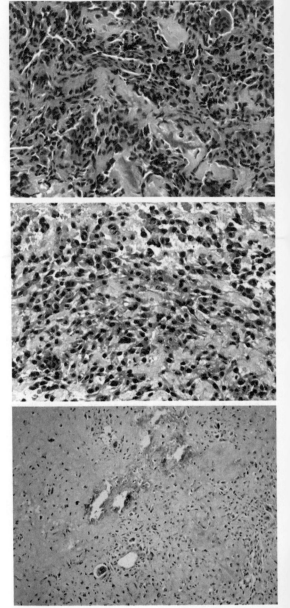

Fig. 2. Conventional osteosarcoma demonstrates haphazardly arranged, partly mineralized osteoid rimmed by osteoblastic tumor cells (*upper panel*). An epithelioid osteosarcoma exhibits minimal osteoid production (*middle panel*). Chondroblastic osteosarcoma shows prominent chondroid matrix intimately associated with randomly arranged mineralized osteoid (*lower panel*) (H&E, original magnification [*A*] ×200; [*B*] ×200; [*C*] ×40).

Conventional osteosarcomas can be subdivided into osteoblastic, chondroblastic, and fibroblastic subtypes, based on the predominant matrix, although a significant proportion of tumors are mixed type (**Fig. 2**). Other reported histologic subtypes include (but not limited to) giant cell rich, epithelioid, clear cell, osteoblastoma-like, chondroblastoma-like, and chondromyxoid fibroma-like.

Telangiectatic osteosarcoma is composed of numerous blood-filled spaces with no endothelial lining, thus simulating aneurysmal bone cyst. The intervening fibrous septa separating the spaces typically contain abundant reactive multinucleated giant cells and malignant mononuclear cells, producing variable amounts of neoplastic bone (**Fig. 3**). Small cell osteosarcoma characteristically consists of small, blue, round cells with scant cytoplasm, thus, histologically resembling

Ewing sarcoma. Lace-like osteoid production is always present but may be subtle (see **Fig. 3**). Microscopically, periosteal osteosarcoma is indistinguishable from those of conventional chondroblastic osteosarcomas (**Fig. 4**). High-grade surface osteosarcoma shows the same

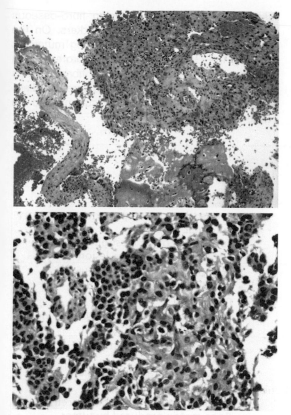

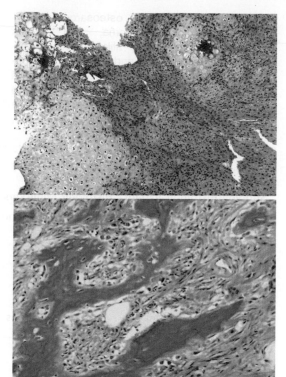

Fig. 3. Telangiectatic osteosarcoma contains large, blood-filled spaces simulating aneurysmal bone cyst (*upper panel*). Small cell osteosarcoma demonstrates subtle osteoid production in a lace-like pattern (*lower panel*) (H&E, original magnification [A] ×100; [B] ×200).

Fig. 4. Periosteal osteosarcoma exhibits a condensation of spindle cells; the cartilage elements display greater nuclear pleomorphism (*upper panel*). Parosteal osteosarcoma shows woven bone spicules in the background of a moderately cellular spindle cell stroma (*lower panel*) (H&E, original magnification [A] ×40; [B] ×200).

spectrum of histologic features seen in conventional osteosarcomas.

Parosteal osteosarcoma and low-grade central osteosarcoma have similar histomorphologic characteristics, both consisting of well-formed bony trabeculae in a mildly cellular fibroblastic stroma. The bone trabeculae commonly are arranged in a parallel manner but also may be haphazard, mimicking that of long-standing fibrous dysplasia. The spindled/fibroblastic cells lack the degree of cytologic atypia seen in conventional osteosarcoma (see **Fig. 4**). Low-grade central osteosarcoma essentially is indistinguishable from parosteal osteosarcoma based solely on the histomorphologic rounds.

DIFFERENTIAL DIAGNOSIS

Differential diagnosis of osteosarcoma largely depends on the histomorphologic features and clinic-radiologic correlation. The distinguishing feature of osteosarcoma over non–bone-forming neoplasms essentially is identification of tumor

osteoid/bone along with cytologic atypia, including nuclear pleomorphism, hyperchromasia, and atypical mitoses. That said, tumor osteoid may be subtle or absent in a small biopsy with limited amount of pathologic tissue. Immunohistochemistry may be helpful in this regard. Although not specific, SATB2 is a marker of osteoblastic differentiation thus has the potential to be a useful adjunct in some settings, particularly in clinically aggressive lesions suspicious for osteosarcoma but lacking identifiable tumor osteoid in a limited biopsy.[17] In parallel, membranous expression of CD138 can be seen in a significant proportion of benign and malignant bone-forming tumors.[18] Thus, CD138 reactivity of neoplastic cells in bone is not a definitive marker for osseous or plasmacytic origin when dealing with a plasmacytoid lesion, and caution is required to interpret CD138-positive cells within a bony lesion for which a hematologic etiology has not been established.

Molecular genetic analysis also play a crucial role in distinguishing a subset of osteosarcomas from their histologic mimickers. Fibro-osseous lesions, namely parosteal osteosarcoma, low-grade central osteosarcoma, and fibrous dysplasia, have seemingly alike histologic features. Detection of MDM2 and CDK4 gene amplification/protein overexpression provides a useful diagnostic tool for parosteal osteosarcoma and low-grade central osteosarcoma (arising on the surface of bone and within the medullary cavity, respectively). In contrast, benign fibro-osseous lesions are negative for these markers. On the other hand, identification of activating mutations involving the G-nucleotide binding protein alpha subunit (GNAS) characterizes a fibro-osseous lesion as fibrous dysplasia. The differential diagnoses of osteosarcoma are summarized in **Table 2**.

Table 2
Differential diagnosis of osteosarcoma

Subtype/Histologic Variant	Histologic Mimickers	Salient Distinguishing Features
Osteoblastic, sclerosing variant	• Reactive new bone formation	• Permeative growth pattern • Cytologic atypia • Tumor cells often most obvious at the advancing edge of the lesion
Chondroblastic	• Chondrosarcoma	• Randomly arranged osteoid/bone • Lace-like pattern of osteoid production
Fibroblastic, malignant fibrous histiocytoma-like	• Malignant fibrous histiocytoma	• Variable amount of tumor-producing osteoid/bone
Osteoblastoma-like	• Osteoblastoma	• Permeative growth pattern • Cytologic atypia • Cellular intertrabecular regions
Giant cell-rich	• Giant cell tumor of bone	• Nonepiphyseal location • Cytologic atypia in neoplastic cells • Bone matrix produced by tumor
Epithelioid	• Epithelioid osteoblastoma • Metastatic carcinoma • Plasmacytoma	• Infiltrate and/or isolate preexisting lamellar bone; lack of large, plump osteoblasts with a prominent nucleus and nucleoli • Presence of tumor osteoid/bone • Presence of tumor osteoid/bone (irrespective of CD138 expression)
Chondroblastoma-like	• Chondroblastoma	• Nonepiphyseal location • Infiltrative growth pattern • Tumor osteoid • Cytologic atypia
Chondromyxoid fibroma–like	• Chondromyxoid fibroma	• Destructive growth pattern • Tumor osteoid • Cytologic atypia
Telangiectatic	• Aneurysmal bone cyst	• Marked cellular pleomorphism, atypical mitoses
Periosteal	• Periosteal chondrosarcoma • Central chondroblastic osteosarcoma	• Osteoid-producing • Intermediate grade osteosarcoma intermixed with cartilaginous elements
Small cell	• Other small, blue, round cell tumor	• Tumor osteoid/bone
Low-grade central	• Fibrous dysplasia	• Permeation of preexisting bone and soft tissue extension • MDM2 and CDK4 amplification/overexpression
Parosteal (juxtacortical)	• Fibrous dysplasia	• Arising on the surface of bone • MDM2 and CDK4 amplification/overexpression

PROGNOSIS

Multiagent chemotherapy followed by complete surgical resection for high-grade osteosarcoma has had a dramatic impact on clinical outcomes. Factors influencing prognosis include age, race, gender, tumor size, location, and stage. Greater than 90% chemotherapy-induced tumor necrosis has been regarded as a significant positive prognostic factor. A more recent large cohort has indicated that previously defined distinctive prognostic factors differed significantly among different age groups, thus providing a rationale for age-based management strategies.[16]

The treatment of low-grade (parosteal and low-grade central) and intermediate grade (periosteal) osteosarcomas is surgical resection with a wide margin. The prognosis for low-grade tumors is excellent whereas that for periosteal osteosarcoma is relatively good.[15]

NONSARCOMA BONE LESIONS

OSTEOMYELITIS

Overview

Osteomyelitis is a rare benign condition and is defined by inflammation of bone and bone marrow secondary to infection that can progress to debilitating osteonecrosis, that is, bone and cartilage destruction. The most common cause is pyogenic infections due to bacteria and mycobacteria. Viral and fungal infections also can be seen. Common causative agents are *Staphylococcus aureus*, *Klebsiella*, *Aerobacter*, *Proteus*, *Pseudomonas*, *Streptococcus pneumonia*, *Neisseria ghonorrhea*, and, particularly in sickle cell disease patients, *Salmonella*. In developed countries, the incidence has decreased with advances in preventive medicine and highly effective antibiotic use. The overall incidence in the Untied States is 22 cases per 1,000,000 persons per year.[19] Osteomyelitis is seen primarily in immunocompromised patients and elderly individuals as a result of an increased prevalence of chronic debilitating diseases, including vascular diseases, peripheral neuropathy, and degenerative joint diseases requiring arthroplasty and diabetes.

Osteomyelitis may occur due to hematogenous spread of infection from another body site, contiguous spread from surrounding soft tissue and joints, or direct inoculation as a result of trauma, insertion of orthopedic hardware, and puncture wounds.[20] Hematogenous osteomyelitis usually affects pediatric and adolescent populations and typically involves the longer bones of the lower extremities.

Clinical and Laboratory Findings

The most common symptoms are high fever and localized pain. Other local symptoms include edema, erythema, and warmth in the infected area. In a subacute clinical presentation, patients may have malaise, mild pain lasting several weeks with minimal fever. In children less than 1 year of age, extension of the infection into the adjacent joint and epiphyseal damage can be seen, whereas in older children the damage often is in metaphyseal region of the bone.

Laboratory findings usually are nonspecific for osteomyelitis. An increased white cell count along with elevation of both the erythrocyte sedimentation rate (ESR) and C-reactive protein levels are common changes. Blood cultures are critical for determining the infectious etiology.

Radiologic Findings

Radiologic imaging is essential in the evaluation of osteomyelitis. Conventional radiographs have low sensitivity and specificity in making a diagnosis, particularly in the acute phase because up to 80% of patients may have normal radiographic findings.[21] A periosteal reaction, abscess formation of soft tissue swelling, can be detected using standard techniques, and fractures can be ruled out. MRI has the highest sensitivity and specificity for osteomyelitis. Bone marrow edema can be detected in early stages of the disease. Triple-phase bone scanning also is sensitive in early stages, particularly when there is no bone destruction. CT is also widely used in diagnosing osteomyelitis. CT is superior to MRI for resolution and demonstrating of bone changes, including cortical destruction, periosteal reactions and sequestrum formation.[22]

Microscopic Features

Biopsy is essential for a definitive diagnosis of osteomyelitis. Osteomyelitis is divided into 3 categories based on histomorphologic characteristics: acute phase, chronic phase, and subacute phase (Brodie abscess). Acute-phase osteomyelitis often demonstrates infiltration of neutrophils accompanied by lymphocytes and plasma cells in the background of marrow fibrosis and thrombosed blood vessels (**Fig. 5**). Microorganisms also can be identified within the lesion. The chronic phase is characterized by necrotic bone along with a chronic inflammatory infiltrate, granulation tissue and periosteal bone proliferation. The subacute phase refers to osteomyelitis with heavy plasma cell infiltrate. Brodie abscess is a rare condition with an indolent disease course. Due to the dense plasmacytic component, it can be confused with SBP and other benign and malignant diseases.

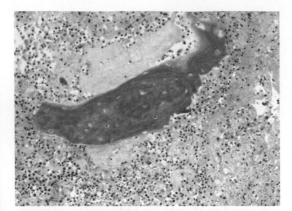

Fig. 5. Acute pyogenic osteomyelitis demonstrates infiltration of neutrophils accompanied by lymphocytes and plasma cells (H&E, original magnification ×40).

Differential Diagnosis

The differential diagnosis includes various malignant and benign conditions[23]:

- Arthritis, including rheumatoid arthritis
- Metastatic bone disease
- Fractures
- Charcot arthropathy
- Gout, avascular necrosis of the bone, and bursitis
- Sickle cell vaso-occlusive crisis
- Synovitis, acne, pustulosis, hyperostosis, and osteitis (SAPHO) syndrome
- Plasma cell neoplasms

Treatment and Prognosis

Treatment of osteomyelitis often is with surgical débridement and prolonged antibiotic use depending on the causative agent. Removal of orthopedic hardware sometimes is necessary in patients with associated osteomyelitis. With aggressive therapy, the prognosis is good. Recurrent infection may be seen in the area of involvement, particularly in immunocompromised patients.

LANGERHANS CELL HISTIOCYTOSIS

Overview

Langerhans cell histiocytosis (LCH), formerly known as histiocytosis X and several dozen other eponyms, is a rare disorder defined by infiltration of various tissues (skeletal and visceral) by abnormal histiocytes. LCH was historically divided into 3 major clinical variants; eosinophilic granuloma (unifocal solitary lesion of bone), Hand-Schüller-Christian disease (skull lesion, exophthalmos, and diabetes insipidus), and the Letterer-Siwe disease (fulminant multisystemic disease). Recent research suggests a clonal and neoplastic nature for the disease.[24,25] and the World Health Organization classifies LCH as a neoplastic disease derived from histiocytic cells. It is still unclear, however, if LCH is a neoplastic or inflammatory disease in all its clinical manifestations. LCH predominantly affects children with an estimated incidence of 4.6 per million in the pediatric population.[26]

Clinical Findings

Symptoms of LCH vary from an asymptomatic solitary bone nodule to multisystem failure. Skin, bone, and central nervous system are the most commonly affected organs. Unifocal bone involvement is the most common presentation in the pediatric population, is found in approximately 75% of LCH patients.[26,27] LCH of bone is exceedingly uncommon in the adult population. It often involves flat bones, including the skull, mandible, and pelvic bones in adults.

Imaging Findings

Imaging findings in LCH are nonspecific. Plain films with or without CT or MRI are necessary for radiologic evaluation. The most common radiologic finding in osseous LCH is that of a lytic lesion with a sclerotic rim detected by conventional imaging or CT.[28] On MRI, the lesions demonstrate a hyperintense signal and enhancement on T1 imaging.[28]

Microscopic Features

The lesion's characteristic features include a diffuse infiltration of Langerhans cells that are oval to round-shaped histiocytoid cells with grooved nuclei, fine chromatin, and inconspicuous nucleoli and a fair amount of eosinophilic cytoplasm (**Fig. 6**). Admixed lymphocytes, giant cells, plasma cells, and eosinophils also can be seen.

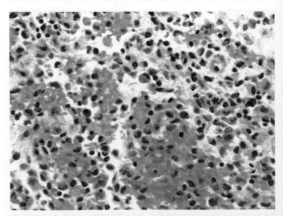

Fig. 6. LCH consists of abundant Langerhans cells with ovoid, coffee bean nuclei with prominent longitudinal nuclear grooves. Collections of eosinophils and other inflammatory cells often are accompanying (H&E, original magnification ×200).

The background stroma often is fibrotic. Langerhans cells typically express S100 protein, CD1a and Langerin. CD21, CD23, and CD35 are negative. Also, Birbeck granules detected by electron microscopy are pathognomonic, although this technique no longer is commonly used.

Molecular Findings

Gene copy number changes and recurrent loss of heterozygosity have been shown in LCH; however, no recurrent cytogenetic abnormalities associated with the disease have been described. A BRAF gain-of-function mutation has been detected in a majority of the patients with severe disease.[29]

Differential Diagnosis

The differential diagnosis for LCH is broad:

- Reactive histiocytosis
- Acute and chronic myelomonocytic leukemia; clonal proliferation of myelomonocytic or monocytic precursors in bone marrow or extramedullary organs
- Histiocytic sarcoma; aggressive, malignant neoplasm of histiocytes
- Primary bone lymphoma
- Mastocytosis
- Chronic osteomyelitis

Treatment and Prognosis

There is no established treatment protocol for LCH. Based on the location and severity of the disease, the accepted treatment approaches for isolated bone lesions include observation, curettage, steroid injections into the lesion, and surgical excision.[30] The prognosis is overall good to excellent when confined to a single bone but nearly uniformly fatal when disseminated to multiple organs in infants.

MASTOCYTOSIS

Overview

Mastocytosis is defined by a clonal proliferation of mast cells involving the various reticuloendothelial system organs, including skin, bone, liver, spleen, gastrointestinal tract, and lymph nodes. Mastocytosis is subclassified based on the involved organs and systems: (1) cutaneous mastocytosis, (2) systemic mastocytosis, and (3) mast cell sarcoma.[31] The etiology of disease is unknown. The cutaneous form is more common in children with a slight male predilection whereas systemic mastocytosis usually occurs in the adult population. Skeletal lesions are seen in 70% to 75% of patients with systemic mastocytosis and the most common bones affected are those of the axial skeleton, pelvis, and proximal ends of the long bones.[32,33] Bone involvement often causes loss in bone density and particularly affects trabecular bone rather than cortical bone.[34] Sclerotic bone lesions also can be seen.

Clinical and Laboratory Findings

There may be systemic symptoms of mastocytosis, including fatigue, fever, weight loss, and night sweats. Skeletal involvement often causes bone pain, osteopenia/osteoporosis, arthralgias, and myalgias. Bone fractures may occur due to fragility and men are more prone to have vertebral fractures.[33,34] Hepatosplenomegaly and lymphadenopathy may be present in severe disease.

Serum tryptase levels are increased in patients with mastocytosis involving bone. The hematology abnormalities include anemia, leukocytosis, eosinophilia, neutropenia, and thrombocytopenia. Increased histamine levels also are a feature of mastocytosis. Increased serum interleukin 6 has been linked to disease progression.[35] Systemic mastocytosis also can be associated with hematopoietic neoplasms.

Imaging Findings

Osteoporosis and bone fractures are common manifestations in systemic mastocytosis. Bone radiographs demonstrate irregular sclerotic lesions in the involved bones. Bone mineral density is assessed using dual-energy x-ray absorptiometry to assess osteoporosis. Bone scintigraphy is helpful in defining asymptomatic lesions.

Microscopic Features

Nonneoplastic mast cells display round to oval nuclei with clumped chromatin, abundant cytoplasm containing small granules and absent nucleoli. Systemic mastocytosis is characterized by proliferation of atypical mast cells showing significant spindling with decreased or absent cytoplasmic granules forming clusters. The mast cells often are associated with dense fibrosis and paratrabecular areas (**Fig. 7**). Bilobation or multilobation of nuclei usually are associated with high-grade aggressive disease. Admixed chronic inflammatory cells, including eosinophils, lymphocytes, and plasma cells, typically are present. Although the morphology is characteristic and the diagnosis can be made on routine stains, immunohistochemistry can be used to support the diagnosis. Neoplastic mast cells express tryptase, chymase, KIT (CD117), CD25, and less commonly CD2 and CD30. Bright CD117 and aberrant CD2 and 25 expression often is detected by flow cytometry as well.

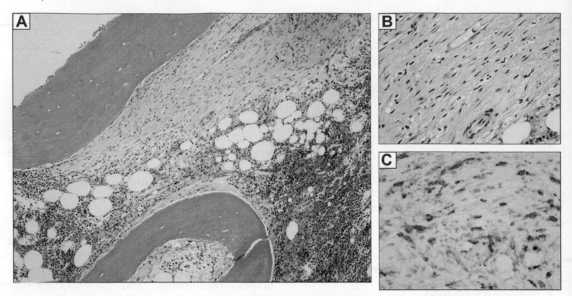

Fig. 7. Systemic mastocytosis with paratrabecular fibrosis and atypical mast cells (*A*) showing spindled morphology (*B*). Mast cells as positive for mast cell tryptase (*C*) (H&E, original magnification [*A*] ×20; [*B*] ×200; [*C*] ×200).

Molecular Findings

Gain-of-function KIT mutations, especially *KIT*D816 V mutations are detected in more than 80% of all patients.[36] Other mutations found in mastocytosis patients include the *TET2, ASXL1, CBL, JAK2V617 F, TP53,* and *RUNX1* genes.[37]

Differential Diagnosis

Mast cell proliferation can be seen in reactive and nonclonal conditions.

- Mast cell hyperplasia can be associated with hypersensitivity conditions, solid tumors, and other hematopoietic malignancies.
- Systemic mast cell activation disease is a nonclonal condition that is characterized by enhanced release of mast cell mediator's accompanied by proliferation of dysfunctional mast cells.[38]

Treatment

Indolent and smoldering systemic mastocytosis often does not require treatment and patients are monitored on a regular basis. Patients with osteoporosis are treated to increase bone density. Aggressive disease is treated with tyrosine kinase inhibitors as well as stem cell transplantation.

ROSAI-DORFMAN DISEASE OF BONE

Overview

Rosai-Dorfman disease (RDD), also known as sinus histiocytosis with massive lymphadenopathy, is a rare benign disease of unknown etiology. It is characterized by a proliferation of histiocytes that frequently accumulate in lymph nodes as well as extranodal sites. The most common extranodal organs involved are those in the region of the orbit, eyelid, upper respiratory tract, salivary gland, skin, bone, and testes.[39] Up to 10% of the RDD cases manifest bone in nature, primarily secondary involvement.[39] Primary involvement of bone is rare. According to published cases series, osseous RDD is seen mostly in young patients, mean age of 28 years, with a female predilection.[40] The most commonly involved bones are the long bones, including the femur, tibia, and humerus, along with the bones of the hands.

Clinical and Imaging Findings

The most common clinical symptom is bone pain in the involved area. Headache and seizures have been noted in patients with skull lesions.[40] Imaging often shows well demarcated or ill-defined lytic bone lesions, primarily within the medullary cavity, whereas a sclerotic pattern is seen only in rare cases. A periosteal reaction and cortical thickening adjacent to the lesion can be seen. RDD rarely involves multiple systems and organs but when present is linked to fatal disease.

Microscopic Findings

Morphologically the medullary cavity of bone is the site demonstrating classic features of RDD consisting of a proliferation of large, irregularly shaped histiocytes filled with an abundant eosinophilic and vacuolated cytoplasm, oval to kidney-shaped nuclei, and inconspicuous nucleoli. The histiocytes typically show lymphocytophagocytosis, referred to as emperipolesis. Background stroma shows the presence of inflammatory cells, including lymphocytes, plasma cells, rare eosinophils, and neutrophils. Foci of necrosis surrounded by histiocytes mimicking granulomas have been reported.[40] The involved bone may show mixed osteoclastic and osteoblastic activity with new bone formation in some cases.

RDD histiocytes are positive for S100 protein by immunohistochemistry as well as, in some cases, CD68. CD1a often is negative.

Differential Diagnosis

- Reactive histiocytosis, that is, Chronic osteomyelitis and infectious osteomyelitis with granulomatous inflammation
- Histiocytic sarcoma; often characterized by marked cytologic atypia and frequent mitosis as well as necrosis
- LCH; histiocytes characterized by nuclear grooves

SARCOIDOSIS

Overview

Sarcoidosis is a granulomatous inflammatory disease that involves multiple organ systems, including lungs, lymph nodes, skin, visceral organs, and the musculoskeletal system. The etiology for sarcoidosis is still unknown. Bone involvement in sarcoidosis has been reported in 1% to 15% of patients, and a majority of the cases can result in dactylitis and/or osteolysis.[41] Any bone can be affected by sarcoidosis, including the skull, facial bones, ribs, and long bones and small bones of the hands and feet. In rare cases, sarcoidosis can involve the sacroiliac bones and joints and can be associated with ankylosing spondylitis, particularly in patients who are positive for HLA-B27.[41]

Clinical and Imaging Findings

Sarcoidosis often involves adults. The disease usually present with systemic symptoms, including fever, weight loss, and mediastinal lymphadenopathy. Bone involvement by sarcoidosis often is asymptomatic but hematology manifestations, such as cytopenia, can be seen. Symptomatic cases often present with dactylitis. Multiple cystic lesions of bone are a typical finding that can be diagnosed easily by radiography. Single cystic lesions are rare. Unifocal or multifocal osteosclerotic lesions rarely are reported.

Sarcoidosis of the small bones of the hands and feet also is called Perthes disease or Jüngling

disease. The axial skeleton and long bones uncommonly are involved.

Microscopic Findings

Diagnosis of sarcoidosis requires a tissue biopsy and histomorphologic examination. Bone and bone marrow involvement in sarcoidosis shows features similar to sarcoidosis elsewhere, including well-demarcated noncaseating granulomas formed by epithelioid histiocytes and associated multinucleated giant cells along with asteroid and Schaumann bodies. Necrosis in granulomas rarely is seen. The granulomas often are surrounded by reactive T lymphocytes and B lymphocytes, plasma cells, and fibroblasts. In early stages of disease, there is an increased CD4:CD8 ratio, which can be detected by immunohistochemistry or flow cytometry. The epithelioid histiocytes in granulomas usually are positive for lysozyme.

Differential Diagnosis

- Mycobacterial infection, including tuberculosis and Mycobacterium avium-intracellulare complex. Mycobacterium tuberculosis causes ill-demarcated caseating granulomas. Nontuberculosis mycobacterial granulomas often are noncaseating. Staining for acid-fast bacteria shows rod-shaped organisms. Culture is definitive.
- Fungal infections, including histoplasma and cryptococcus. Histoplasmosis causes large necrotizing granulomas, and Gomori methenamine silver stain highlights yeasts. Cryptococcus often is associated with nonnecrotizing granulomas, and Gomori methenamine silver and periodic acid–Schiff stains highlight the organisms, which vary in size. The cell walls in cryptococcus can be highlighted by use of a mucicarmine stain. Culture is positive for both microorganisms but is slowly being replaced by molecular techniques, as is true for the rest of microbiologic identification and speciation.

SMALL, ROUND CELL TUMORS

Primary small, round cell tumors of bone are a divergent group of neoplasms that largely constitute Ewing sarcoma/primitive neuroectodermal tumor (PNET), small cell osteosarcoma, and mesenchymal chondrosarcoma. Furthermore, there are 2 recently identified round cell sarcomas characterized by harboring CIC-DUX4 and BCOR-CCNB3 fusions, respectively. Often encountered in the differential diagnosis are hematopoietic malignancies (lymphoma and plasmacytoma/myeloma), along with metastatic round cell tumors, including (but not limited to) neuroblastoma, rhabdomyosarcoma, medulloblastoma, desmoplastic small round cell tumor, Wilms tumor, and small cell carcinoma.[42] Rarely, small, round cell morphology may represent an unusual variant/component of a primary or metastatic tumor (ie, synovial sarcoma). Thus, a clinical and pathologic correlation is required during the work-up of a small, round cell tumor involving the bone. Importantly, hematologic malignancies of bone, including myeloid sarcoma, can present as a small, round cell tumor in the biopsy but are outside of the scope of this article.

EWING SARCOMA

The Ewing sarcoma/PNET family of tumors originally was believed separate entities, with the latter demonstrating neuroectodermal differentiation. It now is generally accepted that Ewing sarcoma of bone, extraosseous Ewing sarcoma, PNET, and Askin tumor (PNET arising in the chest wall) are histologic variants of the same tumor spectrum sharing common genetic abnormalities.[42,43] Accounting for 6% to 8% of primary malignant bone tumors, Ewing sarcoma is the second most common bone malignancy in children and young adults after osteosarcoma. The tumor occurs more commonly in whites, with a slight male predominance. It predominantly affects patients between 5 years and 20 years. The patient most commonly presents with pain with or without a mass. Intermittent fever, anemia, and pathologic fracture are uncommon clinical presentations. The classic location is in the diaphysis or metaphysis of long, tubular bones, although it may arise in any bone of the skeleton.[42] An ill-defined, osteolytic (sometimes osteosclerotic) lesion involving the diaphysis of a long tubular bone with an onion skin–like multilayered periosteal reaction is the most characteristic radiologic feature.

The gross pathologic features of Ewing sarcoma (typically seen post–neoadjuvant chemotherapy) are those of an ill-defined, tan-gray mass with destructive borders. Geographic regions of necrosis and hemorrhage often are discernible, reflecting a treatment response to the therapeutic agents. Microscopically, the tumor typically exhibits solid sheets of uniform small, blue, round cells embedded within a vascular-rich stroma with minimal extracellular matrix. The tumor cells are slightly larger than normal lymphocytes and have scant cytoplasm and indistinct cell membranes (Fig. 8). The cytoplasm typically is rich in

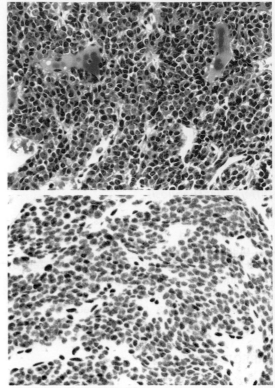

Fig. 8. Ewing sarcoma demonstrates solid sheets of round cells with minimal cytoplasm (*upper panel*, H&E). The lesional cells show diffuse nuclear expression of FLI1 protein (*lower panel*) (original magnification, [*A*] ×200; [*B*] ×200).

glycogen, thus can be highlighted by a periodic acid–Schiff stain. Perivascular rosettes and Homer Wright pseudorosettes may be seen in some cases. Some uncommon morphologic variants reportedly include large cell (atypical Ewing sarcoma), adamantinoma-like, sclerosing, and spindle cell sarcoma-like.[42,44]

Immunophenotypically, diffuse membranous CD99 expression is the most sensitive marker for Ewing sarcoma but is not specific. Nuclear FLI1 and ERG expression is characteristically seen in a majority of Ewing sarcoma cases harboring the t(11;22) (q24;q12) and t(21;22) (q22;q12) chromosomal translocations, respectively. Focal expression of cytokeratin is not an uncommon finding (up to 30% of cases). Importantly, FLI1 expression is not specific for Ewing sarcoma. In addition to its utility as a vascular marker, the molecule is also expressed in a majority of lymphoblastic lymphomas (also CD99-positive), anaplastic large cell lymphomas, and angioimmunoblastic T-cell lymphomas. FLI1 also can be expressed in a small subset of melanomas, Merkel cell carcinomas, synovial sarcomas, and carcinomas of various origins. FLI1 may be convenient, however, in distinguishing Ewing sarcoma from small cell osteosarcoma and mesenchymal chondrosarcoma, both devoid of the molecule, in limited biopsy specimens.

The molecular genetic hallmark of Ewing sarcoma family tumors is the somatic reciprocal chromosomal translocations that lead to fusions of the *EWSR1* gene on chromosome 22 with a member of the *ETS* transcription factor family of genes. An overwhelming majority of Ewing sarcomas are characterized by EWSR1-FLI1 (85%) followed by EWSR1-ERG (approximately 10%) fusions, whereas a large number of other rare alternative fusions have been reported, including EWSR1-ETS, TET-ETS, and non–TET-ETS fusions.[42,43]

Important pathologic prognostic factors include tumor stage, anatomic location, and response to induction chemotherapy (percent tumor necrosis).

MESENCHYMAL CHONDROSARCOMA

Mesenchymal chondrosarcoma most commonly occurs in the craniofacial bones, the ribs, the ilium, and the vertebrae. The peak incidence is in the second and the third decades of life. The cardinal clinical signs are pain and swelling. Skeletal lesions are primarily lytic and destructive with poor margins, often not significantly different from conventional osteosarcoma on imaging studies.[45]

Mesenchymal chondrosarcoma is characterized by a biphasic appearance composed of sheets of primitive small, round, blue cells admixed with islands of well-differentiated hyaline cartilage (**Fig. 9**). The small cell component simulates the histomorphologic features seen in Ewing sarcoma or lymphoma. A hemangiopericytoma-like

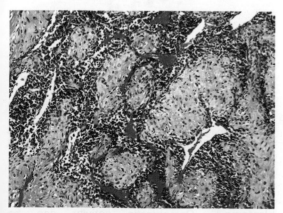

Fig. 9. Mesenchymal chondrosarcoma is characterized by a biphasic appearance composed of islands of well-differentiated hyaline cartilage and sheets of primitive small, round, blue cells (H&E, original magnification ×40).

vascular pattern can be seen in the hypercellular, small cell zones as is subtle osteoid production. The cartilage nodules may mimic normal chondrogenesis in the growth plate or can be indistinguishable from a well-differentiated chondrosarcoma. The transition between the 2 components may be abrupt or gradual.[46] The small cell component is variably positive for CD99. SOX9, a principal regulator of chondrogenesis, is positive in both small cell and cartilaginous components in nearly 100% of cases but negative in other small cell malignancies. Thus, the marker may serve as a useful tool in the differential diagnosis of small, blue, round cell tumors. Recent molecular genetic studies have demonstrated that a HEY1-NCOA2 fusion is the defining molecular signature and is diagnostic at least for a majority of mesenchymal chondrosarcomas, although an *IRF2BP2-CDX1* fusion as the sole chromosomal abnormality has also been reported in mesenchymal chondrosarcoma lacking a HEY1-NCOA2 fusion. On the other hand, *IDH1* or *IDH2* mutations frequently harbored in chondromas and chondrosarcomas have not been identified in mesenchymal chondrosarcoma.[42]

Mesenchymal chondrosarcoma is an aggressive disease generally associated with a dismal outcome. The patient is generally treated with surgical resection followed by adjuvant chemotherapy. Young age and involvement of gnathic bones reportedly are associated with a slightly better prognosis.[45]

OTHER PRIMARY SMALL, ROUND CELL SARCOMAS

A small subset of sarcomas that clinically and histologically mimic Ewing sarcoma but fail to demonstrate any of the reported cytogenetic abnormalities, described previously, exist. These tumors also have been historically designated as Ewing-like sarcomas. Recent studies to that end have led to identifying a few novel molecular genetic abnormalities other than rearrangement of EWSR1 or other TET family members in tumors with primitive round cell morphology.

Round cell sarcoma harboring a CIC-DUX4 fusion, resulting from the chromosomal translocation t(4;19) (q35;q13), mostly arises in deep or superficial soft tissue, but also rarely may involve viscera and bone, with a wide age distribution.[42,47] It has been suggested that some morphologic features, such as myxoid stromal change, nuclear atypia and clear cell cytology, may predict the presence of a CIC–DUX4 translocation.[47] Rare alternative fusion partners also have been identified, including t(18;19) (q23;q13.2) and t(4;22) (q35;q12) [EWSR1–DUX4]. It remains unclear how to classify these variants due to their rarity. Patients with CIC-DUX4 fusion-positive sarcomas generally are aggressive tumors with high disease-associated mortality.[42,47]

A new subtype of bone sarcoma also has been defined by the presence of a BCOR-CCNB3 gene fusion. Most of these tumors were localized to bone with rare cases involving soft tissue.[42] The tumor occurs exclusively in adolescents or young adults. BCOR-CCNB3–positive tumors typically exhibit nuclear CCNB3 immunoreactivity, thus highlighting the potential utility of this marker as a diagnostic tool. BCOR-CCNB3 fusion-positive tumors generally have an unfavorable prognosis.

METASTATIC SMALL, ROUND CELL TUMORS

Virtually all small, round cell tumors of extraskeletal origin may relapse in bone. These tumors include, but are not limited to, neuroblastoma, rhabdomyosarcoma (**Fig. 10**), small cell carcinoma, desmoplastic small round cell tumor, Wilms tumor, medulloblastoma, retinoblastoma, and hepatoblastoma. The differential diagnosis of small round cell tumors is particularly challenging due to their undifferentiated and primitive nature. Moreover, some of the cytomorphologic characteristics of the primary tumor may not be seen in the metastasis, because chemotherapy may induce differentiation in some of the primitive cells.[44] Therefore, a careful clinical-radiologic-pathologic correlation is needed to reach a correct diagnosis. Some of the more commonly encountered small, round cell tumors of bone are summarized in **Table 3**.

METASTASES TO BONE

Bone is the third most frequent site for metastatic disease after lung and liver.[48] The most common metastatic tumors of bone are prostate, breast, thyroid, lung, bladder, and renal cell carcinoma along with melanoma.[49] Rarely sarcoma can metastasize to bone and bone marrow. Bone metastases can be osteolytic, osteoblastic, or mixed.

Osteolytic metastasis is characterized by destruction of normal bone by osteoclasts stimulated through receptor activator of nuclear factor κB pathway.[50] Parathyroid hormone–related peptide also has a major role in osteolytic metastatic disease.[51] Osteolytic metastasis often seen in plasma cell myeloma, non–small cell lung cancer, renal cell carcinoma, melanoma, and thyroid carcinomas.

Osteoblastic and osteosclerotic metastases typically show formation of new bone (**Fig. 11**),

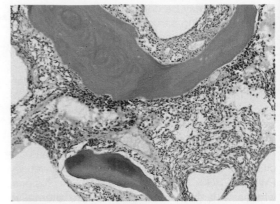
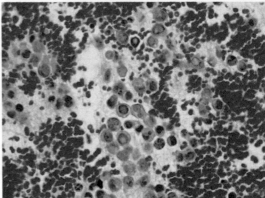
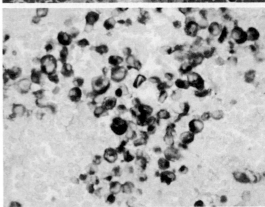

Fig. 10. Metastatic rhabdomyosarcoma in the bone with crush artifact (*upper panel*, [H&E, original magnification ×40]). The clot section exhibits abundant rhabdomyoblasts containing eccentric nuclei in an eosinophilic cytoplasm (*middle panel*, [H&E, original magnification ×200]). The lesional cells show strong desmin expression (*lower panel*, original magnification ×200).

commonly seen in prostate cancer, small cell carcinoma of lung, Hodgkin lymphoma, and medulloblastoma.[49] Osteoblastic activity can be stimulated by transforming growth factor, bone morphogenic protein, and endothelin-1.[52] Runx-2, the core binding protein, also is linked to osteoblastic differentiation of stem cells.[53] Mixed

Table 3
Salient histologic features, key immunophenotypes and molecular genetic characteristics of selected round cell tumors

Tumor Type	Salient Histologic Features	Key Immunophenotype/Molecular Studies
Ewing sarcoma	Uniform small round cells	• CD99, FLI-1 or ERG • t(11;22) (q24;q12) ESWR1-FLI1; t(21;22) (q22;q12) EWSR1-ERG
Mesenchymal chondrosarcoma	Biphasic pattern composed of poorly differentiated small round cells and well-differentiated hyaline cartilage	• SOX9 • HEY1-NCOA2
Small cell osteosarcoma	Small cells with variable degree of osteoid production	• SATB2
Rhabdomyosarcoma	Primitive cells with round or spindled nuclei and variable content of rhabdomyoblasts	• Desmin, myogenin, MyoD1 • t(2;13) (q35;q14) PAX3-FOXO1 or t(1;13) (p36;q14) PAX7-FOXO1 (alveolar rhabdomyosarcoma)
Desmoplastic small round cell tumor	Small round cells with prominent stromal desmoplasia with polyphenotypic differentiation	• Epithelial (keratins/EMA), muscular (dotlike desmin) and neural (NSE) differentiation; WT1 (antibody to the C-terminus) • t(11;22) (p13;q12) EWSR1-WT1
Small cell carcinoma	Small cells with scant cytoplasm and salt-and-pepper chromatin	• Keratin (dotlike, paranuclear or diffuse cytoplasmic staining), neuroendocrine markers, TTF1
Neuroblastoma	Primitive-appearing small round cells in the background of neuropil (Homer-Wright pseudorosettes)	• Neuroendocrine markers
Wilms tumor	Triphasic combination of blastemal, stromal and epithelial cell types	• WT1
Medulloblastoma	Small round undifferentiated cells, Homer-Wright pseudorosettes	• Neuroendocrine markers

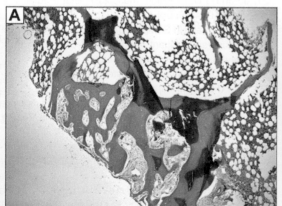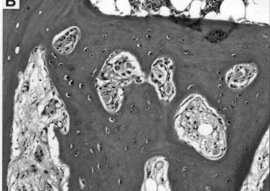

Fig. 11. Low (*A*) and high power (*B*) views of metastatic prostate cancer in the marrow spare showing an osteosclerotic pattern (H&E, original magnification [*A*] × 20; [*B*] × 100).

osteolytic and osteoblastic lesion can be seen in breast cancer, gastrointestinal carcinomas, and squamous cell carcinoma.

SUMMARY

Many primary or metastatic bone diseases demonstrate largely overlapping histomorphologic features with hematologic disorders, thus resulting in diagnostic challenges. Correlation with the clinical and radiologic characteristics of the lesion is critical to reach the correct diagnosis. Immunohistochemical and molecular genetic analyses provide useful tools in accurately characterizing these lesions.

REFERENCES

1. International Myeloma Working Group. Criteria for the classification of monoclonal gammopathies, multiple myeloma and related disorders: a report of the International Myeloma Working Group. Br J Haematol 2003;121(5):749–57.

2. Dores GM, Landgren O, McGlynn KA, et al. Plasmacytoma of bone, extramedullary plasmacytoma, and multiple myeloma: incidence and survival in the United States, 1992-2004. Br J Haematol 2009; 144(1):86–94.

3. Thumallapally N, Meshref A, Mousa M, et al. Solitary plasmacytoma: population-based analysis of survival trends and effect of various treatment modalities in the USA. BMC Cancer 2017;17(1):13.

4. Grammatico S, Scalzulli E, Petrucci MT. Solitary plasmacytoma. Mediterr J Hematol Infect Dis 2017; 9(1):e2017052.

5. de Waal EG, Leene M, Veeger N, et al. Progression of a solitary plasmacytoma to multiple myeloma. A population-based registry of the northern Netherlands. Br J Haematol 2016;175(4):661–7.

6. Rodallec MH, Feydy A, Larousserie F, et al. Diagnostic imaging of solitary tumors of the spine: what to do and say. Radiographics 2008;28(4):1019–41.

7. Caers J, Paiva B, Zamagni E, et al. Diagnosis, treatment, and response assessment in solitary plasmacytoma: updated recommendations from a European Expert Panel. J Hematol Oncol 2018; 11(1):10.

8. Dingli D, Kyle RA, Rajkumar SV, et al. Immunoglobulin free light chains and solitary plasmacytoma of bone. Blood 2006;108(6):1979–83.

9. Rajkumar SV, Dimopoulos MA, Palumbo A, et al. International Myeloma Working Group updated criteria for the diagnosis of multiple myeloma. Lancet Oncol 2014;15(12):e538–48.

10. Ely SA, Knowles DM. Expression of CD56/neural cell adhesion molecule correlates with the presence of lytic bone lesions in multiple myeloma and distinguishes myeloma from monoclonal gammopathy of undetermined significance and lymphomas with plasmacytoid differentiation. Am J Pathol 2002; 160(4):1293–9.

11. Seegmiller AC, Xu Y, McKenna RW, et al. Immunophenotypic differentiation between neoplastic plasma cells in mature B-cell lymphoma vs plasma cell myeloma. Am J Clin Pathol 2007;127(2):176–81.

12. Knobel D, Zouhair A, Tsang RW, et al. Prognostic factors in solitary plasmacytoma of the bone: a multicenter Rare Cancer Network study. BMC Cancer 2006;6:118.

13. Warsame R, Gertz MA, Lacy MQ, et al. Trends and outcomes of modern staging of solitary plasmacytoma of bone. Am J Hematol 2012;87(7): 647–51.

14. Dispenzieri A, Kyle R, Merlini G, et al. International Myeloma Working Group guidelines for serum-free light chain analysis in multiple myeloma and related disorders. Leukemia 2009;23(2):215–24.

15. Osteogenic tumours. In: Fletcher DMC, Bridge JA, Hogendoorn PCW, et al, editors. WHO classification of tumours of soft tissue and bone. Lyon (France): International Agency for Research on Cencer; 2013. p. 275–96.

16. Xing D, Qasem SA, Owusu K, et al. Changing prognostic factors in osteosarcoma: analysis of 381 cases from two institutions. Hum Pathol 2014;45(8): 1688–96.

17. Conner JR, Hornick JL. SATB2 is a novel marker of osteoblastic differentiation in bone and soft tissue tumours. Histopathology 2013;63(1):36–49.

18. Nunez AL, Siegal GP, Reddy VV, et al. CD138 (syndecan-1) expression in bone-forming tumors. Am J Clin Pathol 2012;137(3):423–8.

19. Kremers HM, Nwojo ME, Ransom JE, et al. Trends in the epidemiology of osteomyelitis: a population-based study, 1969 to 2009. J Bone Joint Surg Am 2015;97(10):837–45.

20. Schmitt SK. Osteomyelitis. Infect Dis Clin North Am 2017;31(2):325–38.

21. Jaramillo D. Infection: musculoskeletal. Pediatr Radiol 2011;41(Suppl 1):S127–34.

22. Lee YJ, Sadigh S, Mankad K, et al. The imaging of osteomyelitis. Quant Imaging Med Surg 2016;6(2): 184–98.

23. Momodu II, Savaliya V. Osteomyelitis. Treasure Island (FL): StatPearls; 2018.

24. Weitzman S, Egeler RM. Langerhans cell histiocytosis: update for the pediatrician. Curr Opin Pediatr 2008;20(1):23–9.

25. Leonidas JC, Guelfguat M, Valderrama E. Langerhans' cell histiocytosis. Lancet 2003;361(9365): 1293–5.

26. Guyot-Goubin A, Donadieu J, Barkaoui M, et al. Descriptive epidemiology of childhood Langerhans cell histiocytosis in France, 2000-2004. Pediatr Blood Cancer 2008;51(1):71–5.

27. Haupt R, Minkov M, Astigarraga I, et al. Langerhans cell histiocytosis (LCH): guidelines for diagnosis, clinical work-up, and treatment for patients till the age of 18 years. Pediatr Blood Cancer 2013;60(2): 175–84.

28. Christopher Z, Binitie O, Henderson-Jackson E, et al. Langerhans cell histiocytosis of bone in an adult: a case report. Radiol Case Rep 2018;13(2): 310–4.

29. Badalian-Very G, Vergilio JA, Degar BA, et al. Recurrent BRAF mutations in Langerhans cell histiocytosis. Blood 2010;116(11):1919–23.

30. Rizzo FM, Cives M, Simone V, et al. New insights into the molecular pathogenesis of langerhans cell histiocytosis. Oncologist 2014;19(2):151–63.

31. Swerdlow SH, Campo E, Harris NL, et al. WHO classification of tumours of haematopoietic and lymphoid tissues. Lyon: International Agency for Research on Cancer; 2008.

32. Delsignore JL, Dvoretsky PM, Hicks DG, et al. Mastocytosis presenting as a skeletal disorder. Iowa Orthop J 1996;16:126–34.

33. Rossini M, Zanotti R, Viapiana O, et al. Bone involvement and osteoporosis in mastocytosis. Immunol Allergy Clin North Am 2014;34(2):383–96.

34. Orsolini G, Viapiana O, Rossini M, et al. Bone disease in mastocytosis. Immunol Allergy Clin North Am 2018;38(3):443–54.

35. Mayado A, Teodosio C, Garcia-Montero AC, et al. Increased IL6 plasma levels in indolent systemic mastocytosis patients are associated with high risk of disease progression. Leukemia 2016;30(1): 124–30.

36. Chatterjee A, Ghosh J, Kapur R. Mastocytosis: a mutated KIT receptor induced myeloproliferative disorder. Oncotarget 2015;6(21):18250–64.

37. Pardanani A, Lasho T, Elala Y, et al. Next-generation sequencing in systemic mastocytosis: derivation of a mutation-augmented clinical prognostic model for survival. Am J Hematol 2016;91(9):888–93.

38. Haenisch B, Nothen MM, Molderings GJ. Systemic mast cell activation disease: the role of molecular genetic alterations in pathogenesis, heritability and diagnostics. Immunology 2012;137(3):197–205.

39. Foucar E, Rosai J, Dorfman R. Sinus histiocytosis with massive lymphadenopathy (Rosai-Dorfman disease): review of the entity. Semin Diagn Pathol 1990; 7(1):19–73.

40. Demicco EG, Rosenberg AE, Bjornsson J, et al. Primary Rosai-Dorfman disease of bone: a clinicopathologic study of 15 cases. Am J Surg Pathol 2010;34(9):1324–33.

41. Nessrine A, Zahra AF, Taoufik H. Musculoskeletal involvement in sarcoidosis. J Bras Pneumol 2014; 40(2):175–82.

42. Wei S, Siegal GP. Round cell tumors of bone: an update on recent molecular genetic advances. Adv Anat Pathol 2014;21(5):359–72.

43. de Alava E, Lessnick SL, Sorensen PH. Ewing sarcoma. In: Fletcher DMC, Bridge JA, Hogendoorn PCW, et al, editors. WHO classification of tumours of soft tissue and bone. Lyon (France): International Agency for Research on Cencer; 2013. p. 305–9.

44. Small, round cell lesions. In: Wei S, Siegal GP, editors. Atlas of bone pathology. New York: Springer; 2013. p. 237–82.

45. Nakashima Y, de Pinieux G, Ladanyi M. Mesenchymal chondrosarcoma. In: Fletcher DMC, Bridge JA, Hogendoorn PCW, et al, editors. WHO classification of tumours of soft tissue and bone. Lyon (France): International Agency for Research on Cencer; 2013. p. 271–2.

46. Cartilage-forming tumors. In: Wei S, Siegal GP, editors. Atlas of bone pathology. New York: Springer; 2013. p. 101–56.

47. Gambarotti M, Benini S, Gamberi G, et al. CIC-DUX4 fusion-positive round-cell sarcomas of soft tissue and bone: a single-institution morphological and molecular analysis of seven cases. Histopathology 2016;69(4):624–34.

48. Coleman RE. Metastatic bone disease: clinical features, pathophysiology and treatment strategies. Cancer Treat Rev 2001;27(3):165–76.

49. Macedo F, Ladeira K, Pinho F, et al. Bone metastases: an overview. Oncol Rev 2017;11(1):321.

50. Dougall WC, Glaccum M, Charrier K, et al. RANK is essential for osteoclast and lymph node development. Genes Dev 1999;13(18):2412–24.

51. Southby J, Kissin MW, Danks JA, et al. Immunohistochemical localization of parathyroid hormone-related protein in human breast cancer. Cancer Res 1990;50(23):7710–6.

52. Keller ET, Zhang J, Cooper CR, et al. Prostate carcinoma skeletal metastases: cross-talk between tumor and bone. Cancer Metastasis Rev 2001;20(3–4): 333–49.

53. Yang X, Karsenty G. Transcription factors in bone: developmental and pathological aspects. Trends Mol Med 2002;8(7):340–5.

Castleman Disease

Wei Wang, MD, PhD, L. Jeffrey Medeiros, MD*

KEYWORDS

- Castleman disease • Lymphoproliferative disorder • Unicentric hyaline-vascular Castleman disease
- Multicentric Castleman disease • Human herpes virus type 8

Key Points

- From a clinical point of view, Castleman disease (CD) is divided into unicentric and multicentric types. Histologically, CD is divided into hyaline-vascular and plasma cell variants.

- Unicentric CD is most common and the majority of these cases are hyaline-vascular type. Surgical excision is often curative.

- Multicentric CD is a heterogeneous group composed of HHV8-associated, idiopathic and cases associated with POEMs syndrome. Although there is no consensus approach, therapy is often required for patients in this group.

ABSTRACT

Castleman disease (CD) is divided clinically into unicentric or multicentric type. Pathologically, CD is divided into hyaline-vascular and plasma cell variants. Unicentric CD is most common, about 75% of these cases are hyaline-vascular variant, and surgical excision is often curative. In contrast, there are a number of types of multicentric CD including HHV8-associated, idiopathic, and a subset of cases that arise in association with POEMS syndrome. Therapy is required for most patients with multicentric CD, but there is no consensus approach currently. As is evidence, the designation Castleman disease encompasses a heterogeneous group of diseases of varied pathogenesis and which require different therapies.

OVERVIEW

Benjamin Castleman initially described a large, benign, asymptomatic mass involving mediastinal lymph nodes.[1,2] He later described a series of similar cases and refined the concept. A number of synonyms were used to designate these cases, such as angiofollicular lymph node hyperplasia, giant lymph node hyperplasia, angiomatous lymphoid hamartoma, and benign giant lymphoma.[3,4] However, these terms are currently rarely used or they are obsolete and this disease came to be known as the hyaline-vascular variant of Castleman disease (HV-CD). Subsequently, the plasma cell (PC) variant of CD[3,5] and multicentric CD were described.[6,7]

CLASSIFICATION

CD is a lymphoproliferative disorder that primarily involves lymph nodes. From a clinical point of view, CD is subdivided into unicentric and multicentric types (**Fig. 1**). Unicentric CD is localized involving a single lymph node or a group of closely located lymph nodes at the same anatomic site. Multicentric CD is a systemic lymphoproliferative disorder involving multiple lymph nodes at different sites, often associated with B-type symptoms, body cavity effusions, hepatosplenomegaly, and laboratory abnormalities. Several subtypes of multicentric CD have been identified (**Fig. 2**) and include (1) cases attributable to human herpes virus type 8 (HHV8) infection; (2) cases associated with POEMS (*p*olyneuropathy, *o*rganomegaly, *e*ndocrinopathy, *m*onoclonal immunoglobulin in serum, and *s*kin changes) syndrome; and (3)

The authors declare no conflict of interest.
Department of Hematopathology, The University of Texas MD Anderson Cancer Center, 1515 Holcombe Boulevard, Houston, TX 77030, USA
* Corresponding author.
E-mail address: ljmedeiros@mdanderson.org

Castleman Disease

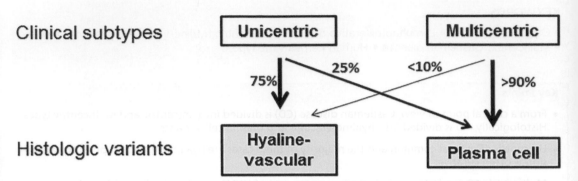

Clinical subtypes

| Unicentric | | Multicentric |

75%   25%   <10%   >90%

Histologic variants

| Hyaline-vascular | Plasma cell |

Fig. 1. The clinical subtypes (unicentric vs multicentric) and histologic variants (hyaline vascular and PC) of CD.

idiopathic multicentric CD including a subset associated with TAFRO (*t*hrombocytopenia, *a*nasarca, *f*ever, *r*enal insufficiency, and *o*rgano-megaly) syndrome.[8] Depending on the study, uni-centric CD represents about up to 80% of all cases of CD,[8–10] and multicentric CD represents 20% to 25% of all cases of CD. Histologically, there are 2 morphologic variants of CD (see **Fig. 1**): HV and PC. There is a clear correlation between the morphologic variants of CD and their clinical pre-sentation. Depending on the study, 65% to 80% of cases of unicentric CD have histologic features of HV variant,[9,10] and the remaining 20% to 35% of cases have histologic features of the PC variant. In contrast, more than 90% of cases of multicentric CD have morphologic features of the PC variant.

CLINICAL FEATURES

UNICENTRIC CASTLEMAN DISEASE

Unicentric HV-CD is usually discovered in adults with a median age in the fourth decade, but can

arise in children or the elderly.[5,10–13] Males and fe-males are equally affected. Patients with HV-CD are often completely asymptomatic and a single or unicentric lesion is detected as an incidental finding during routine physical examination and/or imaging studies performed as part of the workup of an unrelated disease. HV-CD usually in-volves lymph nodes, especially mediastinal lymph nodes, but the spleen can be involved and other extranodal sites, such as soft tissue can be involved rarely. In most patients, HV-CD occurs in lymph nodes above the diaphragm, but abdom-inal lymph nodes can be involved in a subset of cases, particularly in stromal-rich cases.[14] Symp-toms, when present, are often related to the size of the mass and compression of adjacent struc-tures, such as airway compression with shortness of breath or vascular compression that can lead to esophageal varices.[5,11,15] HV-CD is associated with paraneoplastic pemphigus, but in less than 5% patients.[16] Rare patients with HV-CD involving the mediastinum also have had myasthenia

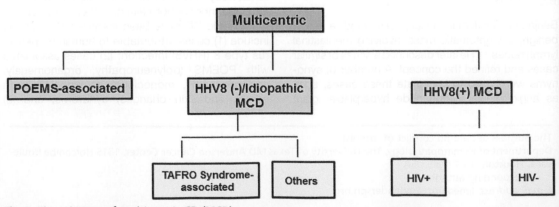

Fig. 2. The subtypes of multicentric CD (MCD).

gravis.[17] Laboratory abnormalities and systemic symptoms are rare in patients with unicentric HV-CD, although serum lactate dehydrogenase (LDH) levels can be elevated in a subset of patients.[11,12]

Unicentric PC-CD occurs over a broad age range, but patients tend to be older than those with HV-CD. No gender preference is noted. It can involve any lymph node, but the mediastinum is involved less frequently than in patients with HV-CD. Patients are often asymptomatic, but systemic symptoms and laboratory abnormalities have been reported in a small subset of patients.[8,10,13] In cases with systemic symptoms, multicentric CD must be excluded because it is possible that some patients diagnosed with unicentric PC-CD in the past may, in fact, have had multicentric disease. This misinterpretation also may be true for some cases of symptomatic unicentric PC-CD reported in the literature. The symptoms most commonly reported in these patients include fever, night sweats, weight loss, and malaise. Laboratory studies most commonly show anemia or thrombocytopenia. Serum IL-6 levels are increased and dysregulation of IL-6 is likely involved in the pathogenesis of unicentric PC-CD.[8]

MULTICENTRIC CASTLEMAN DISEASE

Patients with multicentric CD can be of any age.[13,18] Physical examination and/or imaging studies show lymphadenopathy, either peripheral or abdominal. Mediastinal lymph nodes can be involved, but less often than in patients with unicentric HV-CD.[10,13,18] Splenomegaly (~75%) and hepatomegaly (~50%) are common in patients with multicentric CD. Edema, body cavity effusions, skin rash, and neurologic changes can occur in a small subset of patients.[10,13,18] Fever, night sweats, and/or weight loss (B-type symptoms) occur in more than 95% of patients.[10,13,18,19] The symptoms of multicentric CD are often episodic. Laboratory abnormalities also occur in most patients with multicentric CD. Anemia, thrombocytopenia, polyclonal hyper-gammaglobulinemia, an increased erythrocyte sedimentation rate, and elevated serum levels of IL-6, LDH, γ-interferon, and C-reactive protein are common.[10,18,20]

Human Herpes-8–Positive Multicentric Castleman Disease

Approximately 50% to 60% of cases of multicentric CD are caused by HHV8 infection.[10,13,18] Immunodeficiency of various causes in these patients allows HHV8 to reactivate. These patients can be further subdivided into 2 subsets: those associated with human immunodeficiency virus (HIV) infection and HIV-negative patients. In the United States, HHV8-positive multicentric CD is highly associated with HIV infection and, therefore, the epidemiologic features of this patient group are predominantly those of patients with AIDS. In contrast, HHV8+ multicentric CD in the absence of HIV infection is more common in HHV8 endemic regions and patients tend to be older. The seroprevalance rate of *HHV8* is estimated to be 5% or less in the United Kingdom, up to 25% in some areas of the United States, 10% to 35% in Mediterranean countries, and approximately 50% in sub-Saharan Africa.[21]

Idiopathic Multicentric Castleman Disease

Depending on the study, idiopathic multicentric CD represents about 30% to 50% of all multicentric CD cases. There is a wide age range with a median age in the fourth decade. There is either a slight male predominance or no sex preference. Within the idiopathic group, there is a subgroup of patients who have TAFRO syndrome.[13,19,22] The median age of patients with TAFRO is in the sixth decade, but there is a wide age range.[22] The clinical course can be acute or subacute, but is generally more aggressive than patients with non-TAFRO idiopathic multicentric CD. The presence of thrombocytopenia, normal serum immunoglobulin levels, and severe fluid accumulation in body cavities or massive peripheral edema distinguishes TAFRO from non-TAFRO idiopathic multicentric CD.[22,23] Lymphadenopathy tends to be more prominent in patients with idiopathic multicentric CD of non-TAFRO type.[22] Kawabata and colleagues[24] have suggested the term idiopathic plasmacytic lymphadenopathy with polyclonal hyperimmunoglobulinemia for non-TAFRO cases of idiopathic multicentric CD.

POEMS Syndrome

This disease was first described in 1938, but became much better known after the acronym POEMS was introduced by Bardwick and colleagues.[25] Patients with POEMS syndrome have a constellation of clinical and laboratory abnormalities. Peripheral neuropathy (symmetric and both sensory and motor) and a monotypic PC neoplasm (usually lambda light chain) are present in all patients; Plasma cell variant CD is present in 25% to 50% of patients. Other features of POEMS include sclerotic bone lesions, hepatosplenomegaly, lymphadenopathy, peripheral edema or body cavity effusions, abnormalities in endocrine organ function (eg, hypogonadism, glucose metabolism abnormalities, adrenal insufficiency, etc), papilledema, thrombocytosis and/or polycythemia, and many skin changes including hyperpigmentation, hypertrichosis, acrocyanosis, white nails, and a distinctive skin neoplasm, glomeruloid hemangioma.[26,27]

PATHOGENESIS

UNICENTRIC CASTLEMAN DISEASE

Unicentric HV-CD is likely a benign neoplasm of follicular dendritic cells (FDC) and this theory is supported by the absence of monoclonal immunoglobulin and T-cell receptor gene rearrangements, the presence of dysplastic FDCs, subsequent risk of developing FDC sarcoma in a small subset of HV-CD cases, identification of clonal cytogenetic abnormalities in a small number of HV-CD cases, and loss of heterozygosity as determined by assessing the human androgen receptor alpha (HUMARA) gene in most cases.[28–30]

The neoplastic nature of unicentric HV-CD does not necessarily explain other histologic findings identified in this disease, such as the prominent lymphoid infiltrate and vascular proliferation with sclerosis. Cytokines and adhesion molecules such as vascular endothelial growth factor (VEGF), intercellular adhesion molecule-1 (ICAM1, CD54), and CXCL13 are likely involved in pathogenesis, whereas IL-6, a key player in multicentric CD, may play little or no role in HV-CD.[8,31] The effects of cytokines are likely amplified by the obliteration of lymph node sinuses, which impairs the flow of lymph and makes the lymph node a closed system. The poorly developed or atrophic follicles observed in HV-CD suggest that follicle formation is impaired or disorganized. A disturbance of B-cell and FDC interaction or a block in development or maturation of type 2 dendritic cells (also known as plasmacytoid monocytes) has been proposed, but is unproven.[14,31]

Based on the histologic resemblance of unicentric PC-CD to multicentric CD, it seems likely that the pathogenesis of PC-CD also may be related to an overproduction of IL-6.[8] Unicentric PC-CD also can share some similar morphologic features with lymph nodes in autoimmune diseases, such as rheumatoid arthritis; therefore, unicentric PC-CD may arise as part of an autoimmune reaction pattern.

MULTICENTRIC CASTLEMAN DISEASE

IL-6 plays a key role in the development of multicentric CD. Serum IL-6 levels are elevated in patients with multicentric CD during symptomatic episodes.[32] Cells within lymph nodes from patients with multicentric CD express and produce high levels of IL-6 as detected by in situ hybridization and immunohistochemical methods.[33] Accordingly, B lymphocytes from patients with CD overexpress the IL-6 receptor CD126 and, thus, autocrine and paracrine mechanisms may be involved.[34] IL-6 is a pleiotropic lymphokine involved in differentiation of B lymphocytes to PCs.[35] IL-6 also plays a role in T-cell regulation, stimulates the production of acute phase reactants from hepatocytes, and is an endogenous pyrogen.[35,36] IL-6 overproduction may explain the presence of B-type symptoms.[32,37] Using animal models, mice injected with bone marrow cells genetically engineered to overexpress IL-6 develop a syndrome that resembles multicentric CD,[38] further supporting a pathogenic role for IL-6 in multicentric CD.

In addition to IL-6, other cytokines are likely involved in the pathogenesis of multicentric CD. VEGF, a potent angiogenic factor found to be elevated in the serum of patients with multicentric CD, is likely to be responsible for hypervascularity. There is also some evidence to suggest that immune dysregulation may be involved in the pathogenesis of multicentric CD. Many patients with multicentric CD have autoimmune-type phenomena.[39] Laboratory abnormalities commonly associated with immune dysfunction can occur in patients with multicentric CD, including elevated levels of IL-6, IL-2 receptor, LDH, beta-2-microglobulin, hypergammaglobulinemia (IgA, IgG, and IgE), and cytopenias.[10,19] Multicentric CD can occur in patients with inherited immunodeficiency, such as Wiskott-Aldrich syndrome, as well as acquired immunodeficiency, most often HIV infection.[40]

Human Herpes Virus Type 8–Positive Multicentric Castleman Disease

Infection by HHV8, also known as Kaposi sarcoma herpes virus, is the most common known cause of multicentric CD. HHV8 is a γ-herpes virus with at least 11 open reading frames and encodes a number of homologs of cellular proteins involved in cell cycle regulation, control of apoptosis, immune modulation, and signal transduction.[41] HHV8 encodes for viral IL-6, a homolog of human IL-6, which can stimulate human IL-6–induced cellular pathways and, by this mechanism, plays a role in pathogenesis.[42] The role of other viral homologs of cellular proteins in disease pathogenesis is unknown, but it seems likely some of these viral proteins also may be involved. In *HHV8*-associated multicentric CD, human IL-6 levels are also increased. HHV8 load in peripheral blood mononuclear cells correlates with aggressiveness of disease.[43]

Idiopathic Multicentric Castleman Disease

In contrast with the well-known HHV8-induced IL-6 production in HHV8-associated multicentric CD, the mechanisms of IL-6 elevation in idiopathic multicentric CD are unknown. A number of hypotheses have been suggested as potential causes, including infection by a virus that is as yet undiscovered; an autoimmune etiology as a result of autoantibodies or germline mutations in genes involved in cell pathways normally involved in inflammation; or a paraneoplastic syndrome.[8] The end result is thought to result in cytokine dysregulation involving IL-6 and/or VEGF as well as other cytokines in patients with idiopathic multicentric CD.

POEMS Syndrome

These patients have a monoclonal PC neoplasm and the PCs (possibly other cells as well) likely secrete cytokines or stimulate other cells to secrete cytokines including VEGF, IL-6, IL-1β, IL-12, and tumor necrosis factor-α, resulting in a cytokine storm, similar to other types of multicentric CD.[26]

HISTOPATHOLOGY

UNICENTRIC CASTLEMAN DISEASE

Grossly, HV-CD presents as a mass in lymph node that is commonly large and firm. The cut surface is white and may be calcified. The size of involved lymph nodes is variable, ranging from 1.5 to 20.0 cm with a median of 5.8 cm in an early study[5] and 7.0 cm in a more recent study.[14]

The overall lymph node architecture is distorted. The histologic findings in HV-CD can be divided into 2 broad groups: follicular changes and interfollicular/stromal changes. Follicular changes are characterized by an increased number of follicles, scattered throughout the cortex and medulla, and often contain 2 or more small germinal centers (so-called twinning)[4,5,14] (Fig. 3). The follicles can be round or irregular

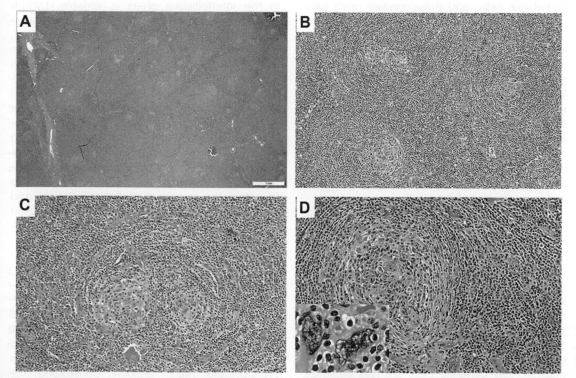

Fig. 3. HV-CD, follicular variant. (A) The lymph node architecture is distorted with obliteration of the sinuses. Background fibrosis is present. Follicles are increased in numbers with atrophic germinal centers surrounded by expanded mantle zones. (B) Germinal centers show decreased numbers of lymphocytes (lymphocyte depletion) and increased numbers of FDCs. Mantle zones are expanded, composed of concentric rings of small lymphocytes (onion skin pattern). Vascular proliferation is present in the follicles and interfollicular areas with sclerotic blood vessels penetrating the germinal centers (lollipop lesions). (C) The follicle shown contains 2 germinal centers (so-called twinning), a feature commonly seen in HV-CD. (D) Large and bizarre cells consistent with dysplastic FDCs are present in germinal centers, mantle zones, and interfollicular areas.

and variably sized, but these follicles are usually of approximately the same size within an individual case. The germinal centers are depleted of small lymphocytes and are composed of increased numbers of FDCs. Hyaline deposits, highlighted by the periodic acid–Schiff reaction, can be prominent within germinal centers. Sclerotic blood vessels radially penetrate the germinal centers, forming HV lesions (also known as lollipop lesions). In some cases, FDCs or other stromal cells can be large and bizarre, consistent with dysplastic features[5,31,44] (see **Fig. 3D**). Dysplastic FDCs can be present as single scattered cells or small nodules and can be found in germinal centers, mantle zones, or interfollicular regions. The mantle zones of these follicles are broad and in many cases, the mantle zones are composed of concentric rings of small lymphocytes (the so-called onion skin pattern).[4,5,14] At low power, these changes in the follicles impart a target-like appearance (see **Fig. 3**). The expanded follicles can compress or obliterate contiguous structures. The interfollicular regions in HV-CD are composed of numerous high endothelial venules with plump endothelial cells, and these vessels often have sclerotic walls. Clusters of plasmacytoid dendritic cells are often (but not invariably) present in the interfollicular regions, usually as clusters with a starry sky pattern.[4,5,14] Scattered PCs, immunoblasts, and eosinophils can be seen in the interfollicular regions; sheets of PCs (as seen in PC-CD) are absent. Lymph node sinuses are characteristically absent in fully developed HV-CD and obliteration of the subcapsular sinuses is often an early morphologic change in HV-CD. Usually, the capsule is thickened and dense bands of sclerosis traverse throughout the lymph node parenchyma and surround large blood vessels.

Importantly, the proportions of the follicular and interfollicular changes described are variable in different cases and form a spectrum, ranging from cases characterized mostly by abnormal follicles, so-called follicular HV-CD, to cases with an equivalent degree of changes in the follicles and interfollicular regions, to cases characterized mostly by changes in the interfollicular regions, so-called stroma-rich CD.[14] Arbitrarily, follicular HV-CD can be defined as having follicles that represent more than 50% of the lymph node[14]; plasmacytoid dendritic cells are less common, and the interfollicular areas have less abundant or few sclerotic blood vessels. In the stroma-rich variants of HV-CD, in which interfollicular abnormalities represent more than 50% of the lymph node, the lymph node can be subtotally replaced by numerous sclerotic blood vessels and other spindle cells.[14] These interfollicular

areas, based on their variable cell composition as determined by immunohistochemical reactivity for actin, CD68, or dendritic cell markers, have been referred to as angiomyoid, histiocytic reticulum cell, or FDC stromal proliferations.[14,45] The diagnosis of stroma-rich variant of HV-CD can sometimes be challenging, especially in cases of limited sampling, such as needle core biopsies, which are a popular method for diagnosis in current clinical practice. The diagnostic clues in this scenario include stroma-rich proliferation with many sclerotic blood vessels and spindle cell proliferation including many FDCs (**Fig. 4**).

Unicentric PC-CD is less common and it is important to exclude multicentric CD when the diagnosis is considered, especially in patients with systemic symptoms. In unicentric PC-CD, the interfollicular areas and medulla are occupied by sheets of mature PCs, with occasional binucleated forms (**Fig. 5**).[5,14,46] The PCs are polytypic by immunohistochemical assessment for kappa and lambda, although rare cases with light chain restricted PCs occur. Vascular proliferation in the interfollicular areas is variable. Lymph node sinuses are usually present and can be distended. Follicles in PC-CD are widely scattered, and may contain reactive germinal centers with polarization. Typically, a subset of follicles has HV features, although usually less well-developed than those observed in HV-CD.[5,14] The mantle zones are sharply defined from the interfollicular areas. In the older literature, a subset of cases of CD was described as having mixed histologic features.[3] However, because most cases of PC-CD have some histologic features of HV-CD, many consider mixed cases to fit within the spectrum of the PC variant and the designation mixed type is seldom used currently.

MULTICENTRIC CASTLEMAN DISEASE

All multicentric CD cases share common morphologic features regardless of etiology. Lymphoid follicles can be hyperplastic, but often a subset of follicles show some HV changes, including small germinal centers with lymphocyte depletion and onion skin–like mantle zones. Different from HV-CD, the radial arteriole penetrating the germinal center usually does not have sclerotic walls. In addition, dysplastic FDCs are uncommon.[4,10,19] The interfollicular areas and medulla are expanded by variable numbers of PCs that show a range of maturation, from mature to atypical, the latter associated with HHV8 infection. Vascular proliferation is also present in the

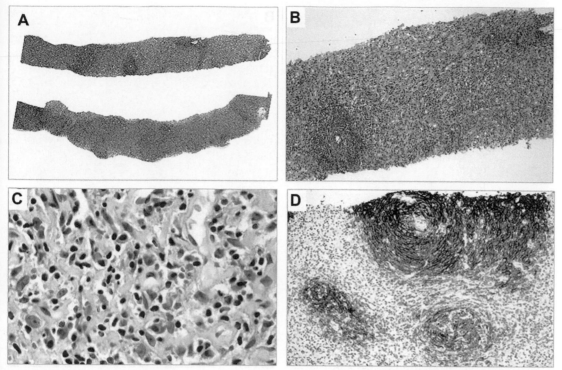

Fig. 4. HV-CD, stroma-rich variant in a needle core biopsy. (*A*) Two needle-shaped fragments of tissue composed of a few follicles with markedly expanded interfollicular areas. (*B, C*) the interfollicular areas are rich in vasculature and composed of many spindle to elongated cells. Many cells are oval to elongated, large in size, with thin nuclear membrane, pale chromatin, and each cell has a small but distinct eosinophilic nucleolus, consistent with FDCs. Scattered small lymphocytes are present in the background. (*D*) in the areas with follicles, anti-CD21 highlights the onion skin appearance of mantle zones.

interfollicular areas.[10,46] Lymph node sinuses are usually patent.

In HHV8+ cases of multicentric CD (**Fig. 6**), the histologic findings are those of PC variant of CD with coexistent evidence of HHV8 infection. The boundary between the mantle zones and the surrounding interfollicular areas is blurred. HHV8+ cells are most often located in the mantle zones of follicles, but also can be scattered in the interfollicular regions.[47] These HHV8+ cells are often large with features of immunoblasts or plasmablasts. Patients with HHV8+ multicentric CD have a higher risk of coexistent HHV8-associated neoplasms such as Kaposi sarcoma (see **Fig. 6**) and HHV8-diffuse large B-cell lymphoma.

In patients with TAFRO, lymph nodes have a mixture of HV and PC variant features that fit, in part, within the spectrum of findings seen in mixed type as described in the older literature. The interfollicular areas and medulla are occupied by variable numbers of mature PCs, which may be present in lesser numbers compared with other subtypes of multicentric CD.[4,19,22] The bone marrow in patients with TAFRO shows increased reticulin fibrosis, increased megakaryocytes that

may show separated nuclear lobes, and, in some cases, emperipolesis. In idiopathic multicentric CD of non-TAFRO type, lymph nodes show features of the PC variant, or less often mixed features of the HV and PC variant. In general, the features of PC variant are better developed in patients without TAFRO syndrome. Unlike HHV8+ multicentric CD, mantle zones are sharply defined from the interfollicular areas in idiopathic multicentric CD.

In POEMS syndrome, most cases of CD show features of the PC variant, but a few HV follicles can be also present. Bone marrow in patients with POEMS usually shows increased monotypic PCs and osteosclerotic bone lesions are common.

There are also unusual cases of multicentric CD in which the histologic features of HV-CD have been reported.[19] These cases represent, at most, about 10% of cases. Because many investigators consider HV variant to occur only in unicentric CD, others have proposed the terminology "hypervascular" to designate multicentric CD cases with HV-like histologic features, but often lacking dysplastic FDC and sclerotic blood vessels.[19]

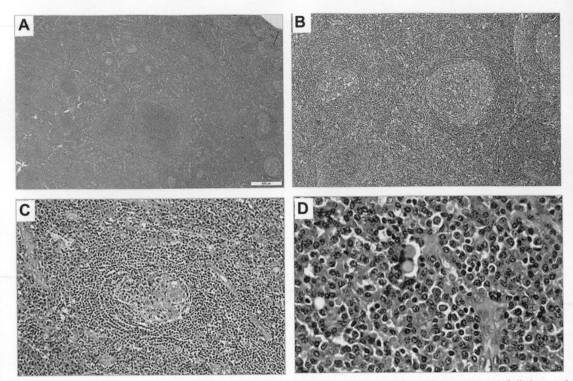

Fig. 5. Unicentric PC-CD. (*A*) the lymph node architecture is distorted with widely scattered follicles and expanded interfollicular regions. (*B*) Some follicles are hyperplastic with polarized germinal centers. (*C*) Other follicles show atrophic germinal centers with increased FDCs and expanded mantle cells. (*D*) The interfollicular areas are occupied by sheets of PCs that are small to intermediate sized with mature appearance.

IMMUNOPHENOTYPE

In HV-CD, the follicles show numerous concentric rings of FDCs that can be highlighted with various markers (CD21, CD23, CD35, epidermal growth factor receptor). These dendritic cells are also commonly positive for vascular cell adhesion molecule (VCAM-1, CD106).[31] The small germinal centers are often variably lymphocyte-depleted, but the B cells that remain are positive for CD10 and BCL-6 and negative for BCL-2. In contrast, the mantle zones of the follicles are expanded and are composed of many B cells positive for polytypic light chains, CD19, CD20, IgD, and BCL-2 and are negative for CD10 and BCL-6; other investigators have reported that these mantle zone B cells are weakly positive for CD5 in a subset of cases using a sensitive rabbit monoclonal antibody.[48] B cells in HV-CD do not express, or express only low levels, of IL-6. In the interfollicular regions, numerous blood vessels are present, and their endothelial cells express vascular markers such as CD31 and factor VIII-related antigen. However, these cells are often negative for HLA-DR and inducible adhesion molecules (eg, VCAM-1 and ICAM-1) and, therefore, are thought to be poorly activated.[31] Clusters of

plasmacytoid dendritic cells are also often present in the interfollicular region, positive for CD68, CD123, and TCL1. T cells with a normal immunophenotype and scattered polytypic PCs are present between the follicles. In stroma-rich variants of HV-CD, numerous CD21-positive cells are present; histiocytes and actin-positive cells also can be numerous.[14,45] There is no evidence of Epstein-Barr virus or HHV8.

In PC-CD, the interfollicular regions are composed of polytypic PCs and T cells without aberrancy. Some follicles often show HV lesions that immunohistochemically seem to be similar to the follicles in HV-CD. The reactive follicles without HV changes in PC-CD resemble those of nonspecific follicular hyperplasia, and the germinal center cells are positive for CD10 and BCL6 and are negative for BCL2. Sinuses, which are usually patent, may be expanded by histiocytes highlighted by CD68 or other histiocyte-associated markers. HHV8 is usually negative in unicentric PC-CD. Epstein-Barr virus is negative.

In HHV8+ multicentric CD, the virus can be shown using monoclonal antibodies specific for viral components. An antibody specific for latent nuclear antigen (LNA-1) is commercially available and is used most often. HHV8 is present in

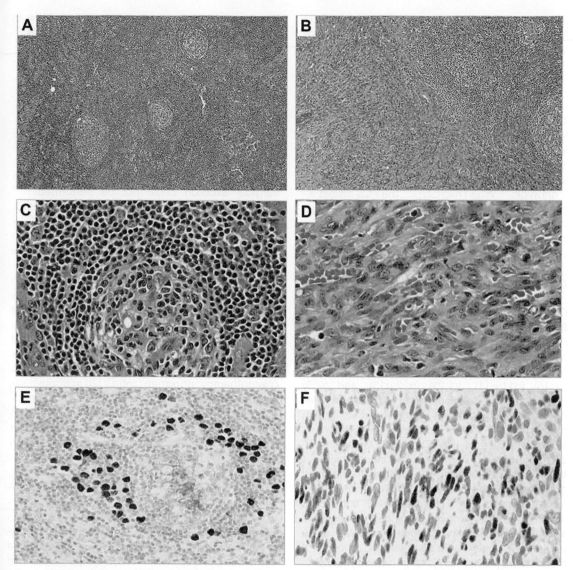

Fig. 6. HHV8-positive multicentric CD (*A*, *C*, and *E*) with concurrent Kaposi sarcoma (*B*, *D*, and *F*). (*A*) The lymph node is composed of scattered follicles with expanded interfollicular zones. Some follicles show some HV changes, including lymphocyte depleted germinal centers with onion-skin like mantle zones. (*B*) There is a spindle cell proliferation adjacent to hyperplastic follicles, consistent with Kaposi sarcoma. (*C*) There are scattered large cells in mantle zones and some have distinct nucleoli, consistent with immunoblasts/plasmablasts. (*D*) High-power view of spindle cell proliferation with vascular channels. (*E*) HHV8 immunostain highlights large cells in mantle zones surrounding atrophic follicles. (*F*) HHV8 immunostain highlights spindle cells.

atypical cells with features of plasmablasts or immunoblasts that are most common in the mantle zones of follicles (see **Fig. 6**). These HHV8+ cells almost always express lambda light chain and can form small nodules that have been referred to as microlymphomas. This term, however, has fallen out of favor because the cells in these small nodules are usually polyclonal at the molecular level, do not correlate with prognosis and likely only rarely progress to become a true HHV8+ large B-cell lymphoma. Other HHV8 lytic

proteins are also expressed in infected lymph nodes.[49,50] Abundant IL-6 in germinal center B cells and immunoblasts in the mantle zones and interfollicular regions has been shown and viral IL-6 and HHV8 have been colocalized in a subset of lymphocytes.[49] Epstein-Barr virus has been detected rarely in multicentric CD, most often in HHV8+ cases.[51] The exclusive expression of lambda light chain in HHV8-infected B cells is intriguing. A recent study explored a potential mechanism toward this biased expression and demonstrated that HHV8 virus can induce lambda light chain expression in mature B cells by triggering V(D)J rearrangement, a phenomenon normally restricted to early B-cell development in the bone marrow.[52]

The PCs in cases of HHV8+ and HHV8-negative types of multicentric CD are most often polytypic. The PCs express a mixture of heavy chains, with IgM+ cells more common around follicles and IgG+ and IgA+ cells mainly occurring within the interfollicular areas.[53,54] However, in up to one-third of cases of multicentric CD the PCs may be monotypic.[54] When monotypic, the PCs almost always express cytoplasmic lambda as well as IgG or IgA. The frequency of monotypic PCs is higher in cases of HHV8+ and POEMS-associated cases of multicentric CD.

CYTOGENETIC AND MOLECULAR FINDINGS

Conventional cytogenetic analysis has been performed on a small number of cases of HV-CD. A subset of these cases has been associated with clonal cytogenetic abnormalities. The following translocations have been identified: t(1;16) (p11;p11), t(1;22) (p22;q13), and t(7;8) (qter;q12).[28,30] Cokelaere and colleagues[29] reported rearrangement of the gene encoding high mobility group protein isoform C (*HMGIC*) within FDCs in a case of HV-CD using fluorescence in situ hybridization methods. The clonal status of the lymphocytes in HV-CD has been assessed and there is no evidence of *IGH* or *TRG* or *TRB* rearrangements.[30,55] Thus, the B cells and T cells in HV-CD are polyclonal. Chang and colleagues[30] analyzed the human androgen receptor alpha (HUMARA) gene in 29 women and showed a monoclonal pattern (ie, loss of heterozygosity) in about three-quarters of the cases assessed. Combined with the absence of monoclonal antigen receptor gene rearrangements, these data suggest that HV-CD is a monoclonal neoplasm of lymph node stromal cells, with FDCs being suspected based on other data, as discussed elsewhere in this article.

Very few cytogenetic abnormalities have been identified in cases of multicentric CD. One case has been reported with a t(7;14) (p22;q22) involving the IL-6 locus.[56] This patient also had a very high serum level of IL-6. Molecular analysis has shown monoclonal *IGH* rearrangements in a subset of cases of multicentric CD.[51,55,57] Soulier and colleagues[57] reported monoclonal *IGH* rearrangements in 4 of 34 cases of CD, of which 30 cases were multicentric CD. Three of 4 cases with monoclonal *IGH* rearrangement were associated with non-Hodgkin or Hodgkin lymphomas.

T-cell receptor gene rearrangements are rare in multicentric CD, in less than 10% of cases.[57] Gene rearrangements are more common in patients with evidence of HIV infection, usually associated with HHV8+ infection.

TREATMENT AND PROGNOSIS

The localized nature of HV-CD usually allows complete surgical excision, which is usually curative.[11,12] Radiation therapy also has been used in patients in whom relapse occurred or complete surgical excision could not be performed.[11,58] For asymptomatic patients with localized PC-CD, surgical excision seems to be adequate.[11–13] Surgical excision alone for symptomatic patients with PC-CD is often inadequate and therefore these patients require systemic therapy.[4,13]

In comparison with unicentric CD, patients with multicentric CD have a poorer prognosis. This is particularly true in HIV-positive patients and those with POEMS syndrome. Therefore, patients with multicentric CD require therapy and agents used include corticosteroids, other immunosuppressive agents, immunomodulator agents, cytotoxic chemotherapy, rituximab (anti-CD20 antibody), siltuximab (anti–IL-6 antibody), and tocilizumab (anti-gp80 antibody; anti–IL-6 coreceptor).[19,59–61] Although these approaches have resulted in some success, they are not curative and novel therapies are needed.

NEOPLASMS ASSOCIATED WITH CASTLEMAN DISEASE

Patients with CD are prone to developing a variety of neoplasms. In patients with HV-CD, FDC sarcoma can develop within HV-CD lymph nodes[62,63] (**Fig. 7**). The dysplastic-appearing FDCs within the HV follicles, commonly observed in these lesions, may be the precursor lesion[44,62] (see **Figs. 3** and **7**). Distinguishing FDC sarcoma from stroma-rich variants of HV-CD can be problematic, and biologic and histologic overlap may occur.[14] Vascular neoplasms also have been reported in HV-CD.[64] In rare cases of HV-CD, a clinically indolent T-lymphoblastic proliferation without clonal T-cell receptor rearrangements has been reported rarely.[65,66] Patients with HV-CD have no risk, or at most a minimally increased risk, of developing simultaneous or subsequent lymphomas compared with the general population.

Patients with HHV8+ multicentric CD have a higher risk of Kaposi sarcoma, which can coexist with multicentric CD in the same lymph node biopsy specimen[49,50] (see **Fig. 6**). These patients also have an increased risk of HHV8-positive large

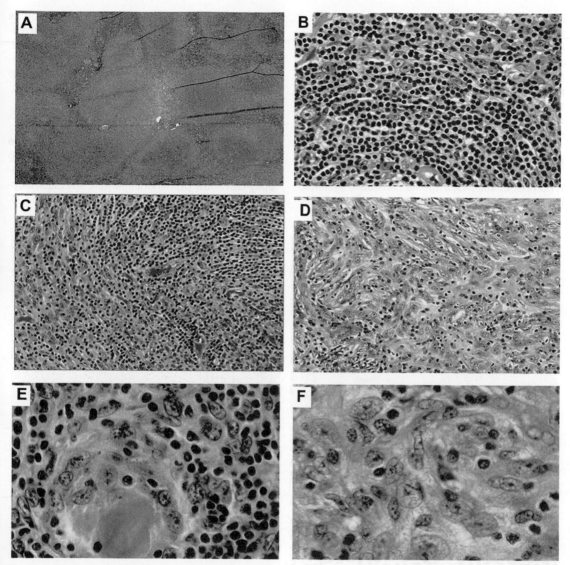

Fig. 7. Follicular dendritic sarcoma in a case of HV-CD. (*A*) A particular area with Castleman features including increased follicles with small germinal centers and expanded mantle zones. (*B* to *D*) Different numbers and locations of FDCs, from scattered FDCs in mantle zones (*B*) to loosely clustered FDCs in interfollicular areas (*C*) to areas composed of sheets of FDCs forming a mass. FDCs in germinal centers and mantle zones (*E*) show similar morphologic features to those in the area of follicular dendritic sarcoma (F).

B-cell lymphoma and primary effusion lymphoma.[50,67] Patients with HHV8-negative types of multicentric CD have an increased risk of developing lymphomas, with classical Hodgkin lymphoma (most often mixed cellularity type), diffuse large B-cell lymphoma, mantle cell lymphoma, and peripheral T-cell lymphoma most often reported.[68]

DIFFERENTIAL DIAGNOSIS

Unicentric HV-CD shows unique clinicopathologic features and the diagnosis is often straightforward.

In contrast, many reactive conditions such as autoimmune and infections can present with some morphologic features shared by PC-CD. In addition, some T-cell or B-cell lymphomas can show a prominent plasmacytic component, a feature seen in PC variant of CD. In these cases, the differential diagnosis can be challenging.

AUTOIMMUNE LYMPHADENOPATHY

Lymph nodes in patients with autoimmune diseases including rheumatoid arthritis, systemic lupus erythematosus, adult-onset Still disease, and juvenile idiopathic arthritis can show features of PC-CD.[69,70] This observation suggests that a subset of cases of unicentric or multicentric PC-CD cases have an autoimmune etiology, or at least an autoimmune component in their pathogenesis. The diagnosis of rheumatoid arthritis or systemic lupus erythematous usually can be established based on the patient's symptoms, physical findings, and laboratory studies such as rheumatoid factor and antinuclear antibody.

INFECTIOUS LYMPHADENOPATHY

A number of infectious agents can cause systemic lymphadenopathy that may be confused clinically with multicentric CD. These infectious etiologies include Epstein-Barr virus, cytomegalovirus, toxoplasmosis, HIV, and *Mycobacterium tuberculosis*. Biopsy is very helpful because these infections uncommonly cause histologic features that overlap with the findings in multicentric CD lymph nodes.

IgG4-RELATED LYMPHADENOPATHY

Some patients with IgG4-related disease can have systemic lymphadenopathy that clinically can mimic multicentric CD. In addition, lymph node biopsy can show prominent interfollicular plasmacytosis overlapping with the PC of multicentric CD.

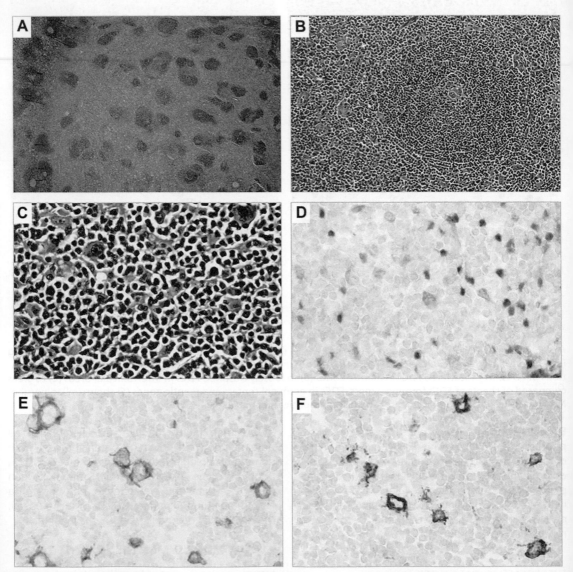

Fig. 8. Classic Hodgkin lymphoma with Castleman-like features. (*A*) A low-power view shows many follicles with atrophic germinal centers and expanded mantle zones. Interfollicular areas are pink with vascular proliferation. (*B*) An atrophic follicle with expanded mantle zones and vascular proliferation in interfollicular areas. (*C*) Scattered Hodgkin cells are present, positive for PAX5 (*D*), CD30 (*E*), and CD15 (*F*).

Features that are helpful to distinguish IgG4-related lymphadenopathy from multicentric CD include high serum IgG4 levels; variable presence of follicular hyperplasia with intrafollicular PCs within germinal centers; an increased ratio of IgG4/IgG PCs; normal serum levels of IL-6, LDH, and C-reactive protein; and an absence of HHV8 or HIV infection.[71]

CLASSIC HODGKIN LYMPHOMAS

In lymph nodes involved by classic Hodgkin lymphoma (**Fig. 8**), histologic changes that resemble HV-CD or PC-CD also can be present. These changes are detected as HV changes in follicles or as interfollicular plasmacytosis.[72,73] In general, these changes are often only focal or they only partially involve lymph nodes, and the complete constellation of histologic findings that occur in CD is usually absent. Furthermore, patients do not have symptoms attributable to CD. For these reasons, we use the designation "Castleman-like" for these changes and their importance is not letting these changes distract from the recognition of Hodgkin lymphoma.

NON-HODGKIN LYMPHOMAS

As stated elsewhere in this article, Castleman-like changes can coexist in cases of non-Hodgkin lymphoma. In a report of 6 cases of follicular lymphoma by Pina-Oviedo and colleagues,[74] the biopsy specimens showed 1 or more of the following features: prominent radial arterioles penetrating into the follicles mimicking HV lesions, onion skin–like mantle zones, twinning follicles, and increased vascular stroma in the interfollicular regions. In addition, needle biopsy specimens of HV-CD sometime are composed predominantly of expanded mantle zone B-cells that may be misconstrued as chronic lymphocytic leukemia/small lymphocytic lymphoma or mantle cell lymphoma, particularly if the B cells are CD5-positive, or as a marginal zone lymphoma. Flow cytometry immunophenotypic or molecular analysis showing no evidence of a monoclonal cell population is helpful in this differential diagnosis.

REFERENCES

1. Castleman B, Iverson L, Menendez VP. Localized mediastinal lymph node hyperplasia resembling thymoma. Cancer 1956;9:822–30.
2. Castleman B, Towne VW. Case records of the Massachusetts General Hospital: case no. 40231. N Engl J Med 1954;250:1001–5.
3. Flendrig J, Schillings P. Benign giant lymphoma: the clinical signs and symptoms and the morphological aspects. Folia Med 1969;12:119–20.
4. Menke DM, Camoriano JK, Banks PM. Angiofollicular lymph node hyperplasia: a comparison of unicentric, multicentric, hyaline vascular, and plasma cell types of disease by morphometric and clinical analysis. Mod Pathol 1992;5:525–30.
5. Keller AR, Hochholzer L, Castleman B. Hyaline-vascular and plasma-cell types of giant lymph node hyperplasia of the mediastinum and other locations. Cancer 1972;29:670–83.
6. Gaba AR, Stein RS, Sweet DL, et al. Multicentric giant lymph node hyperplasia. Am J Clin Pathol 1978; 69:86–90.
7. Frizzera G, Banks PM, Massarelli G, et al. A systemic lymphoproliferative disorder with morphologic features of Castleman's disease. Pathological findings in 15 patients. Am J Surg Pathol 1983;7:211–31.
8. Fajgenbaum DC, Shilling D. Castleman disease pathogenesis. Hematol Oncol Clin North Am 2018; 32:11–21.
9. Simpson D. Epidemiology of Castleman disease. Hematol Oncol Clin North Am 2018;32:1–10.
10. Yu L, Tu M, Cortes J, et al. Clinical and pathological characteristics of HIV- and HHV-8-negative Castleman disease. Blood 2017;129:1658–68.
11. Wong RSM. Unicentric Castleman disease. Hematol Oncol Clin North Am 2018;32:65–73.
12. Talat N, Belgaumkar AP, Schulte KM. Surgery in Castleman's disease: a systematic review of 404 published cases. Ann Surg 2012;255:677–84.
13. Oksenhendler E, Boutboul D, Fajgenbaum D, et al. The full spectrum of Castleman disease: 273 patients studied over 20 years. Br J Haematol 2018; 180:206–16.
14. Danon AD, Krishnan J, Frizzera G. Morpho-immunophenotypic diversity of Castleman's disease, hyaline-vascular type: with emphasis on a stroma-rich variant and a new pathogenetic hypothesis. Virchows Arch A Pathol Anat Histopathol 1993;423: 369–82.
15. Serin E, Ozer B, Gumurdulu Y, et al. A case of Castleman's disease with "downhill" varices in the absence of superior vena cava obstruction. Endoscopy 2002;34:160–2.
16. Wang L, Bu D, Yang Y, et al. Castleman's tumours and production of autoantibody in paraneoplastic pemphigus. Lancet 2004;363:525–31.
17. Day JR, Bew D, Ali M, et al. Castleman's disease associated with myasthenia gravis. Ann Thorac Surg 2003;75:1648–50.
18. Liu AY, Nabel CS, Finkelman BS, et al. Idiopathic multicentric Castleman's disease: a systematic literature review. Lancet Haematol 2016;3:e163–75.
19. Fajgenbaum DC, Uldrick TS, Bagg A, et al. International, evidence-based consensus diagnostic

criteria for HHV-8-negative/idiopathic multicentric Castleman disease. Blood 2017;129:1646–57.

20. Winter SS, Howard TA, Ritchey AK, et al. Elevated levels of tumor necrosis factor-beta, gamma-interferon, and IL-6 mRNA in Castleman's disease. Med Pediatr Oncol 1996;26:48–53.

21. Simpson GR, Schulz TF, Whitby D, et al. Prevalence of Kaposi's sarcoma associated herpesvirus infection measured by antibodies to recombinant capsid protein and latent immunofluorescence antigen. Lancet 1996;348:1133–8.

22. Igawa T, Sato Y. TAFRO syndrome. Hematol Oncol Clin North Am 2018;32:107–18.

23. Iwaki N, Fajgenbaum DC, Nabel CS, et al. Clinicopathologic analysis of TAFRO syndrome demonstrates a distinct subtype of HHV-8-negative multicentric Castleman disease. Am J Hematol 2016;91:220–6.

24. Kawabata H, Kadowaki N, Nishikori M, et al. Clinical features and treatment of multicentric Castleman's disease : a retrospective study of 21 Japanese patients at a single institute. J Clin Exp Hematop 2013;53:69–77.

25. Bardwick PA, Zvaifler NJ, Gill GN, et al. Plasma cell dyscrasia with polyneuropathy, organomegaly, endocrinopathy, M protein, and skin changes: the POEMS syndrome. Report on two cases and a review of the literature. Medicine (Baltimore) 1980; 59:311–22.

26. Dispenzieri A. Poems syndrome: 2017 update on diagnosis, risk stratification, and management. Am J Hematol 2017;92:814–29.

27. Chan JK, Fletcher CD, Hicklin GA, et al. Glomeruloid hemangioma. A distinctive cutaneous lesion of multicentric Castleman's disease associated with poems syndrome. Am J Surg Pathol 1990;14: 1036–46.

28. Pauwels P, Dal Cin P, Vlasveld LT, et al. A chromosomal abnormality in hyaline vascular Castleman's disease: evidence for clonal proliferation of dysplastic stromal cells. Am J Surg Pathol 2000;24: 882–8.

29. Cokelaere K, Debiec-Rychter M, De Wolf-Peeters C, et al. Hyaline vascular Castleman's disease with hmgic rearrangement in follicular dendritic cells: molecular evidence of mesenchymal tumorigenesis. Am J Surg Pathol 2002;26:662–9.

30. Chang KC, Wang YC, Hung LY, et al. Monoclonality and cytogenetic abnormalities in hyaline vascular Castleman disease. Mod Pathol 2014;27:823–31.

31. Ruco LP, Gearing AJ, Pigott R, et al. Expression of ICAM-1, VCAM-1 and ELAM-1 in angiofollicular lymph node hyperplasia (Castleman's disease): evidence for dysplasia of follicular dendritic reticulum cells. Histopathology 1991;19:523–8.

32. Oksenhendler E, Carcelain G, Aoki Y, et al. High levels of human herpesvirus 8 viral load, human interleukin-6, interleukin-10, and C reactive protein correlate with exacerbation of multicentric Castleman disease in HIV-infected patients. Blood 2000; 96:2069–73.

33. Hsu SM, Waldron JA, Xie SS, et al. Expression of interleukin-6 in Castleman's disease. Hum Pathol 1993;24:833–9.

34. Ishiyama T, Koike M, Nakamura S, et al. Interleukin-6 receptor expression in the peripheral B cells of patients with multicentric Castleman's disease. Ann Hematol 1996;73:179–82.

35. Akira S, Taga T, Kishimoto T. Interleukin-6 in biology and medicine. Adv Immunol 1993;54:1–78.

36. Kawano MM, Mihara K, Huang N, et al. Differentiation of early plasma cells on bone marrow stromal cells requires interleukin-6 for escaping from apoptosis. Blood 1995;85:487–94.

37. Foussat A, Fior R, Girard T, et al. Involvement of human interleukin-6 in systemic manifestations of human herpesvirus type 8-associated multicentric Castleman's disease. AIDS 1999;13:150–2.

38. Brandt SJ, Bodine DM, Dunbar CE, et al. Dysregulated interleukin 6 expression produces a syndrome resembling Castleman's disease in mice. J Clin Invest 1990;86:592–9.

39. Frizzera G. Castleman's disease and related disorders. Semin Diagn Pathol 1988;5:346–64.

40. Oksenhendler E, Duarte M, Soulier J, et al. Multicentric Castleman's disease in HIV infection: a clinical and pathological study of 20 patients. AIDS 1996; 10:61–7.

41. Boshoff C, Chang Y. Kaposi's sarcoma-associated herpesvirus: a new DNA tumor virus. Annu Rev Med 2001;52:453–70.

42. Osborne J, Moore PS, Chang Y. KSHV-encoded viral il-6 activates multiple human il-6 signaling pathways. Hum Immunol 1999;60:921–7.

43. Grandadam M, Dupin N, Calvez V, et al. Exacerbations of clinical symptoms in human immunodeficiency virus type 1-infected patients with multicentric Castleman's disease are associated with a high increase in Kaposi's sarcoma herpesvirus DNA load in peripheral blood mononuclear cells. J Infect Dis 1997;175:1198–201.

44. Medina EA, Fuehrer NE, Miller FR, et al. Dysplastic follicular dendritic cells in hyaline-vascular Castleman disease: a rare occurrence creating diagnostic difficulty. Pathol Int 2016;66: 535–9.

45. Lin O, Frizzera G. Angiomyoid and follicular dendritic cell proliferative lesions in Castleman's disease of hyaline-vascular type: a study of 10 cases. Am J Surg Pathol 1997;21:1295–306.

46. Amin HM, Medeiros LJ, Manning JT, et al. Dissolution of the lymphoid follicle is a feature of the HHV8+ variant of plasma cell Castleman's disease. Am J Surg Pathol 2003;27:91–100.

47. Dupin N, Fisher C, Kellam P, et al. Distribution of human herpesvirus-8 latently infected cells in Kaposi's sarcoma, multicentric Castleman's disease, and primary effusion lymphoma. Proc Natl Acad Sci U S A 1999;96:4546–51.

48. Liu Q, Pittaluga S, Davies-Hill T, et al. Increased cd5-positive polyclonal B cells in Castleman disease: a diagnostic pitfall. Histopathology 2013;63:877–80.

49. Brousset P, Cesarman E, Meggetto F, et al. Colocalization of the viral interleukin-6 with latent nuclear antigen-1 of human herpesvirus-8 in endothelial spindle cells of Kaposi's sarcoma and lymphoid cells of multicentric Castleman's disease. Hum Pathol 2001;32:95–100.

50. Katano H, Sato Y, Kurata T, et al. Expression and localization of human herpesvirus 8-encoded proteins in primary effusion lymphoma, Kaposi's sarcoma, and multicentric Castleman's disease. Virology 2000;269:335–44.

51. Hanson CA, Frizzera G, Patton DF, et al. Clonal rearrangement for immunoglobulin and T-cell receptor genes in systemic Castleman's disease. Association with Epstein Barr virus. Am J Pathol 1988;131:84–91.

52. Totonchy J, Osborn JM, Chadburn A, et al. Kshv induces immunoglobulin rearrangements in mature b lymphocytes. PLoS Pathog 2018;14:e1006967.

53. Hall PA, Donaghy M, Cotter FE, et al. An immunohistological and genotypic study of the plasma cell form of Castleman's disease. Histopathology 1989;14:333–46, [discussion: 429–32].

54. Radaszkiewicz T, Hansmann ML, Lennert K. Monoclonality and polyclonality of plasma cells in Castleman's disease of the plasma cell variant. Histopathology 1989;14:11–24.

55. Al-Maghrabi J, Kamel-Reid S, Bailey D. Immunoglobulin and T-cell receptor gene rearrangement in Castleman's disease: molecular genetic analysis. Histopathology 2006;48:233–8.

56. Nakamura H, Nakaseko C, Ishii A, et al. Chromosomal abnormalities in Castleman's disease with high levels of serum interleukin-6. Rinsho Ketsueki 1993;34:212–7, [in Japanese].

57. Soulier J, Grollet L, Oksenhendler E, et al. Molecular analysis of clonality in Castleman's disease. Blood 1995;86:1131–8.

58. Chronowski GM, Ha CS, Wilder RB, et al. Treatment of unicentric and multicentric Castleman disease and the role of radiotherapy. Cancer 2001;92:670–6.

59. Deisseroth A, Ko CW, Nie L, et al. FDA approval: siltuximab for the treatment of patients with multicentric Castleman disease. Clin Cancer Res 2015;21:950–4.

60. Song SN, Tomosugi N, Kawabata H, et al. Down-regulation of hepcidin resulting from long-term treatment with an anti-il-6 receptor antibody (tocilizumab) improves anemia of inflammation in multicentric Castleman disease. Blood 2010;116:3627–34.

61. van Rhee F, Voorhees P, Dispenzieri A, et al. International, evidence-based consensus treatment guidelines for idiopathic multicentric Castleman disease. Blood 2018;132:2115–24.

62. Chan JK, Tsang WY, Ng CS. Follicular dendritic cell tumor and vascular neoplasm complicating hyaline-vascular Castleman's disease. Am J Surg Pathol 1994;18:517–25.

63. Chan AC, Chan KW, Chan JK, et al. Development of follicular dendritic cell sarcoma in hyaline-vascular Castleman's disease of the nasopharynx: tracing its evolution by sequential biopsies. Histopathology 2001;38:510–8.

64. Gerald W, Kostianovsky M, Rosai J. Development of vascular neoplasia in Castleman's disease. Report of seven cases. Am J Surg Pathol 1990;14:603–14.

65. Ohgami RS, Zhao S, Ohgami JK, et al. Tdt+ T-lymphoblastic populations are increased in Castleman disease, in Castleman disease in association with follicular dendritic cell tumors, and in angioimmunoblastic T-cell lymphoma. Am J Surg Pathol 2012;36:1619–28.

66. Quesada AE, Young KH, Medeiros LJ, et al. Indolent T-lymphoblastic proliferation associated with low grade follicular dendritic cell sarcoma and Castleman disease. Pathology 2018;50:351–2.

67. Ascoli V, Signoretti S, Onetti-Muda A, et al. Primary effusion lymphoma in HIV-infected patients with multicentric Castleman's disease. J Pathol 2001;193:200–9.

68. Larroche C, Cacoub P, Soulier J, et al. Castleman's disease and lymphoma: report of eight cases in HIV-negative patients and literature review. Am J Hematol 2002;69:119–26.

69. Kojima M, Motoori T, Nakamura S. Benign, atypical and malignant lymphoproliferative disorders in rheumatoid arthritis patients. Biomed Pharmacother 2006;60:663–72.

70. Kojima M, Nakamura S, Itoh H, et al. Systemic lupus erythematosus (SLE) lymphadenopathy presenting with histopathologic features of Castleman' disease: a clinicopathologic study of five cases. Pathol Res Pract 1997;193:565–71.

71. Sato Y, Kojima M, Takata K, et al. Systemic igg4-related lymphadenopathy: a clinical and pathologic comparison to multicentric Castleman's disease. Mod Pathol 2009;22:589–99.

72. Zarate-Osorno A, Medeiros LJ, Danon AD, et al. Hodgkin's disease with coexistent Castleman-like histologic features. A report of three cases. Arch Pathol Lab Med 1994;118:270–4.

73. Maheswaran PR, Ramsay AD, Norton AJ, et al. Hodgkin's disease presenting with the histological features of Castleman's disease. Histopathology 1991;18:249–53.

74. Pina-Oviedo S, Miranda RN, Lin P, et al. Follicular lymphoma with hyaline-vascular Castleman-like features: analysis of 6 cases and review of the literature. Hum Pathol 2017;68:136–46.

Moving?

Make sure your subscription moves with you!

To notify us of your new address, find your **Clinics Account Number** (located on your mailing label above your name), and contact customer service at:

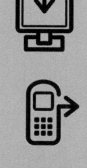

Email: journalscustomerservice-usa@elsevier.com

800-654-2452 (subscribers in the U.S. & Canada)
314-447-8871 (subscribers outside of the U.S. & Canada)

Fax number: 314-447-8029

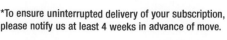

Elsevier Health Sciences Division
Subscription Customer Service
3251 Riverport Lane
Maryland Heights, MO 63043

*To ensure uninterrupted delivery of your subscription, please notify us at least 4 weeks in advance of move.